SECOND EDITION

## SITE-SPECIFIC CANCER SERIES

# Breast Cancer

**Edited by**
**Suzanne M. Mahon, RN, DNSc, AOCN®, APNG**

Oncology Nursing Society
Pittsburgh, Pennsylvania

**ONS Publications Department**

Executive Director, Professional Practice and Programs: Elizabeth M. Wertz Evans, RN, MPM, CPHQ, CPHIMS, FACMPE
Publisher and Director of Publications: Barbara Sigler, RN, MNEd
Managing Editor: Lisa M. George, BA
Technical Content Editor: Angela D. Klimaszewski, RN, MSN
Staff Editor II: Amy Nicoletti, BA
Copy Editor: Laura Pinchot, BA
Graphic Designer: Dany Sjoen

Library of Congress Cataloging-in-Publication Data

Breast cancer / edited by Suzanne M. Mahon. -- 2nd ed.
    p. ; cm. -- (Site-specific cancer series)
  Includes bibliographical references and index.
  ISBN 978-1-935864-11-0 (alk. paper)
  1. Breast--Cancer--Nursing.  I. Mahon, Suzanne M. II. Oncology Nursing Society. III. Series: Site-specific cancer series.
  [DNLM: 1. Breast Neoplasms.  WP 870]
  RC280.B8B6655623 2011
  616.99'449--dc23
                                                                              2011014469

**Publisher's Note**

This book is published by the Oncology Nursing Society (ONS). ONS neither represents nor guarantees that the practices described herein will, if followed, ensure safe and effective patient care. The recommendations contained in this book reflect ONS's judgment regarding the state of general knowledge and practice in the field as of the date of publication. The recommendations may not be appropriate for use in all circumstances. Those who use this book should make their own determinations regarding specific safe and appropriate patient-care practices, taking into account the personnel, equipment, and practices available at the hospital or other facility at which they are located. The editor and publisher cannot be held responsible for any liability incurred as a consequence from the use or application of any of the contents of this book. Figures and tables are used as examples only. They are not meant to be all-inclusive, nor do they represent endorsement of any particular institution by ONS. Mention of specific products and opinions related to those products do not indicate or imply endorsement by ONS. Web sites mentioned are provided for information only; the hosts are responsible for their own content and availability. Unless otherwise indicated, dollar amounts reflect U.S. dollars.

ONS publications are originally published in English. Publishers wishing to translate ONS publications must contact ONS about licensing arrangements. ONS publications cannot be translated without obtaining written permission from ONS. (Individual tables and figures that are reprinted or adapted require additional permission from the original source.) Because translations from English may not always be accurate or precise, ONS disclaims any responsibility for inaccuracies in words or meaning that may occur as a result of the translation. Readers relying on precise information should check the original English version.

Printed in the United States of America

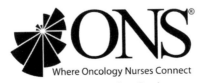

Oncology Nursing Society
Integrity • Innovation • Stewardship • Advocacy • Excellence • Inclusiveness

# Contributors

## Editor

Suzanne M. Mahon, RN, DNSc, AOCN®, APNG
Professor
Saint Louis University
St. Louis, Missouri
*Chapter 1. Introduction; Chapter 2. Risk Factors for Breast Cancer; Chapter 3. Prevention and Detection;*
*Chapter 6. Breast Restoration Options Utilizing Prostheses; Chapter 10. Psychosocial Issues*

## Authors

Michelle A. Casey, CFA
Patient Care Coordinator
Medical West Healthcare Center
St. Louis, Missouri
*Chapter 6. Breast Restoration Options Utilizing Prostheses*

Phillip J. Catanzaro, MD, PhD
Director
Cleveland Clinic Cancer Center
Cleveland, Ohio
*Chapter 7. Radiation Therapy*

Seth Eisenberg, RN, ADN, OCN®
Professional Practice Coordinator, Infusion Services
Seattle Cancer Care Alliance
Seattle, Washington
*Chapter 8. Systemic Therapy*

Connie J. Ferraro, RN, BSN, OCN®
Radiation/Oncology Regional Nurse Leader
Cleveland Clinic Foundation
Cleveland, Ohio
*Chapter 7. Radiation Therapy*

Judith Hatch, RN, MSN, OCN®, CBCN®, FPMH-NP
Breast Cancer Nurse Navigator
Central Baptist Hospital
Lexington, Kentucky
*Chapter 5. Surgical Management and Reconstruction*

Katina Kirby, MS, OTR/L, CLT-LANA
Board Member
Lymphology Association of North America
Wilmette, Illinois
*Chapter 9. Symptom Management*

Carole H. Martz, RN, MS, AOCN®, CBCN®
Clinical Coordinator, Living in the Future
  Cancer Survivorship Program
Northshore University Health System
Highland Park, Illinois
*Chapter 9. Symptom Management*

Elaine Sein, RN, BSN, OCN®, CBCN®
Senior Project Manager
Fox Chase Cancer Center
Fox Chase Cancer Center Partners Division
Philadelphia, Pennsylvania
*Chapter 11. Building Breast Centers of Excellence Through Patient Navigation and Care Coordination*

Susan G. Yackzan, APRN, MSN, AOCN®
Oncology Clinical Nurse Specialist
Central Baptist Hospital
Lexington, Kentucky
*Chapter 4. Pathophysiology and Staging; Chapter 5. Surgical Management and Reconstruction*

## Disclosure

Editors and authors of books and guidelines provided by the Oncology Nursing Society are expected to disclose to the readers any significant financial interest or other relationships with the manufacturer(s) of any commercial products.

A vested interest may be considered to exist if a contributor is affiliated with or has a financial interest in commercial organizations that may have a direct or indirect interest in the subject matter. A "financial interest" may include, but is not limited to, being a shareholder in the organization; being an employee of the commercial organization; serving on an organization's speakers bureau; or receiving research from the organization. An "affiliation" may be holding a position on an advisory board or some other role of benefit to the commercial organization. Vested interest statements appear in the front matter for each publication.

Contributors are expected to disclose any unlabeled or investigational use of products discussed in their content. This information is acknowledged solely for the information of the readers.

The contributors provided the following disclosure and vested interest information:

Seth Eisenberg, RN, ADN, OCN®: Medical Learning Institute, ProCE, honoraria

Connie J. Ferraro, RN, BSN, OCN®: Cephalon, speaker, honoraria; Cogenix, honoraria

# Contents

# Preface

Knowledge and progress regarding the prevention, early detection, treatment, and long-term needs of people diagnosed with breast cancer are ever-changing and expanding. Oncology nurses are constantly challenged to incorporate this knowledge into their care and to respond to questions about breast cancer. The importance of this role should not be underestimated. In 2009, the Oncology Nursing Certification Corporation began to offer certification for the title of certified breast care nurse (CBCN®), further supporting this specialized role. This second edition provides oncology nurses with current, comprehensive information about the care and needs of patients and families affected by breast cancer across the trajectory.

This book provides detailed information about the epidemiology, prevention, and early detection of breast cancer. This is a growing and sometimes controversial area of knowledge that often is influenced by public policy and requires the nurse to interpret this information to individuals in a meaningful way. Oncology nurses guide patients diagnosed with breast cancer through the diagnostic and treatment phases; therefore, the text provides detailed state-of-the-art information on diagnostic procedures, staging, pathophysiology, surgical approaches, radiation therapy, and systemic therapy. Because treatment of the entire person diagnosed with breast cancer is necessary to achieve an optimal outcome, the book includes information about symptom management, breast restoration, complementary medicine, psychosocial adjustment, and the role of the nurse navigator.

The first part of the book is organized to provide information across the cancer trajectory. This includes chapters on epidemiology, risk factors, prevention and early detection, pathophysiology and staging, surgical approaches, radiation therapy, and systemic therapy. This is followed by a chapter on symptom management, which provides detailed information about short- and long-term symptoms that may require intervention. Breast restoration can be an ongoing challenge in care, and an entire chapter is dedicated to the issues of breast restoration, both short and long term, regardless of the surgical approach. The chapter on psychosocial adjustment provides information for all phases of the breast cancer journey along with emerging data on complementary and alternative medicine.

This second edition provides new chapters on radiation therapy and the rapidly emerging role of nurse navigation not found in the first edition, as well as more detailed information about surgical approaches, systemic therapy, and complementary approaches. This textbook imparts the efforts of several breast cancer nursing experts to synthesize scientific information on care across the breast cancer trajectory. The authors of each chapter have carefully researched the literature and updated the content from the first edition. This information can be used to provide evidence-based knowledge in patient care to those affected by breast cancer.

# CHAPTER 1

# Introduction

Suzanne M. Mahon, RN, DNSc, AOCN®, APNG

## Overview

The very term *breast cancer* sends a message of fear to many, if not all, women. With an estimated 207,090 new cases of invasive breast cancer and an additional 54,010 cases of in situ breast cancer diagnosed in 2010 (American Cancer Society [ACS], 2010), it is not surprising that women and their loved ones fear the disease. Unfortunately, an estimated 40,230 women would die from breast cancer in 2010 (ACS, 2010). Most people know someone who has been affected by the diagnosis. Excluding skin cancer, breast cancer is the most common cancer among U.S. women, accounting for one out of every three cancers diagnosed in women (ACS, 2009).

The cultural and psychological significance of the breast in modern society, in addition to the large number of people affected by the disease, may explain much of the fear associated with the diagnosis. The female breast plays a significant role in nurturing and motherhood. Symbolically, it often is associated with femininity and sexuality. Threats to the health of the breast potentially influence a woman's perceptions of her body and her role in society.

Although breast cancer primarily affects women, an estimated 1,970 men are diagnosed each year. This accounts for about 1% of all cases of breast cancer diagnosed (ACS, 2010). The needs of this special population cannot be ignored (Al-Haddad, 2010). Although this text focuses on breast cancer in women with regard to diagnostic, surgical, and adjuvant therapy, many of the strategies used to treat male breast cancer are similar to those used in women. For many men diagnosed with breast cancer, the psychosocial issues are complex and require much sensitivity and care from oncology health professionals (Onami, Ozaki, Mortimer, & Pal, 2010).

Every October, numerous groups promote breast cancer awareness, including Susan G. Komen for the Cure and ACS, as well as professional societies and local healthcare institutions. The color pink is universally associated with breast cancer, and during these special awareness programs, constant reminders are set against a background of pink about the need for improved detection and treatment of the disease. Many breast cancer survivors have become activists and advocates for other women to prevent the disease and promote early detection.

The impact of this advocacy and promotion of breast cancer awareness should not be underestimated. During the 1980s and 1990s, breast cancer advocates in the United States rallied around the Mammography Quality Standards Act and for expansion of the Breast and Cervical Cancer Early Detection Program (Braun, 2003). Both of these acts, along with significant increases in federal funding for breast cancer research (from $81 million to more than $400 million in the 1990s), dramatically changed the screening and treatment of breast cancer in the United States.

Public awareness and desire to decrease the morbidity and mortality associated with breast cancer is significant. Since Congress first enacted the breast cancer postage stamp program in 1997, the National Cancer Institute (NCI) has received more than $35 million from stamp sales, which funded more than 50 grants and one clinical trial (Savage, 2007). The stamp not only heightens public awareness of breast cancer but also provides significant funding for a variety of research programs.

This awareness of breast cancer has dramatically changed the outlook and treatment for those diagnosed with breast cancer. In the past three decades, thousands of women have participated in awareness races, raised money for research and screening, undergone screening, and enrolled in clinical trials with the hope of improving the outcomes for those diagnosed with breast cancer.

## Historical Perspectives

An examination of the history of breast cancer treatment enables women and healthcare providers to understand how much progress has been made, yet it also leaves questions about what still needs to be done. As early as 400 BC, Hippocrates speculated on the systemic nature of the disease (Foster, 2003). Galen (AD 130–200) believed breast cancer to be a local-regional disease requiring complete excision for cure. The early Romans performed a type of mastectomy that included removal of the pectoralis muscle. Throughout the Middle Ages and Renaissance periods, crude types of mastectomies often were attempted to potentially eradicate disease. These early physicians initiated the debate about whether breast cancer is a systemic disease, local-regional disease, or both.

During the middle of the 18th century, William Hunter identified and described the importance of the lymphatic system in the spread of cancer (Foster, 2003). Surgical techniques greatly improved in the mid-19th century with the introduction of general anesthetics and more antiseptic techniques. In the late 19th century, Thomas Beatson of Scotland reported that oophorectomy resulted in the regression of advanced breast cancer. This early finding was just the beginning of hormonal manipulation as an effective adjuvant therapy in the treatment of breast cancer.

Although considered controversial in his time, William Halsted believed that breast cancer was a local-regional disease and is well known for promoting the Halsted radical mastectomy, which quickly became the standard of care for more than the first half of the 20th century. This radical surgical procedure often was combined with radiation therapy, which was also an emerging science at that time (Foster, 2003). Surgical treatment typically involved a "one-step procedure" in which a woman undergoing a biopsy with general anesthesia also would consent to an immediate mastectomy if the frozen section showed malignancy. It was not until the woman woke up that she would know the actual diagnosis and extent of surgery. Women typically were offered little choice in treatment.

The middle of the 20th century brought about a push toward clinical trials and decreasing the morbidity and mortality associated with breast cancer. These trials have had an enormous impact on breast cancer treatment and have led to the view that breast cancer is systemic and not just a local-regional disease. Because of these trials, lumpectomy followed by radiation therapy is now an appropriate local-regional control strategy for many women. The one-step biopsy procedure was gradually eliminated as biopsy techniques became more refined and women could make informed decisions about local-regional management. Adjuvant therapy trials have greatly changed systemic treatment for breast cancer. The National Surgical Adjuvant Breast and Bowel Project (NSABP) has enrolled more than 40,000 women in more than 30 trials (Foster, 2003).

In the 1970s, the concept of screening for early breast cancer gained more acceptance. Women were encouraged to practice breast self-examination. Today the push is toward breast health awareness (ACS, 2009). Mammography gradually became more readily available and more sensitive in detecting early malignancies. Screening continues to be refined with widespread implementation of digital mammography, and breast magnetic resonance imaging (MRI) is showing promise as a detection tool in some high-risk groups. Although more women are engaged in screening programs, much more work remains to be done. If adequate breast cancer screening and care for all women were readily available, an estimated 20% fewer women would die of the disease each year. If 40,000 women are dying of breast cancer each year, 8,000 lives could be saved (Vanchieri, 2007).

Prevention of breast cancer is not yet a reality, although it may eventually be one. The NSABP P-1 trial clearly demonstrated that tamoxifen may be beneficial in some high-risk women to reduce the risk of, delay the development of, or prevent breast cancer. Genetic testing is now readily available for two hereditary breast cancer susceptibility genes (*BRCA1* and *BRCA2*). Women with a known mutation can be offered prophylactic surgeries to prevent the development of breast cancer. Large-scale epidemiologic studies continue. For example, the Sister Study will follow 50,000 women for at least 10 years who have a biologic sister who was diagnosed with breast cancer and will collect information about genes, lifestyle, and environmental factors that may cause breast cancer ("First Sister Study Results," 2009; "The Sister Study," 2010). Enrollment for the Sister Study was completed on March 31, 2009.

Gene expression analysis has led to the identification of molecularly defined subtypes of breast cancer that have distinct biologic features, clinical outcomes, and responses to chemotherapy. Personalized treatment strategies are now being developed based on an individual's tumor characteristics. A woman's response to chemotherapy is influenced not only by the tumor's genetic characteristics but also by inherited variations in genes that affect a woman's ability to absorb, metabolize, and eliminate drugs (Qureshi & Qureshi, 2008). Personalized medicine is a reality in breast cancer treatment, and it is anticipated that future developments will ultimately lead to much more effective treatment and decreases in mortality.

Social movements have influenced the treatment of breast cancer as well. Prior to the 1970s, breast cancer was considered a stigma. It was not discussed. Then, the diagnosis of breast cancer in several prominent women, including Shirley Temple Black, Betty Ford, Happy Rockefeller, and Betty Rollin, changed public opinion about the disease in a relatively short period of time. These women used their popularity to encourage other women to engage in early detection practices and to be open about their diagnosis. They increased public awareness of the disease and, along with many other women, challenged the breast cancer practices of the time (including the Halsted radical mastectomy) and lobbied for increased accountability and accessibility in mammography (Kolker, 2004). These efforts ultimately led to significant federal funding for more research related to breast cancer.

The trend toward shorter hospitalization is another social movement that has dramatically affected breast cancer treatment. Twenty-five years ago, women would recover for 10 days to two weeks in the hospital. Today, for many women, same-day or one-night stays are the norm after surgical management of the disease. These women still go home with physical limitations and emotional concerns, but often with much less support from the healthcare team. This creates new challenges for patients and their families.

Consumerism also has affected breast cancer (Klawiter, 2004). Two decades ago, few resources were available to women, other than ACS and its "Reach to Recovery" program. Minimal printed resources existed, and the Internet had not been developed yet. Women faced the disease and its treatment often with a limited understanding of the pathophysiology of the disease and its treatment. Today, society promotes the concept that women should be active partners in decisions regarding treatment. NCI and numerous other organizations encourage women to ask questions, and they provide educational resources in many formats.

## Epidemiologic Perspectives

Some epidemiologic trends in breast cancer have occurred that merit notice. Breast cancer risk increases with age. During 2002–2006, 95% of the new diagnoses and 97% of breast cancer deaths occurred in women age 40 and older (ACS, 2009). During this same time period, the median age at diagnosis was 61.

Many women believe that breast cancer has become increasingly more common. Since 1975, three basic incidence trends have occurred (ACS, 2009). From 1975 to 1980, the incidence was relatively constant. Between 1980 and 1987, the incidence increased by 4% per year. This increased incidence is attributed to more widespread use of mammography and the detection of nonpalpable lesions. Between 1987 and 1994, the incidence was essentially constant. Between 1994 and 1999, incidence rates increased by 1.6% per year. Epidemiologists speculate that this increase in incidence is related to changing reproductive patterns, including delayed childbearing and fewer pregnancies. Between 1999 and 2006, however, incidence rates decreased by 2% per year. This decrease is attributed to decreased use of hormone replacement therapy following the publication of the results of the Women's Health Initiative randomized trial in 2002, as well as a decrease in mammography screening (thus, detecting fewer cancers earlier) (ACS, 2009). Despite the increasing incidence, mortality rates are decreasing. Between 1990 and 2006, the mortality rate decreased by 3.2% annually (ACS, 2009). Recent estimates suggest that at least 2.3 million women are alive with a diagnosis of breast cancer (ACS, 2009). Long-term survival rates continue to improve. Currently, of all the women diagnosed, 89% are alive 5 years after the diagnosis; 82% are alive 10 years after the diagnosis; 75% are alive after 15 years; and after 20 years, 63% are still alive (ACS, 2009).

## Clinical Perspectives

Women understandably worry about their risk for developing breast cancer. Understanding this concept is a challenge both for women to comprehend and for healthcare professionals to communicate. Multiple means are available to express risk. Healthcare providers are encouraged to find a risk assessment that correctly conveys risk and is appropriate for the woman. This usually includes a combination of figures including relative, absolute, and, in some cases, attributable risk. The primary reason for conducting a risk assessment is to use it to guide decisions about screening.

The Human Genome Project has greatly changed risk assessment processes, especially in the area of breast cancer risk. Approximately 10% of all breast cancers likely have a hereditary component (Daly et al., 2006). The identification of women with hereditary risk is an ever-emerging role in oncology. Once identified through risk assessment, these women need comprehensive, balanced counseling so that they can make an informed decision about genetic testing. Genetic testing has major ramifications for both the individual tested and for other relatives. For those who test positive for a known mutation, difficult choices can arise regarding prevention, including the possibility of prophylactic surgery.

For all women, the risk assessment guides screening recommendations. Multiple screening recommendations are available from numerous organizations. These recommendations usually include some combination of breast self-examination, a professional clinical breast examination, and mammography. For women with significant risk, other modalities such as MRI may be added, as well as more frequent screening. When making screening recommendations, healthcare providers need to inform women about why a particular guideline is being utilized, as well as the potential risks, benefits, and limitations associated with a particular screening modality.

In an ideal world, all breast cancer would be prevented. However, limited strategies currently exist that are routinely used in the prevention of breast cancer. All women should be counseled about the benefits of a low-fat diet, weight control, and regular exercise. The role of exogenous hormone use in the development of breast cancer is still poorly understood. Tamoxifen and raloxifene, however, have shown some promise for the prevention of breast cancer (ACS, 2009). Clearly, more chemoprevention trials are needed to identify agents, the ideal age at which to begin taking them, and the best administration schedules to ultimately offer women some choice for the prevention of breast cancer. For women with an identified hereditary predisposition for developing breast cancer, recommended prevention measures may include prophylactic mastectomy and oophorectomy, but both of these surgeries are not without significant physiologic and psychological consequences.

The diagnostic process for evaluating any breast abnormality can be terrorizing for women, thereby necessitating the need for compassionate support and honest, comprehensive, understandable education. On a positive note, biopsy techniques continue to become less invasive. For most, the workup will result in a benign finding. These women usually feel a great sense of relief and ideally a heightened awareness of the importance of the early detection of breast cancer. For those with a positive finding, they are suddenly thrown into an unfamiliar and potentially frightening arena of health care. Being sensitive to the needs of these women is critical to promote their overall adjustment to the diagnosis.

Treatment for breast cancer has changed greatly and is continually evolving. Mastectomy is no longer the only choice for many women. The Halsted radical mastectomy is no longer the norm. For many women, breast-sparing procedures are more than adequate treatment. Lymph node sampling techniques have improved, especially with sentinel lymph node procedures, with the potential benefit of reducing lymphedema and other complications. Women, however, must make often complicated decisions about which treatment (or treatments) to undergo, and this decision-making process can be extremely stressful for some, especially for those with limited abilities to understand complex medical information and terminology.

Breast restoration also has improved dramatically. Women have many options in breast and reconstructive surgery. Patients with breast cancer need much guidance, support, and education as they make choices about reconstructive surgery. Although often forgotten, prosthetics can be an appropriate and satisfactory choice for women. They should not be considered as a "second-rate" choice or reserved simply for women who are not good surgical candidates. The choices in prosthetics are numerous. Similarly, bras, undergarments, and swimsuits no longer need to be ugly, and all women, regardless of their breast restoration choices, should be offered access to these items. Women need to be counseled and encouraged to learn about these different options before making a decision about breast restoration.

The past decades have demonstrated great strides in understanding the pathology of breast cancer and how it influences treatment. Two decades ago, systemic treatment was limited to a few chemotherapeutic agents and tamoxifen combined with surgery. Treatment now includes multiple chemotherapeutic agents, breast-sparing surgery, immunomodulating agents, radiation therapy, and hormonal manipulation. Each of these areas continues to expand, and many active research trials are currently available. Most recently, targeted therapies are becoming available for those with some types of breast cancer.

These advances in treatment, however, have not come without a price. The acute toxicities associated with surgery and adjuvant therapy can be significant. Many research efforts are ongoing to determine how to more accurately as-

sess, prevent, and manage these side effects. In addition to short-term side effects, many breast cancer survivors must cope with long-term consequences. The pool of survivors is steadily increasing, and with longer survival rates comes the increased possibility of long-term complications. Most notably, the past decade has seen a significant number of survivors coping with the consequences of early menopause, osteoporosis, and mental changes. Addressing the needs of this patient population through tertiary prevention practices is an ever-expanding role for nurses.

Breast cancer can be an overwhelming diagnosis for both patients and those close to them. Many women cope with the diagnosis and ultimately may have a renewed sense of purpose in life. For others, it can be devastating. The psychological ramifications of the diagnosis are significant. It forces women to confront mortality. The body image changes that result from surgery and related treatments serve as a constant reminder of the diagnosis. Role changes during treatment disrupt many family routines. After treatment, women need to adjust to a new normalcy.

Women worry about hereditary susceptibility and whether a child has inherited an increased risk for developing the disease. Genetic testing is becoming increasingly available. Although genetic testing enables women to better understand their risks and choices available to manage the risk, it also brings about intense psychosocial reactions and ramifications.

The diagnosis of breast cancer is accompanied by many unknowns, including prognostic factors, treatment issues, and how family and friends will react to the diagnosis. These unknowns contribute to stress with the diagnosis. The psychological care of these women and their families requires ongoing intervention by healthcare providers. For women whose breast cancer cannot be cured and who will ultimately die from the disease, there is an ongoing need to recognize and implement palliative care interventions in a timely fashion.

Research in breast cancer and its treatment continues. Researchers are actively looking for ways to detect breast cancer as early as possible. Much effort is being made to find effective and tolerable prevention strategies. Genetic markers continue to be identified to better stratify risk. Management of the long-term complications of surgery and treatment continues to provide challenges to healthcare providers. Women need to continue to be offered clinical trials to build an evidence-based practice for the management of breast cancer.

## Conclusion

This book seeks to address issues related to cancer control, breast cancer treatment, psychosocial concerns, and the management of complications related to cancer and its treatment in depth. Many issues in breast cancer are controversial. Patients and healthcare providers need to consider all issues, and then each woman needs to make choices that are consistent with her value system and place in life. In some cases, no single correct answer exists. New questions and challenges will continue to arise.

Many resources are available to healthcare providers who care for women with breast cancer. Healthcare providers also need to continually be aware of the recommendations and position statements of respected professional organizations. The Oncology Nursing Society has published several position statements on topics that are especially relevant for the care of women with breast cancer. These include breast cancer screening, cancer predisposition genetic testing and risk assessment counseling, rehabilitation of people with cancer, and prevention and early detection of cancer in the United States (see www.ons .org/publications/positions).

For many women diagnosed with breast cancer, nurses truly make an enormous difference in how they cope with the treatment and its associated complications. Different needs and concerns accompany each phase of the breast cancer trajectory. Nurses are challenged to consider the history of breast cancer treatment and to provide information and care in a way that promotes health, hope, and well-being for the women and families affected by the diagnosis of breast cancer.

# References

Al-Haddad, M. (2010). Breast cancer in men: The importance of teaching and raising awareness. *Clinical Journal of Oncology Nursing, 14,* 31–32. doi:10.1188/10.CJON.31-32

American Cancer Society. (2009). *Breast cancer facts and figures 2009–2010.* Atlanta, GA: Author.

American Cancer Society. (2010). *Cancer facts and figures 2010.* Atlanta, GA: Author.

Braun, S. (2003). The history of breast cancer advocacy. *Breast Journal, 9*(Suppl. 2), S101–S103.

Daly, M.B., Axilbund, J.E., Bryant, E., Buys, S., Eng, C., Friedman, S., ... Weitzel, J.N. (2006). Genetic/familial high-risk assessment: Breast and ovarian. *Journal of the National Comprehensive Cancer Network, 4,* 156–176.

First Sister Study results reinforce the importance of healthy living. (2009). *Alternative Therapies in Women's Health, 11*(5), 40.

Foster, R.S., Jr. (2003). Breast cancer detection and treatment: A personal and historical perspective. *Archives of Surgery, 138,* 397–408. doi:10.1001/archsurg.138.4.397

Klawiter, M. (2004). Breast cancer in two regimes: The impact of social movements on illness experience. *Sociology of Health and Illness, 26,* 845–874. doi:10.1111/j.0141-9889.2004.00421.x

Kolker, E.S. (2004). Framing as a cultural resource in health social movements: Funding activism and the breast cancer movement in the US 1990–1993. *Sociology of Health and Illness, 26,* 820–844. doi:10.1111/j.0141-9889.2004.00420.x

Onami, S., Ozaki, M., Mortimer, J.E., & Pal, S.K. (2010). Male breast cancer: An update in diagnosis, treatment and molecular profiling. *Maturitas, 65,* 308–314. doi:10.1016/j.maturitas.2010.01.012

Qureshi, S.Y., & Qureshi, N. (2008). Genetic profiling in primary care can enhance personalized drug therapy: Reality or myth? *Personalized Medicine, 5,* 311–316. doi:10.2217/17410541.5.4.311

Savage, L. (2007). Breast cancer stamp funds new NCI program. *Journal of the National Cancer Institute, 99,* 587–589. doi:10.1093/jnci/djk172

The Sister Study: A study of the environmental and genetic risk factors for breast cancer. (2010). Retrieved from http://www.sisterstudy .org/English/index1.htm

Vanchieri, C. (2007). National Cancer Act: A look back and forward. *Journal of the National Cancer Institute, 99,* 342–345. doi:10.1093/jnci/djk119

# CHAPTER 2

# Risk Factors for Breast Cancer

Suzanne M. Mahon, RN, DNSc, AOCN®, APNG

## Introduction

A risk factor is a trait or characteristic that is associated with a statistically significant increased likelihood of developing a disease. In the case of breast cancer, the presence of a risk factor does not absolutely mean that a woman will develop breast cancer, nor does the absence of a risk factor make her immune to developing the breast cancer.

Many women are very worried about developing breast cancer. This stems from extensive media coverage of the topic, which often is confusing and conflicting. Most women know someone who has been affected by the diagnosis of breast cancer. This pervasive worry is compounded by the fact that the best way to assess and manage breast cancer risk is not always completely clear. Women who receive breast cancer screening and other health care would like to better understand their risk for developing breast cancer and what specifically can be done to reduce their risk, as well as their anxiety about the disease. Breast cancer risk assessment is the critical initial step in helping women to better comprehend the ramifications of the disease and to take appropriate steps to prevent it or detect it early, when it is most treatable. The outcome of risk assessment has different implications for each woman because risk is different for every woman, and every individual has different capacities to understand risk figures. Unfortunately, breast cancer risk assessment often is ignored or minimized, resulting in inappropriate or ineffective prevention and detection strategies.

The basic elements of a breast cancer risk assessment generally include a review of medical history, a history of exposures to carcinogens in daily living, and a detailed family history. Once all information is gathered, it must be interpreted for the patient in reasonable and understandable terms. This is paramount in communicating breast cancer risk. Risk assessment guides not only screening decisions but also, in some cases, treatment decisions. For example, genetic testing (a tool for breast cancer risk assessment) affects and guides treatment decisions. Decisions based on genetic testing often are significant,

are emotionally laden, and can have many ramifications, such as prophylactic surgery. This underscores the importance of constructing an accurate risk assessment so that genetic testing and prophylactic measures can be implemented appropriately in individuals who stand to gain the most benefit.

Because risk communication alters screening and treatment decisions, nurses need to understand the known and suspected risk factors for breast cancer and their physiologic basis. Genetic predisposition testing for breast cancer susceptibility genes is readily available on a commercial basis, and people need sufficient, accurate information to make appropriate choices about testing based on their own individual situation. To provide effective education and support for women who are concerned about breast cancer risk and genetic testing, nurses must use clear communication strategies regarding cancer risk. This chapter will provide a discussion of conceptual issues in risk assessment, a review of risk factors associated with the development of breast cancer, considerations in genetic testing for breast cancer susceptibility genes, and issues in breast cancer risk communication.

## Types of Risk Used in Breast Cancer Risk Counseling

### Absolute Risk

*Absolute risk* is a measure of the occurrence of cancer, by either incidence (new cases) or mortality (deaths), in an identified population. Absolute risk is helpful when patients need to understand what the chances are for all individuals in a population of developing a particular disease. Absolute risk can be expressed either as the number of cases for a specified denominator (for example, 123.6 cases of breast cancer per 100,000 women annually) or as a cumulative risk up to a specified age (for example, one in eight women will develop breast cancer if they live to age 85) (American Cancer Society [ACS], 2010a). Another way to express absolute risk is to discuss the average risk of developing breast cancer at a certain age. For example, a woman's risk of developing breast cancer may be 2.39% at age 50, but at age 85, it might be 12.08%. Risk estimates will be much different for a 50-year-old woman than for an 85-year-old woman, as approximately 50% of breast cancer cases occur after age 65 (ACS, 2010a) (see Table 2-1).

| Table 2-1. Absolute Risk of Developing Breast Cancer Over Time* | |
|---|---|
| **Age** | **Risk** |
| 0–39 years | 0.5% (1 in 206 women) |
| 40–59 years | 3.83% (1 in 27) |
| 60–69 years | 3.4% (1 in 29) |
| 70 or more years | 3.73% (1 in 15) |

*Lifetime risk is 12.08% (one in eight women). Percentages do not add up exactly because of rounding.

*Note.* Based on information from American Cancer Society, 2009a.

Women need to understand that certain assumptions are made to reach an absolute risk figure for breast cancer. For example, the one-in-eight figure describes the average risk of developing breast cancer in Caucasian American women, and its calculation considers other causes of death over the life span. This figure will overestimate breast cancer risk for some people with no risk factors and will greatly underestimate the risk for people with several risk factors or those with a genetic mutation. What this statistic actually means is that the average woman's breast cancer risk is 0.5% until age 40, 3.83% for ages 40–59, 3.4% for ages 60–59, and 3.73% for ages 70 and older. The 12.08% or one-in-eight risk figure is obtained by adding the risk in each age category. When a woman who has an average risk reaches age 40 without a diagnosis of breast cancer, she has passed through 0.49% of her risk, so her lifetime risk is 12.08% minus 0.49%, which equals 11.58%. Time always must be considered for the risk figure to be meaningful.

## Relative Risk

The term *relative risk* refers to a comparison of the incidence or number of deaths among those with a particular risk factor compared to those without the risk factor. By using relative risk factors, patients can determine their risk factors and thus better understand their chances of developing a specific cancer as compared to people without such risk factors. If the risk for a woman with no known risk factors is 1.0, one can evaluate those with risk factors in relation to this figure (see Table 2-2).

The use of relative risk factors can be confusing to some patients. When providing information about relative risk, it is important to specify exactly what comparison is being made. Often, percentages are confusing when used with relative risk. If a news report states that taking a particular hormone therapy after menopause causes a 30%–50% increase in breast cancer risk, in absolute numeric terms this means that 0.6 more cases of breast cancer will occur per 100 women ages 50–70. The same concept applies if a person has a 1% chance of developing cancer. This means that the risk has increased from 1 in 10,000 to 1.3 in 10,000 (Klein & Stefanek, 2007).

Relative risk is sometimes expressed as a ratio. Ratios can create problems because people fail to consider the relevant sample size. For example, individuals may respond differently to a ratio when it is expressed as 1:10 rather than 10:100, even though both ratios express the same probability. People may rate a health problem as riskier if informed that it kills 1,275 of 10,000 people (12.75%) when compared with 12.75 of 100 people (12.75%).

Relative risk figures are only helpful if everyone understands what the baseline group is. If the baseline is unclear, a statement of relative risk can be misleading. Relative risk figures cannot be mathematically added together. Each needs to be considered separately in light of the baseline group or anchor of comparison. Women with multiple risk factors, especially those with higher relative risk figures, should consider that information carefully when making decisions about breast cancer prevention and detection measures.

## Attributable Risk

*Attributable risk* is the amount of disease within the population that could be prevented by alteration or elimination of a risk factor. Attributable risk has enormous implications for public health policy. A risk factor could convey a very large relative risk but be restricted to a few individuals; so, changing it would benefit only a small group. Conversely, some risk factors amenable to change could potentially decrease the morbidity and mortality associated with malignancy in a significant number of people. Little is known about attributable risk in breast cancer, and most gains at this point are probably small. For example, a package insert might report a relative risk of 2.35 for developing breast cancer in women younger than age 35 whose first exposure to an oral contraceptive (OC) drug was within the previous four years. Because the annual incidence rate (absolute risk) for women ages 30–34 is 26.7 per 100,000, a relative risk of 2.35 increases the possible risk from 26.7 to 62.75 cases per 100,000 women. The attributable risk of breast cancer is calculated to be an additional 3.38 per 10,000 women per year. This increase in the number of cases possibly is associated with the use of a pharmacologic agent. Public health policy related to the use of this agent will need to incorporate a harm-versus-benefit analysis to determine whether the recommendation for the agent should be altered to decrease breast cancer risk.

**Table 2-2. Relative Risk Factors for Developing Breast Cancer**

| Risk Factor | Comparison Category | Relative Risk |
|---|---|---|
| Early menarche (before age 12) | Menarche after age 15 | 1.1–2.0 |
| Late menopause (after age 55) | Menopause age 45 or younger | 1.5–2.0 |
| First live birth between ages 25–29 | First live birth before age 25 | 1.5–2.0 |
| First live birth after age 30 | First live birth before age 25 | 1.9 |
| First live birth after age 35 | First live birth before age 25 | 2.0–3.0 |
| Nulliparous | First live birth before age 25 | 3.0 |
| Recent oral contraceptive use | No contraceptive use | 1.1–2.0 |
| Biopsy-proven proliferative disease | No proliferative disease | 1.9–2.5 |
| Biopsy-proven proliferative disease with atypical hyperplasia | No proliferative disease | 4.4–5.3 |
| Lobular carcinoma in situ | No proliferative disease | 6.9–16.4 |
| Alcohol intake (two or more drinks per day) | No alcohol intake | 1.2 |
| Obesity/increased body mass (in 80th percentile or higher at age 55) | Body mass in 20th percentile or less | 1.2 |
| First-degree relative with postmenopausal breast cancer | No first-degree relative with breast cancer | 1.8 |
| First-degree relative with premenopausal breast cancer | No first-degree relative with breast cancer | 3.3 |
| Two first-degree relatives with postmenopausal breast cancer | No first-degree relative with breast cancer | 3.6 |
| Two first-degree relatives with premenopausal breast cancer | No first-degree relative with breast cancer | 7.1 |
| Past history of invasive breast cancer | No past history of invasive breast cancer | 6.8 |
| Radiation exposure for Hodgkin disease | No exposure | 5.2 |
| Current hormone replacement therapy user with estrogen and progesterone for at least five years | No history of use | 1.3–1.8 |
| Age older than 55 years | Age younger than 45 years | 1.2–1.5 |

*Note.* Based on information from American Cancer Society, 2009a; Lee et al., 2003; Singletary, 2003.

## Challenges in Risk Communication

### Rationale for Breast Cancer Risk Assessment

Several important reasons exist for identifying and quantifying breast cancer risks. The identification of risk factors contributes to the understanding of the biology of breast cancer, and when identified, such risk factors may be altered to decrease the number of new cases of or deaths from cancer (Bradbury & Olopade, 2006).

The quantification of risk also guides public policy for the allocation of funds for screening and for utilization of costly services (i.e., genetic testing). Screening is most likely to be recommended for cancer sites in which reasonable screening tests exist, incidence is substantial, and risks are understood and for which screening directly affects the morbidity and mortality associated with the disease. Breast cancer is a perfect example of a cancer in which screening can directly alter morbidity and mortality.

Not all risk factors are amenable to change, however, as is the case with many risk factors for breast cancer. An individual cannot change her gender, age, history, or some of the other cited factors. In such a case, it is appropriate to recommend secondary cancer prevention or screening efforts.

When nurses discuss risk factors with patients, they need to carefully articulate the type of risk (absolute, relative, or attributable) and the physiologic basis of the risk factor, if known. Much research has been conducted to better understand risk factors for the development of breast cancer. Known risk factors are associated with aging, reproductive history, exogenous hormone exposure, family history, and other environmental exposures. Much remains unknown about the influence and interaction of these risk factors, and at present, they provide only a modest explanation at best for the risk of developing breast cancer. Other factors that probably have significantly contributed to the increasing incidence of breast cancer in the past 30 years include better nutrition leading to an earlier menarche, delayed or no childbearing related to career and societal expectations, and increased exogenous hormone use, including OCs and hormone replacement therapy (HRT) (ACS, 2010a). Women would like to have a simple explanation as to why they may be at risk for breast cancer, but the interaction of risk factors makes this nearly impossible (Mahoney, Bevers, Linos, & Willett, 2008). Clearly, some risk factors are under the control of individuals, and others are not. The risk factor assessment for breast cancer is based on past medical history, lifestyle behaviors, and family history.

## Components of a Risk Assessment

The cancer risk assessment should include the patient's past medical history and personal history factors that may increase the risk of developing cancer and should be documented. Many of these risk factors are not within an individual's control and are not amenable to primary prevention efforts (e.g., age at menarche). In contrast, lifestyle factors complete the risk factor assessment and often are within the control of the individual. They provide a framework for providing education about primary prevention efforts.

Past screening activities and findings from such activities contribute to the risk assessment and provide further opportunity to educate the patient about the potential strengths, benefits, and risks associated with screening. The patient's reports of these results may not be accurate. It is important to order pathology reports or actual mammograms for review before determining risk and communicating risk information to the patient. For example, there is a big difference between the risk for development of breast cancer in a woman with a biopsy-proven fibroadenoma and in a woman with biopsy-proven ductal hyperplasia with atypia. *Fibrocystic disease* or *change* is a generic term and should not be equated with an increased risk for developing breast cancer. Obtaining accurate information is necessary to develop the most accurate risk assessment possible, correct misconceptions if indicated, and make the best possible recommendations for cancer screening or select the best model to predict mutation carrier status.

The family history is a critical component of cancer risk assessment. For those with a true hereditary predisposition verified by positive genetic test results, screening and prevention recommendations usually are significantly altered. Hereditary risk is poorly understood by many individuals. Often, individuals fail to understand that risk can be transmitted through both the paternal and maternal sides. The presence of one or two relatives with breast cancer does not necessarily denote hereditary risk, as breast cancer is a relatively commonly diagnosed malignancy. Many factors are con-

sidered, including age at onset and the number of female relatives affected and not affected. Simply stating that a family history of breast cancer is present does not necessarily mean there is true increased risk.

Obtaining a family history in the primary care setting may take 15–30 minutes, depending on the size of the family and the level of reported detail. Pursuing pathology reports to confirm diagnoses takes additional time. Interpreting that information can take even longer. Because risk assessment can be time consuming and is poorly reimbursed, a complete risk assessment is often never completed.

The pedigree provides an organized way to document the risk factors related to family history, such as whether a relative is alive or dead, age at death if applicable, significant medical diagnoses, or a diagnosis of cancer. The pedigree can include space in which to describe the specific type of cancer, age at diagnosis, and other characteristics, such as whether a breast cancer was premenopausal or bilateral. Healthcare providers should ask patients about specific relatives and their health individually rather than asking a more general question such as, "Have any of your relatives been diagnosed with cancer?" After gathering the family history, it is important to recheck whether any of the patient's relatives have been diagnosed with these cancers. It is amazing how often patients forget to provide this information, and reiterating this question may unearth valuable information.

## Communication of Risk Assessment

After completion of the breast cancer risk assessment, the next challenge for healthcare providers is to communicate the information to women who may be anxious or concerned about their risk for developing breast cancer. This anxiety often affects patients' ability to completely grasp and comprehend the meaning of the assessment and their actual risk.

Another reason why risk communication is such a daunting task is that risk can be presented in a variety of ways, and the interpretation of risk measures can be confusing to both healthcare professionals and the public (Akobeng, 2008). Moreover, not all of the various ways of reporting risk clearly show the benefits or risks of treatments or screening maneuvers in a clinically useful way, and many of these measures are frequently misunderstood. This is particularly crucial when the treatment decision confronting the patient is an emotionally charged decision (Fagerlin, Zikmund-Fisher, & Ubel, 2007).

Nurses providing breast cancer risk assessment services need to interpret the assessment so that women can make informed and appropriate choices for prevention and early detection. Central to this communication is selecting an appropriate risk-prediction model.

A major limitation of risk assessment relates to the assessment models, which are based on assumptions and epidemiologic studies. If these assumptions and studies are weak or deficient, the resulting assessment can be inaccurate or inappropriate. Most studies are epidemiologic: they identify an association between exposure or no exposure to an agent and the subsequent occurrence of disease. If a statistically significant correlation is found, researchers can make one conclusion only: that an association (not necessarily a cause-and-effect relationship) exists between the substance and cancer. As with many cancers, the etiology of breast cancer appears to be multifactorial, with endogenous and exogenous risk factors contributing to risk. No model can include all of the risk factors that may apply to each individual. Therefore, another general limitation of risk assessment is that no model completely and accurately explains an individual's risk for developing a particular cancer (Freedman et al., 2005).

In some cancers, such as breast cancer, the central role of risk factor identification is to identify women who are at higher-than-average risk, particularly those with a genetic susceptibility to breast cancer, and to screen them more aggressively. For example, women from families prone to breast cancer may be advised to undergo screening mammograms at a younger age and more than once a year (National Comprehensive Cancer Center [NCCN], 2010; Saslow et al., 2007).

Each risk assessment model has inherent strengths and weaknesses; these will be discussed later in this chapter. Nurses need to be aware of these and provide each client with a balanced discussion that incorporates an understanding of each model's characteristics.

## Risk Factors for Breast Cancer

### Age

The most consistently documented uncontrollable risk factor for the development of breast cancer is increasing age (Vogel, 2008). Table 2-1 illustrates how at different ages women have different statistical risks for developing breast cancer. One way to consider this risk is that if all women younger than 65 years of age are compared with women ages 65 and older, the relative risk of breast cancer associated with increased age is 5.8 (Singletary, 2003).

### Reproductive Factors

A woman's hormone levels normally change throughout her life for a variety of reasons. These hormonal fluctuations can lead to changes in the breast tissue. Hormonal changes occur during puberty, pregnancy, and menopause. Studies have linked the age at menarche, menopause, and first live birth to breast cancer risk (Vogel, 2008). Collectively, the patterns of risk associated with reproductive history suggest that prolonged exposure to ovarian hormones increases breast cancer occurrence. Although results are mixed, research suggests that the number of menstrual cy-

cles during a lifetime may have a greater impact on risk than the number of cycles until the first full-term pregnancy (Chavez-MacGregor et al., 2005). Support for this theory stems from the observation that women who had both ovaries removed before the age of 40 showed a 45% reduction in breast cancer risk compared with women who underwent a natural menopause between ages 50–54 (Singletary, 2003). Thus, women who experience menarche before age 12 or menopause after age 50 are considered at somewhat higher risk because of the total increased number of ovulatory cycles in their lifetime.

Specific pathways involved in estrogen metabolism that may play a role in the etiology of breast cancer are not as well understood. It has been hypothesized that breast tissue damage or aging starts at a constant rate at menarche and continues at that rate until the time of first pregnancy, at which point the rate of tissue aging decreases (Vogel, 2008). This continues until menopause, when an additional decrease occurs, and after menopause, when the rate is more constant but decreased (Colditz, 2005). Researchers speculate that if the first full-term pregnancy is delayed, the proliferation due to pregnancy hormones would be acting on a more damaged or aged set of DNA and would carry a greater adverse effect. Furthermore, when the interval between births is shortened, the rate of tissue aging and incidence of breast cancer are lower. In the United States, the interval between menarche and the first full-term pregnancy has been greatly lengthened because of increasing reproductive education and more effective contraception.

After a transient increase in risk after childbirth, a long-term reduction occurs in breast cancer risk (Collaborative Group on Hormonal Factors in Breast Cancer, 2002). The same is true of miscarriage (Brewster, Stockton, Dobbie, Bull, & Beral, 2005; National Cancer Institute [NCI], 2005). The degree of risk reduction appears to be related to age. Increasing parity is associated with a long-term reduction in breast cancer risk, presumably because of the interruption of estrogen cycling (NCI, 2005).

A large prospective cohort of 60,075 women associated breast-feeding with a decreased risk of premenopausal breast cancer (Stuebe, Willett, Xue, & Michels, 2009). These researchers found a 59% reduction in the incidence of premenopausal breast cancer among women who had ever breast-fed and also had a first-degree relative with breast cancer. It is not clear whether breast-feeding confers protection against postmenopausal breast cancer (Vogel, 2008). Reproductive risk factors also may interact with other predisposing genotypes, placing some women at high risk for developing breast cancer.

Although modulation of reproductive risk factors or hormonal interventions that simulate the preventive effects of early pregnancy or early menopause are theoretically possible, these types of interventions may not be effective for all women, including those with a family history of breast cancer (Colditz, 2005). Chemoprevention is an example of this expanding area of research to modulate risk factors in the development of breast cancer.

## History of Benign Breast Disease

A history of benign breast disease often is reported to be a risk factor for developing breast cancer. The key to understanding the usefulness of this risk factor is to be very careful to review the findings of all pathology reports. Defining this risk is becoming increasingly important as more women undergo breast biopsies for asymptomatic abnormalities found on mammography and, more recently, breast magnetic resonance imaging, which creates a larger pool of "higher risk" women. This risk factor can be stratified only when fibrocystic or benign breast disease is quantified according to a histology or pathology report. Nonproliferative lesions (which account for more than 70% of all breast biopsies [Colditz, 2005]) include adenosis, fibrosis, cysts, mastitis, duct ectasia, fibroadenomas, and mild hyperplasia and confer no added risk for developing breast cancer. Of concern are pathology reports that suggest the presence of atypical hyperplasia or lobular carcinoma, although an accurate risk figure associated with this finding is difficult to quantify (Vogel, 2008).

## Exogenous Hormone Use

The exact risk of breast cancer conferred by the use of OCs is controversial. The composition of OCs has changed greatly over time. Early formulations of OCs used in the 1960s and 1970s contained larger amounts of estrogen and progestin than current formulations. Large randomized controlled trials are not readily available and present many methodologic and ethical concerns that make them very challenging to conduct. Interpretation of these studies is further confused by the different end points. Different risks of specific histologic types may exist based on the type and duration of OC used (Casey, Cerhan, & Pruthi, 2008; Newcomer, Newcomb, Trentham-Dietz, Longnecker, & Greenberg, 2003).

Marchbanks et al. (2002) reported one of the largest case-control studies among former and current users of OCs. These researchers interviewed 4,575 women with breast cancer and 4,682 controls. They concluded that among women ages 35–64, former OC use was not associated with a significantly increased risk of developing breast cancer. OCs have been associated with a small increased risk of breast cancer in current users that gradually diminishes over time.

Similar to OCs, HRT is associated with a slightly increased risk for developing breast cancer, but the amount of risk is not clear. HRT has been readily available since the 1970s, but it was not until the later 1990s that reports began to link HRT use with the development of breast cancer (Vogel, 2008).

Evidence supporting an association between the use of exogenous hormones after menopause and breast cancer is more consistent than that for OC use. The landmark Women's Health Initiative (WHI) study suggested that HRT may not be as safe or as effective as originally thought (Anderson et al., 2004). Combination HRT using an estrogen and progestin is associated with an increased risk of developing breast cancer. The exact risk is unclear because of the multiple forms of HRT available and the varying number of years of use, but it is thought to be approximately a 24% increase overall. The evidence is mixed concerning the association between estrogen-only therapy and breast cancer (Conner, Lundström, & von Schoultz, 2008).

More recently, concern exists about an increased risk of breast cancer associated with fertility medications, which are used with increasing frequency (Sprague et al., 2008). In one study of more than 7,000 British women, the relative risk of breast cancer after using ovulation-stimulating medications was 1.13 (Idos et al., 2009). A study of 1,135 Swedish women using fertility medications did not show any increase in breast cancer risk (Orgéas et al., 2009). Pappo et al. (2008) reported a possible association between in vitro fertilization therapy and breast cancer development, especially in women older than 40. The relationship between the use of ovulation-stimulating medications and the risk of breast cancer is unclear, and more research is needed.

## Alcohol Consumption

Clear, documented evidence shows that the consumption of more than two alcoholic drinks per day increases the risk of developing breast cancer. The proposed mechanisms for this phenomenon are alcohol's stimulation of the metabolism of carcinogens, such as acetaldehyde, and more global mechanisms, such as decreased DNA repair efficiency or poor nutritional intake of protective nutrients (Vogel, 2008). Associated relative risks when compared to women who do not consume alcohol of 1, 2, and 3 drinks per day are estimated to be 1.1, 1.2, and 1.4, respectively (Conner et al., 2008).

Individual data from 53 case-control and cohort studies were included in a British meta-analysis (Hamajima et al., 2002). Results showed that the relative risk of breast cancer increased by approximately 7% for each 10 g (one drink) of alcohol per day. The same result was obtained even after additional stratification for race, education, family history, age at menarche, height, weight, breast-feeding history, OC use, HRT use, and type of and age at menopause.

Breast cancer risk also may be increased in women who began consuming alcohol at a younger age (Berkey et al., 2010). Higher amounts consumed and more frequent consumption of alcoholic beverages in adolescence may increase the occurrence of benign breast disease and possibly breast cancer in young women.

## Increased Body Mass

Increased body mass may be a more important risk factor in postmenopausal women than in premenopausal women.

Adipose tissue is an important source of extragonadal estrogens in postmenopausal women. Theoretically, the more tissue that is available, the higher the circulating levels of these estrogens (Vogel, 2008). Obesity is associated with increased breast cancer risk, especially among postmenopausal women (Conner et al., 2008). The WHI Observational Study looked at 85,917 women ages 50–79 and collected information on weight history, as well as known risk factors for breast cancer (Morimoto et al., 2002). Increased breast cancer risk was associated with weight at entry, body mass index (BMI) at entry, BMI at age 50, maximum BMI, adult and postmenopausal weight change, and waist and hip circumferences. Weight was the strongest predictor, with a relative risk of 2.85. It has been estimated that for every seven pounds of weight gained after age 18, the risk of dying from breast cancer increased 7% (Hede, 2008).

Additionally, women who have lower body mass may exercise more. Exercise can decrease the number of ovulatory cycles. This may offer a small amount of protection against breast cancer in women who are physically active on a regular basis (ACS, 2009a).

Recent preliminary research also suggests that taller women may be at increased risk for developing breast cancer (Vogel, 2008). An increase of 5 cm in height can be associated with a 5% increased risk of breast cancer (Conner et al., 2008). It is hypothesized that tall women have more breast tissue parenchyma. Clearly this is an area of evolving research.

## Ionizing Radiation

Exposure of the breast to ionizing radiation is associated with an increased risk of developing breast cancer, especially when the exposure occurs at a young age (Taylor & Taylor, 2009). The evidence of this emerged from cohort and case-control studies. This finding supports the avoidance of unnecessary breast irradiation. Women treated for Hodgkin lymphoma before age 16 may have a subsequent risk of developing breast cancer by age 40 as high as 35%, with higher doses of radiation (median dose is 40 Gy in breast cancer cases) and treatment between 10–16 years of age corresponding with higher risk (Travis et al., 2003). When radiation therapy was administered after age 16 but before age 30, the risk of developing breast cancer also increased, but to a lesser degree. Unlike the risk for secondary leukemia, the risk of treatment-related breast cancer did not abate with duration of follow-up, and the increased risk persisted for more than 25 years after treatment. The median age of breast cancer diagnosis in this population is 32–35 years of age (Pinkowish, 2009).

In theory, patients with breast cancer who were treated with lumpectomy and radiation therapy may be at increased risk for second breast or other malignancies, compared with those treated by mastectomy. Outcomes of 1,029 patients treated with lumpectomy and radiation therapy were compared with 1,387 patients treated with mastectomy. After a median follow-up of 15 years, results showed no difference in the risk of second malignancies (Fisher et al., 2002). Another study of 701 women randomized to radical mastectomy or lumpectomy and radiation therapy demonstrated the rate of contralateral breast carcinomas per 100 woman-years to be 10.2 versus 8.7, respectively (Veronesi et al., 2002).

## Abortion History

The possibility of an association between induced abortion and subsequent breast cancer development has been suggested, although the exact risk is not clear, and this risk factor is controversial. Initial research was based on studies using recalled information in populations where induced abortion had a negative social or religious stigma (Singletary, 2003). Trials conducted in social environments where abortion is accepted have not shown an increased risk (Committee on Gynecologic Practice, 2009; Mahue-Giangreco, Ursin, Sullivan-Halley, & Bernstein, 2003; Singletary, 2003).

## Diet and Vitamins

A low-fat diet might influence breast cancer risk. Epidemiologic studies show a positive correlation between international age-adjusted breast cancer mortality rates and the estimated per-capita consumption of dietary fat (Cummings et al., 2009). A low-fat diet might reduce the relative risk of breast cancer by approximately 9%. When case-control studies have been used to evaluate the hypothesis that dietary fat is related to breast cancer risk, the results have been mixed (Lof & Weiderpass, 2009).

Fruit and vegetable consumption has been thought to be associated with reduced breast cancer risk. A pooled analysis of adult dietary data from eight cohort studies, which included 351,823 women in whom 7,377 incident cases of breast cancer occurred, provided little support for an association (Smith-Warner et al., 2001). When examining the dietary data treated as continuous variables (based on grams of intake per day), no association was present. These studies suggest that if any decreased risk of breast cancer associated with consumption of fruits and vegetables does exist, the association is probably weak (Pierce, 2009).

Micronutrient intake also may play a small role in the development of breast cancer. Low folate intake has been suggested to increase breast cancer risk, as folate is involved in one-carbon metabolism, which is important for DNA methylation, repair, and synthesis. Current epidemiologic evidence of the association between folate intake and breast cancer risk is inconsistent (Lof & Weiderpass, 2009). Vitamins A (as carotenoids), C, and E may exert a protective effect for breast cancer through their antioxidative properties (Lof & Weiderpass, 2009).

Milk consumption induces a rise in endogenous insulin-like growth factor I levels and may decrease breast cancer risk. Dairy items also are naturally rich in calcium and, because of fortification, vitamin D, both of which may decrease breast cancer risk. Epidemiologic evidence regarding the association between consumption of dairy products or intakes of calcium or vitamin D and breast cancer risk is inconsistent. A recent study indicated that the protective effect of vitamin D and calcium may be restricted to or may be stronger in premenopausal women (Chlebowski et al., 2008).

## Increased Breast Density

Breast density is directly linked to breast cancer risk (Boyd et al., 2007). Breast density has little to do with breast size, although this is a common misconception. Breast density actually refers to the amount of white area on a breast mammogram, which otherwise appears black. The balance of white and black reflects the breast composition and relative amount of glandular tissue, connective tissue, and fat. Different methods of estimating the proportion of white area on the mammogram exist and vary from the perception of the radiologist to using a software program to outline the white area and compare it to the total breast area.

The underlying causes of breast density are mostly inherited. Higher breast density is more common in some ethnic groups, including Caucasian women (Boyd et al., 2007). It also is more common in younger women, beginning when hormones escalate during puberty and continuing through the childbearing years. Breast density decreases during menopause in a process called breast involution, where the milk glands and ducts atrophy and connective tissue disappears. Studies have shown that women who have extremely dense breasts have a three- to five-fold increased risk of breast cancer compared with women who have mostly fatty breasts (Vogel, 2008).

One concern has been whether the breast cancer associated with dense breasts is due to a "masking effect," where the lack of contrast (that is, a breast image that is very white throughout) between normal tissue and tumors in dense breasts makes it difficult to discriminate between the two. Although this may contribute to a delay in detection, it is not truly a risk factor (Boyd et al., 2009). Postmenopausal women with increased breast density should be considered at increased risk for developing breast cancer.

## Family History and Genetic Predisposition

Assessment of risk for breast cancer would be incomplete without an accurate assessment of hereditary risk. This may be the most quantifiable of all the risk factors, as well as the most clinically significant. Assessment of hereditary risk for breast cancer is confusing to many patients. It often is incor-

rectly assumed that any family history of cancer automatically infers a higher risk of developing the disease. In a subgroup of families, this is indeed the case, but for many women, the presence of one or two relatives with breast cancer does not contribute to a substantially increased risk. Breast cancer is a common malignancy in women; consequently, it is plausible that a woman may have one or two relatives with the diagnosis, especially if the age at onset was older. Assessment of the family history is important primarily to determine who may have a genetic predisposition for developing breast or other cancers. These family members should be offered information on the risks and benefits associated with genetic testing.

Traditionally, risk has been assessed for an individual. Because families share a pool of genes, they also share similar risks for inheriting a predisposition to a particular cancer. Genetic risk assessment, therefore, must include not only individuals but also entire families. Genetic testing is one of the tools used in the cancer risk assessment process to accurately quantify risk.

### Biology of Genetic Transmission

Approximately 10% of all cases of breast cancer are related to a hereditary predisposition (ACS, 2010a). This predisposition usually results from the inheritance of a single germ-line mutation, which usually is autosomal dominant. Most commonly this is a mutation in *BRCA1* or *BRCA2*, for which commercial testing is readily available. Other genetic syndromes associated with a family history of breast cancer are shown in Table 2-3. Given the high incidence of breast cancer, even a seemingly small incidence of 10% potentially translates into a large number of affected patients. The overall prevalence of deleterious *BRCA1* mutations is estimated to be 1 in 800 in the general population (Lindor, McMaster, Lindor, & Greene, 2008). The prevalence of *BRCA2* mutations in the general population is unknown (Petrucelli, Daly, Culver, & Feldman, 2007).

*BRCA1* and *BRCA2* are tumor suppressor genes. These genes are normally present in every human and function to suppress tumor cell growth. The presence of a germ-line mutation in either *BRCA1* or *BRCA2* renders an individual significantly more likely than others in the general population to develop breast and/or ovarian cancer. These are autosomal dominant genes, so each first-degree relative has a statistical 50% chance of inheriting the mutation and the associated cancer risk. Because they are located on chromosomes 13 and 17, they can be passed to subsequent generations by either male or female transmission.

Current estimates suggest that *BRCA1* and *BRCA2* mutation carriers have up to an 86% lifetime risk of developing at least one breast cancer and approximately a 30%–50% risk of developing ovarian cancer (Lindor et al., 2008; Petrucelli et al., 2007). Approximately half of the women with a *BRCA1* or *BRCA2* mutation develop breast cancer by age 50.

| Table 2-3. Common Hereditary Breast Cancer Syndromes | | |
|---|---|---|
| Syndrome/Incidence | Gene | Common Features |
| Breast and ovarian cancer syndrome<br>1 in 800–2,500 | BRCA1 at 17q21<br>BRCA2 at 13q21<br>Autosomal dominant<br>Up to 90% penetrant for breast cancer and 24%–40% penetrant for ovarian cancer | • Premenopausal breast cancer<br>• Bilateral breast cancer<br>• Multiple generations with multiple relatives affected<br>• Family history of ovarian cancer |
| Li-Fraumeni syndrome<br>Very rare—an estimated 400 nonrelated families | TP53 at 17p13.1<br>Autosomal dominant<br>Up to 90% penetrant breast cancer<br>Mutation-positive women may be seven times more likely to develop cancer than mutation-positive men | • Premenopausal breast cancer<br>• Uterine sarcomas<br>• Childhood sarcoma, brain tumor, leukemia, and adrenocortical carcinoma |
| Cowden syndrome<br>1 in 200,000–250,000 in Dutch population | PTEN at 10q23<br>Autosomal dominant<br>50% penetrant breast cancer | • Excess of breast, gastrointestinal, endometrial, and thyroid disease, both benign and malignant<br>• Skin manifestations including multiple trichilemmomas, oral fibromas, and acral, palmar, and plantar keratoses |
| Ataxia telangiectasia<br>1 in 30,000–100,000 | ATM at 11q22.3<br>Autosomal recessive<br>Almost 100% penetrant | • Characterized by neurologic deterioration, telangiectasias, immunodeficiency states, and hypersensitivity to ionizing radiation<br>• Increased risk of hematologic and breast cancers |
| Peutz-Jeghers syndrome<br>1 in 120,000 | STK11 at 19p13.3<br>Autosomal dominant<br>50% penetrant | • Characterized by melanocytic macules on the lips, perioral area, and buccal regions<br>• Multiple gastrointestinal polyps<br>• Multiple cases of breast, colon, pancreatic, stomach, and ovarian cancers |

Note. Based on information from Lindor et al., 2008.

## Pedigree Construction

Certain features of a family history should raise suspicion that a hereditary breast cancer syndrome may be present (see Figure 2-1). It is usually best to begin a hereditary assessment by constructing a family tree or pedigree as shown in Figure 2-2.

A pedigree should include the ages and causes of death for three generations. Paternal and maternal sides should both be assessed and recorded, as most hereditary susceptibility genes are located on autosomes and can be passed with equal frequency from either side. For family members diagnosed with cancer, the pedigree also should include the type of primary cancers and ages at diagnosis.

For those with a possible hereditary risk for developing breast cancer, accurate risk assessment is critical. It guides genetic testing, as well as decisions about screening. An accurate pedigree and risk assessment is the first step in applying a prediction model. The pedigree can be suggestive of hereditary risk and provide insight into what model might most accurately predict risk. A family history should focus on primary and secondary relatives. First-degree relatives include parents, siblings, and children. Because first-degree relatives share 50% of their genes, these relatives will be the most likely to inherit similar genetic information. These families often will have multiple cases of cancer at an earlier age than expected in the general population. Information about second-degree relatives also can prove helpful. Second-degree relatives include grandparents, aunts, and uncles. Second-degree relatives have 25% of their genes in common. In particular, older second-degree relatives can provide important information about genetic risk because they would have been expected to manifest an early-onset cancer if a hereditary trait is present in the family. The pedigree also should include nieces and nephews because these younger family members can provide information about childhood cancers, which has implications for the genetic risk assessment. Third-degree relatives (cousins, great-aunts and great-uncles, and great-grandparents) can be included as well, although the accuracy of reports on these relatives is not always high. These relatives share 12.5% of the same genes. Once all of this information is documented, it should be stored in a standard pedigree format. In families with multiple cases of malignancy, this pedigree can help to teach the concepts of genetics, clarify relationships, and provide a quick reference. The availability of software to draw these pedigrees has greatly simplified the process of updating this information. The increased use of electronic medical records in health care also will increase the potential for a health-care provider to collect a family history and visually represent it in a standardized pedigree, as well as calculate risks mathematically.

Reliability of patient information should be considered when both obtaining and communicating the risk assessment. Reports suggest that personal recall of a family history of malignancy may be inaccurate. Family reports may be inaccurate as much as 21% of the time for first-degree relatives and even more frequently for second- and third-degree relatives (Tyler & Snyder, 2006). Furthermore, the documentation of family history is variable in primary care settings. Although as many as 97% of all primary care charts may include a mention of family history, the level of detail about the family history, such as specific cancer site and age at diagnosis, is insufficient and inadequate in more than 65% of the cases to make an accurate risk assessment or appropriate referral for cancer genetics services. With the ever-increasing number of guidelines for the management of people at increased risk for cancer because of their genet-

### Figure 2-1. Key Indicators of Hereditary Breast-Ovarian Cancer

- Several relatives have developed breast and/or ovarian cancer. In general, the pedigree will show two or more first-degree relatives who have developed the same or related cancers.
- Cancers are diagnosed at a younger age than is seen in the general population. Often this is 10–15 years earlier than if it were a sporadic cancer. This is especially true with breast cancer before the age of 40 and ovarian cancer before the age of 60.
- A pattern of autosomal dominant transmission is evident. Usually the cancer is seen in more than one generation, and evidence of vertical transmission is present. First-degree relatives have a 50% statistical chance of developing the cancer.
- Unique tumor site combinations may be present. Individuals with a mutation in one of the *BRCA* genes may have a history of breast and ovarian cancers.
- An excess of multifocal or bilateral cancers may exist. This can include more than one cancer in the same organ or cancers that occur in both paired organs, for example, bilateral breast cancer.
- An excess of multiple primary tumors may be present. After successful treatment of one cancer, individuals from these families might go on to develop a completely new cancer, such as ovarian cancer after breast cancer.
- The family is of an Ashkenazi Jewish background.
- A history of male breast cancer exists in the family.
- The lifestyle history excludes a history of environmental risk factors.
- A confirmed *BRCA1/2* or other known mutation is associated with breast cancer.

*Note.* Based on information from Lindor et al., 2008; National Comprehensive Cancer Network, 2010; Petrucelli et al., 2007.

### Figure 2-2. Three-Generation Pedigree of a Family at Risk for Developing Breast and/or Ovarian Cancer

This is a typical pedigree constructed with the purpose of visually portraying the hereditary risk of developing breast and/or ovarian cancer. The arrow indicates the proband, or the member initiating inquiry about risk. Circles represent women, and squares represent men. Three generations are recorded. Current age or age at death is listed. A slash indicates a deceased family member. Cancer diagnoses and age at diagnosis are listed. This pedigree also illustrates how a male can pass the mutation on to a female because the mutation is on an autosome, not a sex chromosome.

## BRCA1-2 Hereditary Breast Cancer

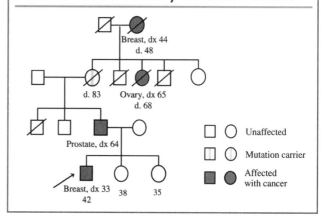

ic background, it is becoming more important for providers to extract a reasonably accurate family history and refer patients accordingly.

In many cases, patients may be unsure of the accuracy of the information. Ideally, they should use pathology reports, medical records, or death certificates to confirm information about cancers. Once such records are collected, the family history often appears very different, and this ultimately may change recommendations regarding testing. For example, when considering testing for *BRCA1* and *BRCA2* in a family, a reported case of ovarian cancer that is later confirmed by report to be cervical cancer might greatly alter the risk assessment. Family members can find this process extremely stressful. An accurate family history also can be challenging to collect if records are lost or if there is a small family size, underlying emotional or psychiatric problems, or cultural or family taboos regarding discussing cancer (Sandler, Wasserman, Fullerton, & Romero, 2004). Nurses need to educate patients on the importance of this activity and encourage them to collect the data. Figure 2-3 describes the limitations of pedigree assessment.

### Founder Effect

Ethnic background also is a consideration when deciding whether testing is appropriate, and this information can alter testing strategies. More than 2% of Ashkenazi Jews are

---

**Figure 2-3. Limitations of Pedigree Assessment**

- Most hereditary cancer syndromes have incomplete penetrance. Most families have carriers of the mutation who have lived to older ages without developing cancer.
- Family histories often are incomplete or inaccurate. Families may have inaccurate information, or family dynamics may lead to incomplete information because family members are unable or unwilling to communicate with each other.
- Sometimes family members who have the mutation may have died early from other causes, such as accidents, infections, or other unexpected deaths.
- There may be false paternity. This creates challenges when counseling family members about the pedigree. The same conflicts arise if an individual learns he or she is adopted. Adoptees may have difficulty obtaining family records.
- There may be a phenocopy in the family. This means that a person develops a sporadic cancer that is the same as the cancer for which the family has hereditary risk. For example, two sisters are diagnosed with breast cancer in their mid-40s. One tests positive for a mutation, and one does not. The sister who tests negative is a phenocopy, meaning that on paper assessment, she appears to have genetic risk because she has early-onset breast cancer, but genetically, she did not inherit the mutation; rather, she developed a sporadic cancer.
- Medical records are sometimes destroyed or impossible to obtain, so an accurate pedigree cannot be constructed.
- The family may be very small or, in the case of assessing breast or ovarian cancer risk, have only a small number of female relatives. A statistical 50% chance of developing hereditary cancers may not be evident.
- Sometimes women who are mutation carriers may have already had prophylactic surgery, especially an oophorectomy, which might mask their risk or may have prevented them from developing the cancer.

*Note.* Based on information from Lynch et al., 2003.

---

estimated to carry *BRCA1* and *BRCA2* mutations associated with an increased risk for breast, ovarian, and prostate cancers (Petrucelli et al., 2007; Struewing et al., 1997). This means 1 in 40 Ashkenazi people carry one of three mutations, which include 185delAG and 5382insC for *BRCA1* and 6174delT for *BRCA2*. This results from a phenomenon referred to as a *founder effect*, when a population has descended from a relatively small number of people without other groups.

### Penetrance

Interpreting family trees is further complicated by the concept of penetrance. Not everyone with a mutation will go on to develop the cancer (or cancers). Mutations in *BRCA1* and *BRCA2* are about 86% penetrant, meaning that approximately 86% of the women with the mutation will go on to develop breast cancer by age 70 (Lindor et al., 2008; Lynch, Snyder, Lynch, Riley, & Rubinstein, 2003). Sometimes a family will have members who have the mutation but for whatever reason have not gone on to develop the cancer. This makes evaluation of family histories challenging.

### Risk Calculations

Women with a potential hereditary risk for developing breast cancer need to understand the risk of developing breast cancer based on their family history, as well as their risk of having a mutation. When providing this information, the nurse needs to differentiate between the two risks. The risk of developing breast cancer usually is expressed as a relative risk figure or a cumulative risk. In some cases, a checklist or group of risk factors may suggest hereditary predisposition.

A number of models have been developed that can be used to calculate the risk of developing breast cancer over time. Usually these attempt to combine risk factors in a mathematical fashion. Often they will provide risk estimates for the present, the next five years, and over the person's lifetime. Common examples include the Gail model or Claus tables. More recently, the NCI Breast Cancer Risk Assessment Tool has become available online at www.cancer.gov/bcrisktool. This tool is based on the Gail model and provides five-year and lifetime risk figures for developing breast cancer. It may underestimate the risk for women who actually have a *BRCA* or other mutation, but it may be useful for identifying women who have an increased risk and therefore may benefit from more aggressive screening. These models do not predict when or where the woman will develop breast cancer.

A variety of models are available to calculate the risk of having a *BRCA1* or *BRCA2* mutation. These calculations typically provide a range of risk calculations because different models are based on different risk factors. The genetics professional then provides a range of risk for having a mutation.

When genetics professionals offer genetic testing, it is important that they provide the rationale for why it is being offered. The decision to offer testing may be based on a clinical checklist, an extensive family history as reflected in a pedigree, and a high probability of having a mutation. Using risk models can be confusing if the range of risk is large. At this point, clinical judgment remains a key component in estimating the risk for having a mutation or hereditary risk.

### Testing Process

The commercial availability of genetic testing for the cancer susceptibility genes associated with these hereditary breast-ovarian cancer syndromes has greatly changed oncology risk assessment practices. Cancer susceptibility genetic testing has the potential to identify whether a person is at increased risk for a particular cancer or cancers associated with a hereditary breast-ovarian cancer syndrome. These tests, however, cannot predict when, where, or if the individual will be diagnosed with the cancer. One of the challenges in the communication of genetic risk information and genetic test results is that probabilities and uncertainties surround genetic information. The benefits of cancer risk assessment are shown in Figure 2-4.

Genetic tests are relatively simple to order. The clinical challenge is to provide patients and their families with enough information regarding genetic testing so that they can make an informed decision that is best for their individual situation and consistent with their values. Whether a patient might benefit from predisposition genetic testing will depend on the patient's degree of genetic risk, whether testing is likely to address his or her needs, the patient's motivation to actively engage in prevention strategies, and the availability of an appropriate cancer predisposition test. Because of the high cost of some genetic tests (approximately $3,500 for full sequencing of *BRCA1/2*), reimbursement factors are a consideration. Most insurers cover some or all of the cost of genetic testing in patients who meet eligibility criteria set by the insurer. There may be additional costs for counseling and education. The final testing decision, however, will depend on patients' understanding of the potential risks and benefits and whether they want to proceed.

Deciding who is the most appropriate candidate to initiate cancer predisposition testing requires clinical judgment because of the complexity of the issues involved. Ideally, an

affected family member will be the first one to be tested. In the case of testing for *BRCA1/2*, a woman who has been diagnosed with breast (particularly premenopausal) or ovarian cancer usually will be the most informative for the rest of the family. If an affected relative has been tested and found to carry a deleterious mutation known to be associated with increased cancer risk, then at-risk unaffected family members are likely to benefit from single-site testing for the same mutation (which is significantly less expensive, usually costing $475–$600).

The Oncology Nursing Society (ONS, 2009a) has issued a position statement outlining considerations for genetic testing. This statement emphasizes that risk assessment and genetic testing are components of comprehensive cancer care and that cancer predisposition genetic testing requires informed consent. Qualified healthcare professionals should provide pre- and post-test counseling and education.

### Informed Consent

When deciding whether to pursue cancer predisposition genetic testing, each patient and family member must weigh the options, risks, and benefits in light of one's own unique situation. The decision is a very personal one, and for each family member the issues will be different. Just because a person has a personal or family history putting him or her at increased risk for carrying a genetic mutation does not mean that the individual will want to know his or her genetic status. For other people, the uncertainty may be causing them great anxiety or interfering with their ability to make informed choices about their health. The physical risks of having a blood sample drawn are minimal. The real risks are those associated with the psychological and psychosocial impact of knowing one's genetic status.

Most healthcare professionals agree that patients should have enough information to make an informed decision about a screening strategy or treatment option. Risk cannot be separated from choice (Tucker & Ferson, 2008). Once an individual comprehends risk, then she can make good informed choices about how to manage it. Thus, the importance of accurate cancer risk communication, not just genetic risk communication, cannot be underestimated.

Pretest counseling may identify potential psychological problems. Patients who are found to carry a cancer susceptibility mutation may experience anxiety, depression, anger, and feelings of vulnerability or guilt about possibly having passed the mutation to their children. Those who are found not to carry a mutation might experience guilt known as *survivor's guilt*, especially if close family members are found to carry the mutation. Psychological issues to be considered also include fear of cancer or medical procedures, past negative experiences with cancer, unresolved feelings of loss and sorrow, feelings of guilt about passing on a mutation to children, anxiety about learning test results, and concern about the effect of results on other family members. Some families

---

**Figure 2-4. Benefits of Breast Cancer Risk Assessments**

- Provide women with informed consent so they can choose appropriate screening recommendations.
- Allow development of a plan for cancer screening and prevention that is consistent with the values and needs of the woman at risk.
- Provide an educational opportunity to instruct women on basic information about breast cancer, including incidence, mortality, survival trends, and signs and symptoms that merit immediate evaluation.
- Detect cancers at an early stage, when treatment is most likely to be effective and less drastic.
- Enable clinicians to identify psychosocial concerns related to cancer risk and provide appropriate support and encouragement.
- Identify families who might be at risk for a hereditary predisposition. If a mutation is identified in a family, predictive testing can be offered to other at-risk members. For those who test positive, a detailed and aggressive plan for cancer prevention and detection needs to be developed. For those who test negative for a known mutation in the family, recommendations for cancer screening and prevention should reflect those used in the general population. This strategy allows financial healthcare resources to be spent in a sound way.

*Note.* Based on information from Bradbury & Olopade, 2006; Lynch et al., 2003.

---

may need information on how to access additional support services such as counseling, social work, or support groups.

The informed consent process for predisposition genetic testing must include both educational and decision-making components. Components of informed consent for genetic testing include the risks, benefits, cost, accuracy, and purpose of the specific genetic test being ordered; alternatives to genetic testing; implications of a positive, negative, or uncertain test result; how results will be communicated; psychosocial implications; confidentiality issues; and options for medical surveillance and risk reduction for both positive and negative results.

### Direct-to-Consumer Marketing

Many genetic testing laboratories have begun to market their tests directly to consumers. This is similar to the marketing that has been done by pharmaceutical companies since the 1980s. Direct-to-consumer marketing is accomplished largely through print and television advertisements and the Internet. Traditionally, genetic tests have been available only through healthcare providers such as physicians, nurse practitioners, and genetic counselors. Typically a healthcare provider orders the appropriate test from a laboratory, collects and sends the sample, and then interprets the test results when available (Geransar & Einsiedel, 2008). More and more women are requesting genetic testing and not fully understanding whether it is appropriate or the long-term consequences (Mahon, 2006).

Sometimes direct-to-consumer genetic testing is referred to as at-home genetic testing, and it provides access to a person's genetic information without necessarily involving a doctor, counselor, or insurance company in the process. In many cases, when a consumer chooses to purchase a genetic test directly, the test kit is mailed to the consumer instead of being ordered through a doctor's office. The test typically involves collecting a DNA sample at home, frequently by swabbing the inside of the cheek, and mailing the sample back to the laboratory. In some cases, the person must visit a health clinic to have blood drawn. Consumers are notified of their results by mail or over the telephone, or the results are posted online. In some cases, a genetic counselor or other healthcare provider is available to explain the results and answer questions. The price for this type of genetic testing ranges from several hundred dollars to more than a thousand dollars depending on the test being done. In other cases, consumers are encouraged to speak with their healthcare provider about ordering a certain test. Often such advertisements do not address the issue of counseling by a trained professional. Depending on the healthcare provider the consumer approaches, pre- and post-test counseling by a trained genetics professional may or may not take place.

Although the complexity and sophistication of genetic testing is increasing, regulatory oversight is limited (Gniady, 2008; Hogarth, Javitt, & Melzer, 2008). Advertising for genetic tests is regulated by the Federal Trade Commission (FTC).

The FTC may take formal action against the creators of fraudulent advertisements; however, the vastness of the Internet makes these advertisements difficult to regulate. The U.S. Food and Drug Administration regulates diagnostic testing kits. Unfortunately, many genetic tests are not kits but rather freestanding tests developed by laboratories and offered directly to patients.

When patients order a genetic test without consultation with a genetics professional, several scenarios are possible: a wrong test may be ordered, the correct test may not be considered, risk assessment will not be comprehensive, consumers or healthcare professionals may be unable to understand or correctly interpret the results, the implications for prevention and early detection may not be evident or recommendations may not be appropriately implemented, there may be intense fear or anxiety, and appropriate management of family members may be overlooked (Mahon, 2009). Most professional organizations, including the American Congress of Obstetricians and Gynecologists, the American College of Medical Genetics, the American Society of Human Genetics, the American College of Clinical Pharmacology, and the National Society of Genetic Counselors, recommend consultations with a genetic healthcare professional when genetic testing is being considered or ordered or when the test results are being interpreted (Ameer & Krivoy, 2009; American College of Medicine Genetics Board of Directors, 2004; American College of Obstetricians and Gynecologists, 2008; Hudson, Javitt, Burke, & Byers, 2007). Recently, ONS (2010) released a position statement on direct-to-consumer genetic testing, which emphasized that nurses need to advocate for the needs of people who are considering and undergoing genetic testing.

The potential benefits of direct-to-consumer marketing of genetic tests include that such marketing may promote an awareness of genetic diseases, encourage consumers to take a more proactive role in their health care, and offer a means for people to learn about their ancestral origins (Hogarth et al., 2008).

The potential risks of direct-to-consumer marketing of genetic tests include that they may mislead an individual who has a limited understanding of genetics with unproven, inappropriate, or invalid tests, which may result in decision making about treatment or prevention that is based on inaccurate, incomplete, or misunderstood information. Consumers may not understand that genetic testing provides only one piece of information about a person's health and potential risk for developing a disease or disorder. Factors such as lifestyle and environmental exposures, as well as genetic risk, are discussed during a consultation with genetics professional but in many cases are not addressed by genetic tests obtained through direct-to-consumer marketing. When consumers order a test without consultation with a genetics professional, they may not adequately communicate what the results of testing mean to other family members and may not ensure that those individuals receive the appropriate education, counseling, and testing if indicated (Mahon, 2009). Completing testing without adequate counseling also may result in negative psychological responses, including fear, anxiety, and depression, depending on the results of the test, the ability of the individual to correctly interpret the information, and the implications for follow-up (Hogarth et al., 2008).

Many groups have published guidelines on who should provide genetic cancer risk assessment services to high-risk individuals (American Society of Clinical Oncology, 2003; Consensus Panel on Genetic/Genomic Nursing Competencies, 2008; NCCN, 2010; ONS, 2009a, 2009b; Trepanier et al., 2004). There is consensus that cancer genetics services should be provided by individuals with expertise in cancer genetics, there should be a reasonable expectation of finding a genetic mutation, and the results of genetic testing will influence management. Few guidelines are available regarding the communication of general cancer risk assessment, and it is even less clear as to who should provide such services (Metcalfe, Haydon, Bennett, & Farndon, 2008; ONS, 2006). Guidelines tend to focus on the management of specific cancer risks, not the cancer risk assessment and communication strategies (ACS, 2010a).

## Outcomes of Testing

The results of cancer predisposition genetic tests generally fall into several categories, including positive, negative, and indeterminate. It is critical that individuals understand the issues associated with predisposition genetic testing along with all the potential testing outcomes prior to initiating the testing process.

A positive result for a *BRCA1* or *BRCA2* mutation is associated with an increased risk for developing both breast and ovarian cancers. If the patient has already been diagnosed with cancer, a positive test result can have implications for the individual's risk of developing a second primary cancer or a cancer recurrence associated with that mutation. Once a positive result or mutation is identified in a family, other at-risk family members can be offered the option of testing.

A negative test result can occur in two situations. The first is where a known mutation exists in the family, and the patient has been tested specifically for that same mutation. The second situation is when no known mutation exists in the family, and the patient is tested for one or more mutations associated with an increased cancer risk.

Ideally, a person who has been diagnosed with cancer is tested first. If a mutation is identified, subsequent family members can be tested for the same mutation. When a known mutation is identified in the family and an unaffected (no cancer diagnosis) person tests negative, his or her risk of developing cancer approaches the risk of the general population. The patient's cancer risk still may be increased, however, because of nonhereditary risk factors related to lifestyle, diet, environment, or carcinogen exposure.

In a patient without a cancer diagnosis and with no known mutation in the family, several possible interpretations of a negative test result exist. The first possibility is that the cancer in the family is caused by a known mutation for which the patient was tested and did not inherit (true negative result). A second possibility is that the cancer in the family is due to a different gene mutation for which the patient was not tested. A third possibility is that the cancer in the family is caused by environmental or other nonhereditary risk factors. Because it is not possible to know which outcome is true for the patient, it is recommended to first test a blood relative who has been diagnosed with cancer for a mutation known to be associated with that type of cancer. The rationale is that if there is a mutation in the family, it will most likely be found in a family member already diagnosed with cancer. If a mutation is found in an affected family member, then the unaffected family members can be tested for that specific mutation. If a mutation is not found, the family still may be at risk and may want to consider more aggressive screening measures and participation in a research study.

A variation of uncertain significance is when the genetic test indicates that a change in the gene was found, but the cancer risk associated with that change is not yet known. This can occur when a new mutation or variant is found or when the variant is uncommon and not enough information is available to determine whether the variant is a deleterious mutation (i.e., associated with an increased cancer risk) or a harmless variant. Some genes, such as *BRCA1* and *BRCA2*, are very large genes with hundreds of known deleterious mutations. Not all gene changes or variants are deleterious, however, and it is possible for a gene change to be present that does not interfere with protein function and therefore does not increase cancer risk.

Patients with this result will need to be informed that the significance of the mutation found is not yet known. These patients may experience disappointment, anxiety, anger, or depression because the test result did not provide the information they expected. They also may feel confused and uncertain about how to make healthcare decisions regarding cancer surveillance. Until a number of families with the same mutation have been studied, it is impossible to know if an increased cancer risk may be associated with the mutation found. This can be a difficult situation for some patients because of the uncertainty. It may be helpful to test more family members to find out whether the mutation is found only in the affected individuals, but this may not necessarily give concrete answers. Another option is to encourage patients to become part of a research study or confidential registry for people who carry genetic variants in hopes that more information about the particular variant will be known as more people are tested. These patients need to be informed that, as more information about specific variants becomes available, it may be possible to determine whether the particular variant for which they tested positive is deleterious or not. Decisions about cancer surveillance, early detection, and risk reduction are based on patients' personal and family history of cancer and nonhereditary cancer risk factors.

### Confidentiality of Genetic Information

Given the sensitivity of genetic information, patients need to know that their genetic information will not be released to any third party without their specific written informed consent. When a healthcare provider refers a patient to a cancer genetics program for predisposition genetic testing, the patient must sign a written consent form before cancer genetic counseling and predisposition testing information can be released to his or her healthcare provider. If the patient has a positive genetic test result and chooses not to release the cancer predisposition test results to his or her healthcare provider, it may be difficult for the healthcare provider to order appropriate cancer screening tests, offer chemoprevention or prophylactic surgery, and provide appropriate clinical examinations.

The genetic counseling process often involves obtaining the patient's medical records from one or more sources, as well as medical records on one or more family members. The presence of these records in the patient's medical chart creates an additional responsibility in relation to maintaining the confidentiality of information about the patient as well as other family members. When a patient's medical record contains secondary records (i.e., medical records on a family member or patient records from another institution), these records should not be released to a third party, even with written informed consent from the patient. The third party needs to go to the original source to obtain those records. This is especially important now that the Health Insurance Portability and Accountability Act privacy rules have been enacted.

Confidentiality is necessary to protect patients from genetic discrimination. Genetic discrimination occurs when individuals experience workplace or insurance discrimination based on information about their genetic makeup. Patients with a positive genetic test are at risk for genetic discrimination based solely on their genetic makeup. Individuals who are asymptomatic but have a positive predisposition genetic test are at the greatest risk for genetic discrimination. Patients should be informed of the risks of discussing their genetic history in the workplace. They also may want to consider purchasing additional life insurance before testing to prevent higher premiums resulting because of a known genetic predisposition.

The Genetic Information Nondiscrimination Act of 2008, also referred to as GINA, is a new federal law that protects Americans from being treated unfairly because of differences in their DNA that may affect their health. The new law prevents discrimination from health insurers and employers and was fully in effect by December 2009. The law does not cover life insurance, disability insurance, or long-term care insurance (Erwin, 2008).

## Selecting a Prediction Model

Several factors influence the selection of a risk prediction model. Different methods may be appropriate in different settings. Simply considering the patient's age may be sufficient for a woman 40–49 years of age to decide about using the screening tool of mammography. Conversely, simply using the patient's age to determine whether tamoxifen may be effective in reducing breast cancer risk in a 45-year-old woman is probably inappropriate because chemoprevention is best used in those with a moderate to high risk of developing breast cancer. Furthermore, decisions about whether to undergo a prophylactic surgical procedure are best made after genetic testing. Prophylactic surgery involves too many physical and psychological risks to be used with those of average or moderate risk for developing cancer. It is reserved only for those with a high risk, which is probably best identified through genetic testing. Clearly, clinicians need to consider which risk-prediction model they should use and whether it is appropriate to provide guidance for selecting a screening or prevention measure or offering genetic testing.

In regard to most cancers, a portion of the cancer diagnoses cannot be explained by recognized risk factors (Freedman et al., 2005). In the case of breast cancer, most models assume it is a homogenous disease, even though many variations or subtypes of breast cancer may be present in one family. Such models fail to account for other modifying factors. Current models of breast cancer risk usually can account for only a few factors. The researchers noted that, ideally, knowledge of risk factors should guide primary prevention efforts. However, in the case of breast cancer, the inability to alter most risk factors limited their relevance for primary prevention. Similarly, models that predict the risk of having a hereditary cancer mutation have limitations. Pedigrees may be difficult to interpret because of adoption, small family size, and inaccurate reports of history (Freedman et al., 2005).

In general, models for prediction of breast cancer risk focus on two separate types of risk. The first type of risk information generally offered to patients describes their chance of developing breast cancer. Often this information is presented as an estimated chance of developing breast cancer both in the next five years and over their lifetime. Bradbury and Olopade (2006) emphasized that patients must be informed of the imprecision of these cancer risk assessment models because risk models may not always be able to capture all salient features of family history or incorporate a significant risk factor. Furthermore, the significance and interaction of all risk factors in the subsequent development of cancer are not known. The Gail and Claus models typically are used to describe an individual woman's risk of developing breast cancer (see Table 2-4).

The second type of risk information usually is given to those with a family history that suggests hereditary susceptibility and is an estimate of the chance that an individual car-

| Table 2-4. Risk Models for Hereditary Breast and Ovarian Cancer | | | | |
|---|---|---|---|---|
| **Model** | **Reference** | **Indications** | **Strengths** | **Limitations** |
| Gail model | Gail et al., 1989 | • Estimates breast cancer risk<br>• Most effectively used in women with a limited to moderate family history of breast cancer<br>• Often used to determine whether the patient should be enrolled in a chemoprevention trial or treatment | • Readily available to use on computers and handheld devices<br>• Inexpensive and simple to use<br>• Considers previous biopsies<br>• Considers previous pregnancies | • Does not consider personal or family history of ovarian cancer<br>• Does not consider the age at which other relatives were diagnosed (the model does not take into account the impact of early-onset breast cancer in the family)<br>• Does not consider paternal side of family with a diagnosis of breast or ovarian cancer<br>• Does not consider second-degree relatives with a diagnosis of breast or ovarian cancer<br>• Has not been used extensively with many ethnic minorities and may have limited usefulness |
| Claus model | Claus et al., 1994, 1996 | • Provides age-specific estimates for the risk of developing breast cancer<br>• Most effectively used in women with a significant family history of breast cancer | • Considers the age at diagnosis of breast cancer<br>• Considers both maternal and paternal family history<br>• Calculates risk in 10-year increments, which is helpful to younger women or when trying to keep risk in perspective | • Does not consider ethnicity<br>• Does not consider ovarian cancer history<br>• Might significantly underestimate risk in people with a *BRCA1/2* mutation |
| Couch model | Couch et al., 1997 | • Estimates the chance of carrying a *BRCA1* mutation<br>• Most effectively used in women with a family history of multiple cases of breast cancer, especially early-onset breast cancer | • Considers the average age at onset of breast cancer in the family<br>• Takes ethnicity factors into consideration | • Predicts *BRCA1* mutations only<br>• Reported to be less sensitive in small families |
| Shattuck-Eidens model | Shattuck-Eidens et al., 1997 | • Estimates the chance of carrying a *BRCA1* mutation<br>• Most effectively used in women with a family history of multiple cases of breast cancer, especially early-onset breast cancer | • Considers the age at onset of breast cancer in family<br>• Considers both first- and second-degree relatives<br>• Considers breast and ovarian cancer history<br>• Considers the significance of Ashkenazi Jewish background | • Predicts *BRCA1* mutations only<br>• Limited data in ethnic minority groups |
| Berry model (Duke model, BRCAPRO model) | Berry et al., 1997, 2002 | • Calculates the chance of having a *BRCA1* or *BRCA2* mutation | • Considers the age at onset of breast cancer in family<br>• Considers both first- and second-degree relatives<br>• Considers breast and ovarian cancer history | • Readily available in the BRCAPRO computer program<br>• Limited data in some minority groups |
| Frank model (Myriad II model) | Frank et al., 1998 | • Calculates the chance of having a *BRCA1* or *BRCA2* mutation<br>• Most effectively used in women with breast cancer diagnosed before the age of 50 | • Considers the age at onset of breast cancer in family<br>• Considers both first- and second-degree relatives<br>• Considers breast and ovarian cancer history | • Most useful in premenopausal women<br>• Less useful in small families<br>• Limited data available in some minority groups<br>• Readily available in the BRCAPRO computer program |

*(Continued on next page)*

| Table 2-4. Risk Models for Hereditary Breast and Ovarian Cancer *(Continued)* | | | | |
|---|---|---|---|---|
| **Model** | **Reference** | **Indications** | **Strengths** | **Limitations** |
| Pedigree assessment tool (PAT) | Hoskins et al., 2006 | • Identifies women at increased risk for hereditary breast cancer and whether to offer genetic testing<br>• Best used with women being seen in primary care settings with multiple family members diagnosed with breast cancer | • Simple point-scoring system based on family history with points weighted according to features associated with *BRCA1/2* mutations | • May over-refer some women for genetic counseling |
| Manchester model | Evans et al., 2004 | • Estimates the risk of carrying a *BRCA1* or *BRCA2* mutation<br>• Targets non-Jewish women with a family history of breast or ovarian cancer | • May be useful in identifying women who have *BRCA2* mutations | • May be less useful in identifying women who have *BRCA1* mutations |

ries a mutation in a particular cancer susceptibility gene (see Table 2-4). Calculating and interpreting this risk figure is important for those who desire genetic testing. Generally, offering genetic testing is appropriate if at least a 10% probability exists for detecting a mutation in a cancer susceptibility gene and the presence of such a mutation ultimately will have an impact on prevention and treatment decisions.

Selection of a proper model is further complicated by genetic heterogeneity (see Table 2-3). Both *BRCA1* and *BRCA2* mutations are associated with hereditary breast and ovarian cancer. Hereditary breast cancer also may be the primary manifestation of Cowden disease or Li-Fraumeni syndrome because of mutations in the *PTEN* gene or the *TP53* gene. Knowledge about differentiating clinical features is important for identifying the correct syndrome and highlights the need for both physical examination and a thorough family history prior to interpreting the risk assessment and possibly selecting a genetic test to order (Freedman et al., 2005).

As Stopfer (2000) noted, these models sometimes can produce inconsistent risk assessments for the same individual. For example, the same woman might have a 29%–48% likelihood of carrying a mutation depending on the model used. Each model is based on unique combinations of information. This can be a source of confusion for both patients and health professionals. Those using risk assessment models need to explain to patients why they are using a particular risk assessment and what it means. They also should distinguish between risk models that calculate a patient's chances for developing a particular cancer and those that assess one's risk of carrying a specific mutation. Because multiple models are used, families often receive conflicting information, which can lead to increased stress and confusion. Some recommend using one model consistently and explaining its inherent strengths and weaknesses; others recommend using multiple models to give a range of risk (Cummings et al., 2009).

Numbers have great potential to confuse and mislead. Furthermore, risk factors do not necessarily increase in a simple mathematical fashion. For example, if one risk factor gives a woman a 12% risk of developing breast cancer and another gives the woman an 18% risk, the two numbers cannot be assumed to mean the woman now has a 30% chance of developing breast cancer. Risk estimates are generally independent predictors that are not additive. The interaction of risk factors is complicated. Like most cancers, breast cancer is a disease that has many causes that interact in ways that researchers do not fully understand. In fact, some researchers have estimated that 70% of breast cancers occur in women without any of the classic risk factors (ACS, 2009a). Furthermore, a numeric result, such as an absolute- or relative-risk figure, can appear highly scientific and be difficult for many clients to understand. Conversely, using verbal terms, such as high risk or low risk, can be equally confusing. A high risk to one woman might mean a 100% chance of developing breast cancer; for another, it might mean a 25% chance (Carey & Burgman, 2008). Numeric data alone are not sufficient in communicating risk because people vary widely in their affective response to the same probability estimates (O'Doherty & Suthers, 2007).

Hierarchies of numeric skills as well as literary skills are also needed for patients to comprehend and use information about the likelihood of risks and benefits of a treatment or screening maneuver (Peters, 2008). First, information must be available, accurate, and timely, and the patient or healthcare provider must be able to acquire it from tables, charts, and text. This may not always be possible with cancer risk information. Next, patients often must make calculations and inferences. For example, given survival rates for chemotherapy versus hormone therapy, a patient with cancer must calculate the difference between therapies and infer the meaning of that difference. Patients must be able to remember information either for a short period (if the decision is made quickly) or after an extended delay (in the case of a lifetime program of screening), and memory ability differs across patient populations. Finally, patients need to be able to weigh factors to match their needs and values and understand that they must make trade-offs, either minor or emotionally and physically devastating, to ultimately arrive at a health decision. This process can be quite difficult.

Communication of cancer risk also is challenging because it includes both a quantitative and qualitative component (Cummings et al., 2009). The quantitative component usually is more straightforward. It typically involves risk figures such as absolute or relative risk or the probability of having a mutation in a cancer susceptibility gene. Numeric data can be presented to patients and families. Some individuals have a greater ability than others to comprehend the meaning of numeric data. Typically, qualitative information should follow the presentation of quantitative data. This includes a discussion of what the quantitative data specifically mean for the patient. Many experts in risk communication believe that all discussions of risk should include both a qualitative and quantitative component (Hopwood, 2005).

Consideration also must be given to an individual's ability to understand risk assessment. Some groups of patients are more likely to seek information about cancer risk assessment. This may be related to a variety of factors, including educational level and the ability to understand complex technical concepts. Communication of risk information should be given according to how much the patient or family wishes to know (Hopwood, 2005). Timing also can be important. Messages suggesting increased susceptibility to breast cancer may be less effective if delivered too soon after the breast cancer diagnosis of a close relative, but they might be appropriate several months after the diagnosis (Hopwood, 2005).

Many factors influence the perception of risk. All individuals have their own perception of risk, and it often is difficult to determine which risks they deem acceptable and which risks are not acceptable. For some, personal beliefs and perceptions of risk are so strong that they prevent many individuals from adopting healthy behaviors (Klein & Stefanek, 2007).

Many women with a family history of breast cancer incorrectly assume that it is not an issue of *whether* they will be diagnosed with breast cancer but *when* they will be diagnosed. As women approach the age at which their mothers were diagnosed with breast cancer, their anxiety often increases (Hopwood, 2005). As they pass that age, they may begin to feel their risk is sufficiently different and believe they might not get breast cancer after all. Unfortunately, some may become overconfident and then fail to get adequate screening. Critical to the process of cancer risk assessment is determination of a person's beliefs about cancer. All people have beliefs about cancer. Some fit with current scientific findings, and others do not. Health professionals must have an understanding of these beliefs because they will in-

fluence what information is understood and how it is interpreted in the risk assessment.

Healthcare providers can obtain a great deal of information by listening carefully to people describe their past experiences with cancer. Individuals may realize intellectually that improved treatments are now available but continue to remember, and dread, the disease as experienced by a friend or relative. For example, a woman whose mother was treated with a Halsted radical mastectomy may fear the same treatment for herself and consequently ignore a breast lump, despite the availability of more cosmetically acceptable forms of treatment. Such fears need to be assessed in order to correct misconceptions.

In addition to understanding patients' perceptions of the disease, it is important to determine their assessment of their own personal risk for a particular cancer. This information can elucidate the patient's level of concern related to developing cancer. In some cases, an individual may have an actual numeric risk in mind. It is also important to understand whether the patient is considering absolute or relative risk. In some cases, people tend to underestimate their risk, which is termed *optimistic bias*. In cancer risk assessment, the opposite phenomenon also occurs, which is known as *pessimistic bias*. Those with pessimistic bias often will suffer unnecessary anxiety and concern (Finkel, 2008). These biases may occur because people have inaccurate information or are unable to comprehend complex technical information, or the preconceptions may reflect a psychologically protective coping mechanism.

## The Challenge of Uncertainty

Uncertainty exists regarding recommended prevention and detection strategies. This may be the most serious limitation of risk assessment and genetic testing (Klein & Stefanek, 2007). No screening strategy is completely effective in detecting cancer early. The sensitivity and specificity of screening tests are widely variable. Furthermore, many of the prophylactic measures, and sometimes the chemoprevention recommendations, are not based on firm, scientific knowledge. Often the data are extrapolated from other studies and information. This means that the certainty with which recommendations can be made often is limited at best.

Testing for genetic predisposition provides information about risk, but much uncertainty still exists for most patients (Hopwood, 2005). For those who test negative, the risk is not completely eliminated. These people still carry the same probability or risk of developing a sporadic cancer as those in the general population. For those who undergo testing that shows they have a change of indeterminate significance, the uncertainty is very large. These individuals have not gained any new or helpful information from the genetic testing process.

Variable penetrance is another feature of uncertainty that must be addressed in cancer genetics counseling (Fagerlin et al., 2007). Penetrance can change with age and specific mutation and may vary considerably among different families. Additional genetic factors are likely associated with different mutations that modify the risks of gene carriers. To date, these additional factors are largely unknown. Thus, patients who test positive trade the uncertainty of not knowing if they really are at significant risk for developing a malignancy for the uncertainty of when (if at all, in some cases) and what type of cancer will develop.

## Techniques for Communicating Breast Cancer Risk Assessments

Those who communicate cancer risk assessments to patients must be aware of the patients' perceptions of risk and remind them of the fundamental purposes for conducting a risk assessment, which include determining appropriate cancer prevention strategies when known and developing a reasonable schedule for cancer screening. Communication of the risk information should begin by reminding patients of the strengths and limitations as well as the purpose of a cancer risk assessment. In most cases, the next step is to provide basic information about the cancer for which the person is at risk (e.g., the number of people affected annually, average age at diagnosis, clinical presentation). A review of basic anatomy and physiology using diagrams and models may be indicated to provide necessary background information. Information about the general population can serve as a baseline against which individuals can measure the magnitude of their increased risk. Adequate opportunity for patients to ask questions and express concerns must be provided to make the cancer risk assessment process effective and the interview truly informative. Depending on the magnitude of the risk and the ability and desire of the patient to understand the content, the nurse can expand the discussion to include a more detailed conversation about absolute or relative risk (perhaps including information such as that found in Tables 2-1 and 2-2). Care should be taken to distinguish between absolute and relative risk and to reinforce that risk factors do not combine in a simple mathematical fashion.

After the data for risk assessment are collected, one must choose the best method to communicate the assessment. Risk can be presented as a numeric risk, a statistical comparison to an average or anchor risk, given as a risk category (low, average, or high), expressed in qualitative terms (e.g., telling a patient she is more likely to develop this disease than a person who does not smoke), or using graphical or pictorial presentations.

The ultimate goal of risk assessment is a decrease in cancer morbidity and mortality. A more immediate goal is to provide informed consent so that an individual can make appropriate decisions about genetic testing, cancer screening, cancer prevention maneuvers, or cancer treatment protocols. Risk information is being used increasingly in treatment de-

cisions. For many women diagnosed with breast cancer, the risk of recurrence is calculated, and this risk often is considered in making decisions about various treatment modalities.

Risk communication receives little attention in basic educational preparation for most nurses, and there are numerous and varied methods in which risk can be presented. The interpretation of risk measures can be confusing to both healthcare professionals and the public (Akobeng, 2008). For example, when considering various environmental risks, people tend to feel most vulnerable to those that are most involuntary and evoke the most dread, such as nuclear reactors or natural catastrophes. Consequently, people greatly overestimate the risk of such exposures yet underestimate the risks of others viewed as voluntary or less dramatic, such as driving a car (Klein & Stefanek, 2007).

As health risk information becomes more available via the Internet and other sources, people are becoming increasingly engaged in decision making together with their healthcare providers. The need to communicate risk in understandable terms is increasing so that individuals can ultimately make appropriate decisions about cancer prevention and early detection strategies or treatment.

Cancer risk perceptions are a key predictor of risk-reduction practices, health behaviors, and processing of information regarding treatment decisions. Nevertheless, patients and the general public (as well as healthcare providers) exhibit a number of errors and biases in the way they think about risk and try to apply the information to healthcare decision making. People who feel at greater risk spend more time seeking out and processing information that might be used to reduce their risk. Risk perception can be a motivator to participation in a screening program, but in the face of too much fear, it can deter individuals from engaging in prevention or detection practices.

The manner in which the information is communicated, in terms of attitude and context, is called *framing*. Framing can have a significant effect on how the client perceives the information (Wang, 2008). If risk information is presented in a negative fashion, the client may assume the risk is more than it actually is. If the discussion is too positive, the client may underestimate or minimize risk. The same is true in discussions of options. Statistical context can constitute framing.

Graphics can be a very effective means to communicate risk. They can be especially effective in communicating numeric risk. Graphics often can reveal data patterns that may otherwise go undetected. Graphs also hold people's attention for longer periods of time, which might increase their understanding of data. To be useful, graphs must communicate the magnitude of risk, relative risk, cumulative risk, uncertainty, and interactions among risk factors. Despite the popularity of using graphics, little research exists on their impact in communicating risk data. In many cases, a combination of different formats is used to present risk, including numeric, visual, and explanatory. Graphs should decrease the number of mathematical computations that the user must make.

Some healthcare providers who provide risk assessment services develop their own tools to enhance risk communication. These tools might include a combination of words, pictures, and statistics. Although research is limited, patients might find such tailored pieces to be an adjunct in risk communication (Lobb et al., 2006). Educational pieces might include pictorial elements, bar graphs, line graphs, pie charts, risk ladders, and stick figures. A bar graph may decrease the number of mathematical computations that the user must make. Graphs can be helpful for showing differences such as the amounts or frequency of occurrence of different types of data. One example might be the difference in risk between people with different risk factors. The data-to-ink ratio should be high—that is, the graph should not contain extra pictures, busy backgrounds, or patterned fills. Line graphs effectively communicate trends and changes in data. They are commonly used to show changes in incidence or mortality over time, and most clients have experience reading them. Pie charts effectively communicate information about proportions. Pie charts can be combined to explain subcategories of data. For example, a pie chart might be a useful way to communicate proportions of the population affected by hereditary predisposition to developing breast cancer. Stick figures often are used to communicate relative risk or to show how many people out of a certain number may develop a particular disease. When a small number of figures are used, the viewer may perceive the risk to be higher (Kurz-Milcke, Gigerenzer, & Martignon, 2008). If the number of figures is increased, the impact may not be as strong, and some will find the presentation busy and difficult to understand. Graphs should not be used to communicate a low-probability event (Kurz-Milcke et al., 2008), such as an event with a 0.0003 chance. Although most people can understand the probability that accompanies a high-probability event, such as the probability of a flipped coin coming up heads (which represents a 0.50 or 50% chance), understanding a low-probability event, such as a 0.0003 chance, is much more difficult. A solution to this problem is to change the probability to a frequency (i.e., 3 out of 10,000). People's reactions to identical risk information, however, can vary by the size of the denominator used to describe the risk statistic (Zikmund-Fisher, Fagerlin, Roberts, Derry, & Ubel, 2008).

## Sources of Risk Data

Each year, ACS publishes *Cancer Facts and Figures* (ACS, 2010a). Publications also are available that describe specific populations and topics (ACS, 2009b, 2009c, 2010b). This helpful resource presents estimates about cancer cases, including the estimated mortality and number of new cases of a specific cancer per year (incidence). Incidence rates are given by state. *Cancer Facts and Figures* also offers detailed data about primary and secondary prevention of the major tumors

and projected survival data by stage. The publication is free and available from local ACS chapters and at the ACS Web site (www.cancer.org).

Another resource is the Surveillance, Epidemiology and End Results (SEER) program, which is continually updated and available at http://seer.cancer.gov. Cancer incidence and survival statistics are available from 1973, the first year SEER began collecting data, to 2008, the most recent year for which data are reported (at the time of this publication). SEER collects data from 17 population-based registries throughout the United States, which represents more than 25% of the U.S. population. Data sorted by race categories (Caucasian, African American, American Indian/Alaska Native, and Asian/Pacific Islander) and ethnic groups (Hispanic and Non-Hispanic) are available from 1992 onward. Information on rates from states is also available, as well as abbreviated summaries of data.

## Communication About the Risks and Benefits of Screening

Patients should receive information about the strengths and limitations of screening tools, including information about the recommended time interval for using each tool. For most patients, the standard recommendations endorsed by an organization such as ACS (2010a) will be appropriate (see Figure 2-5). People with significantly higher risk may need more aggressive screening and should understand the rationale, strengths, and limitations of such a schedule, as well as the strengths and limitations associated with chemoprevention agents and prophylactic surgery. Signs and symptoms that require immediate attention should be discussed.

## Ethical Concerns

Consideration of a number of ethical concerns and principles is important in communicating a risk assessment. Healthcare professionals who are communicating risk assessments

---

**Figure 2-5. American Cancer Society Recommendations* for the Early Detection of Breast Cancer**

- Yearly mammography beginning at age 40 is recommended. The age at which to stop mammography should be individualized based on the potential risks and benefits of screening in light of the overall health of the woman.
- A clinical breast examination is recommended about every three years for women in their 20s and 30s and annually for women age 40 and older.
- Breast self-examination is an option for women to consider on a monthly basis beginning in their 20s.

*These recommendations are for asymptomatic women without significant risk or hereditary risk for developing breast cancer.

*Note.* Based on information from American Cancer Society, 2010a.

have an obligation to honestly disclose any biases or concerns related to the risk assessment.

One concept involved in cancer risk assessment is *autonomy*, which implies that each individual has the right to choose his or her own course. In relation to cancer screening, patients need information to make appropriate choices about lifestyle habits and screening behaviors, and these decisions can be made only after receiving a realistic and accurate assessment of risk.

The concept of *beneficence* applies to the obligation to inform individuals of a real health risk. The principle of *nonmaleficence* applies to the obligation to not hide, cover up, or otherwise fail to communicate risk information. In the case of cancer risk assessment, information should not be overinterpreted to create a climate of fear or anxiety regarding nonexistent risks. Patients must accurately understand their risk for developing a particular cancer, the potential consequences of not changing a particular behavior or having a particular screening test done, and the strengths and limitations of screening tests. Beneficence also applies to families with a known predisposition mutation and the manner in which other potentially at-risk members are informed of their risk.

Those who communicate a risk assessment also have an obligation to convey as clearly as possible any biases or assumptions that have been made in constructing the risk assessment. For example, a risk assessment may be less accurate if a woman reports that a first-degree relative had breast surgery and it is assumed it was for malignancy when, in reality, it was for a benign cyst. The person conveying the risk information is obligated to explain that the risk would be higher if the surgery was for a malignancy, but if the surgery was for a cyst, it means little in terms of the patient's risk of eventually developing breast cancer. One of the most challenging points can be deciding when a risk is significant and therefore should be communicated.

Accurate assessment is very important when explaining risk issues to a family with an apparent genetic predisposition to cancer. These family members need to understand why their risk is elevated, what preventive means are available, the strengths and limitations of available standard screening tests, and what is involved in genetic testing. To make an informed decision about genetic testing for breast cancer susceptibility, a number of points must be communicated to and comprehended by potential patients. Each family member is autonomous and has the right to make an individual decision regarding genetic testing. Healthcare professionals who obtain a family history suggestive of a genetic susceptibility to developing cancer have an obligation to inform the individual and, if possible, other family members.

## Psychological Concerns

Clearly, the overall impact of risk assessment on quality of life is poorly understood. Similarly, it is not clear why two women with similar risk factors for developing breast cancer who receive risk factor information in a similar format can respond so differently to the information.

Performing a risk assessment and giving patients information about risk factors does not affect their risk of developing cancer. However, such information about risk may influence patients' choices regarding screening and may change the way in which some people think about themselves and their lives. A risk factor assessment can potentially improve patients' health care and ultimately their quality of life if it results in regular screenings and possibly the early detection of a malignancy, or if a woman with a known *BRCA* mutation elects for a prophylactic mastectomy and oophorectomy. Conversely, if a person is distressed or upset by the information conveyed in a risk assessment, the individual may ignore recommendations for screening or may experience psychological harm and possibly increased morbidity if a malignancy is not detected early.

The psychosocial impact of risk factor communication has not received much attention (Hopwood, 2005). Some degree of concern or anxiety about breast cancer might heighten a woman's vigilance and motivation to seek reassurance through repetitive breast screenings. Conversely, such notification may result in anxiety and cancer worries with a reduction in breast self-examination and regularly scheduled clinical breast examinations, as well as less frequent mammography. Of concern would be the potential for inappropriate decisions about the use of prophylactic mastectomy in women who overestimate their risk of breast cancer.

Long-term follow-up is essential after a patient's cancer risk is communicated and genetic testing is completed or declined. Early studies suggest that depression might occur 6–12 months after genetic risk counseling and testing is completed (Hopwood, 2005). As more people receive cancer-risk genetic counseling, healthcare providers need to ensure that long-term follow-up includes assessment for depression and other negative sequelae associated with accepting or declining the testing process.

Those who counsel about genetic testing and risk must be aware of underlying beliefs and psychological distress and how these motivate testing decisions. Several unique considerations exist in cancer-risk genetic counseling. Unlike acquired cancer risk factors, such as a poor diet, lack of physical activity, or smoking, patients cannot alter their genetic risk for developing cancer. This can lead to a sense of fatalism (Hopwood, 2005). The risk assessments completed in a genetic counseling session have implications for the entire family, not just one individual. Helping families to find the best way to share this information with other members is very challenging. Test findings can permanently alter relationships within families. Family communication can be distressing, and responses to testing information will vary. Not knowing what to say and fear of upsetting relatives may be significant barriers to disclosure (Hopwood, 2005).

How long a person can retain information after counseling about cancer risk factors is unclear. Information about risk and recommended screening can be reinforced by sending patients a post-visit letter that summarizes the discussion of risk and recommendations for screening or other follow-up. Consideration must be given to how individuals will be retained in cancer screening programs and genetic counseling programs so that risk assessments can be updated, recommendations for screening can be modified if needed, and regular routine screening can be completed (see Figure 2-6).

## Nursing Implications

### Educational Issues

Risk assessment is the responsibility of many different healthcare professionals, including physicians, nurses, psychologists, and genetic counselors. Formal and clinical education regarding risk assessment is limited in many professions (Freedman et al., 2005). Education of healthcare professionals regarding the techniques and tasks of risk assessment is important because clinically, healthcare professionals make

---

### Figure 2-6. Summary of Breast Cancer Risk Communication Considerations

**Gather Information for the Risk Assessment**
- Gather family history. This should include at least three generations, age at onset of cancer, and diagnoses.
- Confirm family history with pathology reports when possible.
- Assess reproductive history (age at menarche, age at first pregnancy, oral contraceptive use, hormone replacement therapy use, number of pregnancies, and age at menopause).
- Assess past history of breast biopsies (confirm with pathology report).
- Assess social risk factors (alcohol use, exercise patterns, dietary patterns).
- Assess what the patient's perceived risk of cancer is and how the perception was formed.

**Construct the Risk Assessment**
- Select a model to predict risk for the individual patient.
- When appropriate, select a model to predict the patient's risk of carrying a mutation.

**Communicate the Risk Assessment**
- Include the patient's absolute risk of developing breast cancer.
- Discuss the relative risk of developing breast cancer.
- Communicate the risk of carrying a mutation in families with a suspected hereditary predisposition including basic concepts of genetics and inheritance.
- Discuss the strengths and limitations of cancer risk assessment.
- Discuss the options available for risk management, including data on the efficacy of different measures for early detection and risk reduction.
- Inform the patient regarding signs and symptoms of cancer.
- Use graphics and written materials when possible.

**Communicate Information About Cancer Prevention and Early Detection**
- Discuss recommended strategies for cancer prevention, including strengths and limitations.
- Discuss recommended strategies for cancer detection, including strengths and limitations.
- Discuss signs and symptoms of malignancy that warrant immediate evaluation.
- Discuss prognosis of cancer when prevention and early detection strategies are implemented.
- Follow the office visit with a written letter summarizing the recommendations made in the office.

**Address Psychosocial Concerns**
- Assess beliefs about the causes of cancer.
- Assess motivations for seeking cancer risk assessment.
- Assess experiences with cancer and feelings, perceptions, concerns, or fears related to those experiences.
- Assess and be aware of the influence of cancer experiences and perceptions on health behaviors and cancer screening practices.
- Consider cultural, religious, and socioeconomic background.
- Provide an opportunity for the patient to describe any fears and concerns.
- Assess for depression, anxiety, or other signs that might suggest difficulty adjusting to the information. Refer the patient for further services when indicated.
- Provide guidance on discussing the risk assessment with family members, especially in the case of a hereditary predisposition.

**Long-Term Follow-Up**
- Assess whether the patient is engaging in the recommended prevention and early detection strategies.
- Update the family history and risk assessment. Revise recommendations as indicated.
- Assist patients with a hereditary risk in contacting and informing other family members who also may have a hereditary risk.

most of the recommendations for screening. Many oncology professionals have learned about genetics through self-study and clinical practice. Although these professionals may understand oncology well, they may be less familiar with the principles of genetics. Knowledge of statistics also is critical.

Specific content regarding cancer risk assessment that should be incorporated into a curriculum includes basic epidemiologic concepts, specific types of risk (absolute and relative), risk factors for specific cancers and etiologic factors if known, basic statistics, information about cancer prevention and early detection measures, and counseling techniques.

## Administrative Issues

Administrators who want to implement cancer risk assessment into a cancer screening program or other oncology programs need to consider a number of issues. First, they must look at the rationale for implementing such a program. If the institution is unable to provide the screening that will be recommended following a risk factor assessment (e.g., genetic testing), what arrangements will be made for patients who desire such services? Administrators cannot overlook the need to hire nursing or other personnel who have the expertise and skills needed to provide this essential and comprehensive service.

Increasing recruitment to health promotion programs is regarded as a major benefit of completing a health risk assessment. Screening programs that include risk assessments also can be incorporated into outreach programs in worksite settings. Ultimately, the success of most screening programs depends on the effort taken at the beginning to completely assess the unique needs of the population or community being served. Other important considerations include where services will be provided, the marketing of services, and reimbursement issues.

## Clinical Considerations

At the clinical level, the delivery of cancer risk information takes time, and how people who provide such information should be reimbursed for their risk assessment and counseling services is unclear. These charges may be bundled with other service charges, such as mammography. Without adequate reimbursement, however, it may be more likely that risk assessment services will not be given adequate attention or will be provided by people with insufficient background and expertise.

When providing genetic services, many providers use a standard protocol that calls for individuals or families to be seen for two visits, each lasting about one to two hours, prior to testing and at least one appointment for results disclosure and discussion of recommendations. In the setting of genetic risk, the use of multidisciplinary teams and multiple interactions is emphasized. The underlying concern is that individuals may be overwhelmed by all the information provided in a single one-hour visit. Such attention usually is not given to people with an average risk of developing a malignancy.

Risk factor profiles should be reviewed at least annually. Patients should be questioned about any change in their family history since the last assessment, development of any new health problems that may be associated with increased risk, and whether they have started new medications that may change the risk profile (e.g., initiating HRT). If significant changes have occurred, screening recommendations may need to be modified. If no significant changes have occurred, an annual review of the risk factor assessment offers an excellent opportunity to reinforce information on cancer prevention and early detection. It also communicates an ongoing concern for the patient as a dynamic individual and identifies the nurse as a resource for further information should a problem develop.

The cancer risk assessment provides the foundation for the educational process related to cancer prevention and early detection. Oncology nurses have the opportunity to teach individuals about the epidemiology, risk factors, and signs and symptoms associated with various cancers. This provides the framework that individuals need to understand the importance of and rationale for primary and secondary cancer prevention strategies, as well as information about signs and symptoms that merit further evaluation.

Once cancer risks and screening recommendations are identified and communicated to the patient, the patient must make a decision as to which screening tests he or she desires. If a patient declines a recommended screening test, he or she will sign a waiver on a consent form acknowledging the patient was informed of the recommendation and is declining the recommended screening at that time. Information about cancer screening recommendations can be reinforced in a post-visit letter that summarizes the discussion of risk, informs the patient of the results of his or her screening tests, reiterates any recommended follow-up, and summarizes the recommendations for cancer prevention and early detection.

Staff nurses can serve as case finders to identify individuals at increased risk for developing cancer who will benefit from a more detailed risk assessment and possibly cancer genetic counseling. Staff nurses who work directly with patients and get to know their families are in the best position to initiate referrals as case finders and initiate the cancer risk assessment process. To be an effective case finder, nurses must understand basic cancer incidence, epidemiology, and the importance of an accurate family history.

Nurses with advanced practice degrees can perform more in-depth risk assessments, recommend cancer screening procedures, explain the risks and benefits of a particular screening examination, and, in many cases, actually perform the screening examination. For those who provide cancer genetic counseling, additional training in genetics and counseling is recommended. Currently, the means to obtain this additional training are variable. The International Society of Nurses in Genetics (www.isong.org) offers a process in which nurses can earn a credential by submitting a detailed portfolio that demonstrates their expertise.

As more and more nurses become involved in cancer risk assessment and genetic risk assessment, the need for nurses who have the background and expertise to provide this counseling will increase (Mahon, 2009). Both undergraduate- and graduate-level nursing programs need to include content on genetics education. At present, there is limited recognition that genetics and risk assessment are relevant to nurses and that content must be included in educational curricula. Continuing education programs may help to bridge this knowledge gap for practicing nurses.

New risk factors seem to emerge every day. An important educational role for nurses is to help patients to understand which risks they should take seriously. Most people accept a wide variety of risks (e.g., driving faster than the posted speed limit, crossing a busy parking lot, riding a bike, flying across the country in an airplane) on a daily basis with little thought. For some reason, small news segments about cancer risk seem to conjure up more fear. Nurses must be aware of public news reports and go to primary sources when new risk factors are presented so that they can interpret this information accurately for patients. Nurses also need to communicate concepts related to breast and other cancer risks carefully when providing information to the media. This may include providing the media with primary sources and reports and more integrated state-of-the-art information. ACS and other resources should be consulted prior to speaking with the media to ensure that accurate statistics and figures are provided.

## Research

Future research should evaluate the process of risk notification; the impact on knowledge, attitudes, emotions, and practices; and outcomes related to health and disease status. This research should include controlled clinical trials to evaluate different counseling protocols and provide information on the impact and effectiveness of cancer risk assessment and counseling. More research is needed to better understand how patients make decisions about genetic testing and how to facilitate positive outcomes.

Clearly, more information is needed on the roles of cognition, the affective state of the individual, developmental differences, personal values, and how these individual qualities affect cancer risk communication (Klein & Stefanek, 2007). More research also is needed on the best people (including an interdisciplinary approach) to communicate cancer and genetic risks (Edwards et al., 2008). The effect of cancer risk assessment on cancer screening behaviors merits more attention.

## Conclusion

Oncology nurses need to consider risk factor assessment as a wonderful opportunity for patient education, not only on cancer risk factors but also on cancer prevention and early detection activities. Cancer risk assessment can be a technical process requiring expertise. Oncology nurses have an ethical responsibility to communicate risk information in understandable terms and as accurately as possible. Risk assessment is more than collecting assessment data from patients. A critical component of the process is communicating the information to patients in a meaningful way.

Breast cancer risk communication is a continuous process. The risk assessment is a large component of this process. It demands communication with women so that they are informed about the best possible choices regarding cancer prevention and early detection activities. Patients will continue to ask when more will be known about the particular risks related to breast cancer and when there will be improvements in treatment. Developments in genetics will undoubtedly change risk assessments for some patients.

Like many cancers, breast cancer is a multifactorial disease. Causes and risk factors come from both endogenous and exogenous sources that interact in ways that are not completely understood. Much of the data about risk factors is seen at the theoretical level. Many risk factors for cancer, including breast cancer, are not within the control of the individual. Helping patients to understand these risks, live with these risks, and make good choices about breast cancer prevention and early detection strategies are important oncology nursing responsibilities.

## References

Akobeng, A.K. (2008). Communicating the benefits and harms of treatments. *Archives of Disease in Childhood, 93,* 710–713. doi:10.1136/adc.2008.137083

Ameer, B., & Krivoy, N. (2009). Direct-to-consumer/patient advertising of genetic testing: A position statement of the American College of Clinical Pharmacology. *Journal of Clinical Pharmacology, 49,* 886–888. doi:10.1177/0091270009335948

American Cancer Society. (2009a). *Breast cancer facts and figures 2009–2010.* Atlanta, GA: Author.

American Cancer Society. (2009b). *Cancer facts and figures for African Americans 2009–2010.* Atlanta, GA: Author.

American Cancer Society. (2009c). *Cancer facts and figures for Hispanics/Latinos 2009–2011.* Atlanta, GA: Author.

American Cancer Society. (2010a). *Cancer facts and figures 2010.* Atlanta, GA: Author.

American Cancer Society. (2010b). *Cancer prevention and early detection facts and figures 2009.* Atlanta, GA: Author.

American College of Medicine Genetics Board of Directors. (2004). ACMG statement on direct-to-consumer genetic testing. *Genetics in Medicine, 6,* 60. doi:10.1097/01.GIM.0000106164.59722.CE

American College of Obstetricians and Gynecologists. (2008). ACOG Committee Opinion No. 409: Direct-to-consumer marketing of genetic testing. *Obstetrics and Gynecology, 111,* 1493–1494. doi:10.1097/AOG.0b013e31817d250e

American Society of Clinical Oncology. (2003). American Society of Clinical Oncology policy statement update: Genetic testing for cancer susceptibility. *Journal of Clinical Oncology, 21,* 2397–2406. doi:10.1200/JCO.2003.03.189

Anderson, G.L., Limacher, M., Assaf, A.R., Bassford, T., Beresford, S.A., Black, H., ... Wassertheil-Smoller, S. (2004). Effects of conjugated equine estrogen in postmenopausal women with hysterectomy: The Women's Health Initiative randomized controlled trial. *JAMA, 291,* 1701–1712. doi:10.1001/jama.291.14.1701

Berkey, C.S., Willett, W.C., Frazier, A.L., Rosner, B., Tamimi, R.M., Rockett, H.R., & Colditz, G.A. (2010). Prospective study of adolescent alcohol consumption and risk of benign breast disease in young women. *Pediatrics, 125,* e1081–e1087. doi:10.1542/peds.2009-2347

Berry, D.A., Iversen, E.S., Jr., Gudbjartsson, D.F., Hiller, E.H., Garber, J.E., Peshkin, B.N., ... Parmigiani, G. (2002). BRCAPRO validation, sensitivity of genetic testing of BRCA1/BRCA2, and prevalence of other breast cancer susceptibility genes. *Journal of Clinical Oncology, 20,* 2701–2712. doi:10.1200/JCO.2002.05.121

Berry, D.A., Parmigiani, G., Sanchez, J., Schildkraut, J., & Winer, E. (1997). Probability of carrying a mutation of breast-ovarian cancer gene BRCA1 based on family history. *Journal of the National Cancer Institute, 89,* 227–238.

Boyd, N., Martin, L., Gunasekara, A., Melnichouk, O., Maudsley, G., Peressotti, C., ... Minkin, S. (2009). Mammographic density and breast cancer risk: Evaluation of a novel method of measuring breast tissue volumes. *Cancer Epidemiology, Biomarkers and Prevention, 18,* 1754–1762. doi:10.1158/1055-9965.EPI-09-0107

Boyd, N.F., Guo, H., Martin, L.J., Sun, L., Stone, J., Fishell, E., ... Yaffe, M.J. (2007). Mammographic density and the risk and detection of breast cancer. *New England Journal of Medicine, 356,* 227–236.

Bradbury, A., & Olopade, O.I. (2006). The case for individualized screening recommendations for breast cancer [Editorial]. *Journal of Clinical Oncology, 24,* 3328–3330. doi:10.1200/JCO.2006.05.8586

Brewster, D.H., Stockton, D.L., Dobbie, R., Bull, D., & Beral, V. (2005). Risk of breast cancer after miscarriage or induced abortion: A Scottish record linkage case-control study. *Journal of Epidemiology and Community Health, 59,* 283–287. doi:10.1136/jech.2004.026393

Carey, J.M., & Burgman, M.A. (2008). Linguistic uncertainty in qualitative risk analysis and how to minimize it. *Annals of the New York Academy of Sciences, 1128,* 13–17. doi:10.1196/annals.1399.003

Casey, P.M., Cerhan, J.R., & Pruthi, S. (2008). Oral contraceptive use and risk of breast cancer. *Mayo Clinic Proceedings, 83,* 86–90. doi:10.4065/83.1.86

Chavez-MacGregor, M., Elias, S.G., Onland-Moret, N.C., van der Schouw, Y.T., Van Gils, C.H., Monninkhof, E., ... Peeters, P.H. (2005). Postmenopausal breast cancer risk and cumulative number of menstrual cycles. *Cancer Epidemiology, Biomarkers and Prevention, 14,* 799–804. doi:10.1158/1055-9965.EPI-04-0465

Chlebowski, R.T., Johnson, K.C., Kooperberg, C., Pettinger, M., Wactawski-Wende, J., Rohan, T., ... Hubbell, F.A. (2008). Calcium plus vitamin D supplementation and the risk of breast cancer. *Journal of the National Cancer Institute, 100,* 1581–1591. doi:10.1093/jnci/djn360

Claus, E.B., Risch, N., & Thompson, W.D. (1994). Autosomal dominant inheritance of early-onset breast cancer: Implications for risk prediction. *Cancer, 73,* 643–651.

Claus, E.B., Schildkraut, J.M., Thompson, W.D., & Risch, N.J. (1996). The genetic attributable risk of breast and ovarian cancer. *Cancer, 77,* 2318–2324.

Colditz, G.A. (2005). Epidemiology and prevention of breast cancer. *Cancer Epidemiology, Biomarkers and Prevention, 14,* 768–772. doi:10.1158/1055-9965.EPI-04-0157

Collaborative Group on Hormonal Factors in Breast Cancer. (2002). Breast cancer and breastfeeding: Collaborative reanalysis of individual data from 47 epidemiological studies in 30 countries, including 50,302 women with breast cancer and 96,973 women without the disease. *Lancet, 360,* 187–195. doi:10.1016/S0140-6736(02)09454-0

Committee on Gynecologic Practice. (2009). ACOG Committee Opinion No. 434: Induced abortion and breast cancer risk. *Obstetrics and Gynecology, 113,* 1417–1418. doi:10.1097/AOG.0b013e3181ac067d

Conner, P., Lundström, E., & von Schoultz, B. (2008). Breast cancer and hormonal therapy. *Clinical Obstetrics and Gynecology, 51,* 592–606. doi:10.1097/GRF.0b013e318180b8ed

Consensus Panel on Genetic/Genomic Nursing Competencies. (2008). *Essentials of genetic and genomic nursing: Competencies, curricula guidelines, and outcome indicators* (2nd ed.). Silver Spring, MD: American Nurses Association.

Couch, F.J., DeShano, M.L., Blackwood, M.A., Calzone, K., Stopfer, J., Campeau, L., ... Weber, B.L. (1997). BRCA1 mutations in women attending clinics that evaluate the risk of breast cancer. *New England Journal of Medicine, 336,* 1409–1415. doi:10.1056/NEJM199705153362002

Cummings, S.R., Tice, J.A., Bauer, S., Browner, W.S., Cuzick, J., Ziv, E., ... Kerlikowske, K. (2009). Prevention of breast cancer in postmenopausal women: Approaches to estimating and reducing risk. *Journal of the National Cancer Institute, 101,* 384–398. doi:10.1093/jnci/djp018

Edwards, A., Gray, J., Clarke, A., Dundon, J., Elwyn, G., Gaff, C., ... Thornton, H. (2008). Interventions to improve risk communication in clinical genetics: Systematic review. *Patient Education and Counseling, 71,* 4–25. doi:10.1016/j.pec.2007.11.026

Erwin, C. (2008). Legal update: Living with the Genetic Information Nondiscrimination Act. *Genetic Medicine, 10,* 869–873. doi:10.1097/GIM.0b013e31818ca4e7

Evans, D.G., Eccles, D.M., Rahman, N., Young, K., Bulman, M., Amir, E., ... Lalloo, F. (2004). A new scoring system for the chances of identifying a BRCA1/2 mutation outperforms existing models including BRCAPRO. *Journal of Medical Genetics, 41,* 474–480. doi:10.1136/jmg.2003.017996

Fagerlin, A., Zikmund-Fisher, B.J., & Ubel, P.A. (2007). "If I'm better than average, then I'm ok?": Comparative information influences beliefs about risk and benefits. *Patient Education and Counseling, 69,* 140–144. doi:10.1016/j.pec.2007.08.008

Finkel, A.M. (2008). Perceiving others' perceptions of risk: Still a task for Sisyphus. *Annals of the New York Academy of Sciences, 1128,* 121–137. doi:10.1196/annals.1399.013

Fisher, B., Anderson, S., Bryant, J., Margolese, R.G., Deutsch, M., Fisher, E.R., ... Wolmark, N. (2002). Twenty-year follow-up of a randomized trial comparing total mastectomy, lumpectomy, and lumpectomy plus irradiation for the treatment of invasive breast cancer. *New England Journal of Medicine, 347,* 1233–1241. doi:10.1056/NEJMoa022152

Frank, T.S., Manley, S.A., Olopade, O.I., Cummings, S., Garber, J.E., Bernhardt, B., ... Thomas, A. (1998). Sequence analysis of BRCA1 and BRCA2: Correlation of mutations with family history and ovarian cancer risk. *Journal of Clinical Oncology, 16,* 2417–2425.

Freedman, A.N., Seminara, D., Gail, M.H., Hartge, P., Colditz, G.A., Ballard-Barbash, R., & Pfeiffer, R.M. (2005). Cancer risk prediction models: A workshop on development, evaluation, and application. *Journal of the National Cancer Institute, 97,* 715–723. doi:10.1093/jnci/dji128

Gail, M.H., Brinton, L.A., Byar, D.P., Corle, D.K., Green, S.B., Schairer, C., & Mulvihill, J.J. (1989). Projecting individualized probabilities of developing breast cancer for white females who are being examined annually. *Journal of the National Cancer Institute, 81,* 1879–1886. doi:10.1093/jnci/81.24.1879

Geransar, R., & Einsiedel, E. (2008). Online direct-to-consumer marketing of genetic tests: Informed choices or buyers beware? *Genetic Testing, 12,* 13–23. doi:10.1089/gte.2007.0024

Gniady, J.A. (2008). Regulating direct-to-consumer genetic testing: Protecting the consumer without quashing a medical revolution. *Fordham Law Review, 76,* 2429–2475.

Hamajima, N., Hirose, K., Tajima, K., Rohan, T., Calle, E.E., Heath, C.W., Jr., ... Meirik, O. (2002). Alcohol, tobacco and breast cancer—Collaborative reanalysis of individual data from 53 epidemiological studies, including 58,515 women with breast cancer and 95,067 women without the disease. *British Journal of Cancer, 87,* 1234–1245. doi:10.1038/sj.bjc.6600596

Hede, K. (2008). Fat may fuel breast cancer growth. *Journal of the National Cancer Institute, 100,* 298–299. doi:10.1093/jnci/djn050

Hogarth, S., Javitt, G., & Melzer, D. (2008). The current landscape for direct-to-consumer genetic testing: Legal, ethical, and policy issues. *Annual Review of Genomics and Human Genetics, 9,* 161–182. doi:10.1146/annurev.genom.9.081307.164319

Hopwood, P. (2005). Psychosocial aspects of risk communication and mutation testing in familial breast-ovarian cancer. *Current Opinion in Oncology, 17,* 340–344.

Hoskins, K.F., Zwaagstra, A., & Ranz, M. (2006). Validation of a tool for identifying women at high risk for hereditary breast cancer in population-based screening. *Cancer, 107,* 1769–1776. doi:10.1002/cncr.22202

Hudson, K., Javitt, G., Burke, W., & Byers, P. (2007). ASHG statement on direct-to-consumer genetic testing in the United States. *Obstetrics and Gynecology, 110,* 1392–1395. doi:10.1097/01.AOG.0000292086.98514.8b

Idos, S.S., Wark, P.A., McCormack, V.A., Mayer, D., Overton, C., Little, V., ... MacLean, A.B. (2009). Ovulation-stimulation drugs and cancer risks: A long-term follow-up of a British cohort. *British Journal of Cancer, 100,* 1824–1831. doi:10.1038/sj.bjc.6605086

Klein, W.M.P., & Stefanek, M.E. (2007). Cancer risk elicitation and communication: Lessons from the psychology of risk perception. *CA: A Cancer Journal for Clinicians, 57,* 147–167. doi:10.3322/canjclin.57.3.147

Kurz-Milcke, E., Gigerenzer, G., & Martignon, L. (2008). Transparency in risk communication: Graphical and analog tools. *Annals of the New York Academy of Sciences, 1128,* 18–28. doi:10.1196/annals.1399.004

Lee, S.H., Akuete, K., Fulton, J., Chelmow, D., Chung, M.A., & Cady, B. (2003). An increased risk of breast cancer after delayed parity. *American Journal of Surgery, 186,* 409–412. doi:10.1016/S0002-9610(03)00272-1

Lindor, N.M., McMaster, M.L., Lindor, C.J., & Greene, M.H. (2008). Concise handbook of familial cancer susceptibility syndromes (2nd ed.). *Journal of the National Cancer Institute Monographs, 2008*(38), 1–93. doi:10.1093/jncimonographs/lgn001

Lobb, E.A., Butow, P.N., Moore, A., Barratt, A., Tucker, K., Gaff, C., ... Butt, D. (2006). Development of a communication aid to facilitate risk communication in consultations with unaffected women from high risk breast cancer families: A pilot study. *Journal of Genetic Counseling, 15,* 393–405. doi:10.1007/s10897-006-9023-x

Lof, M., & Weiderpass, E. (2009). Impact of diet on breast cancer risk. *Current Opinion in Obstetrics and Gynecology, 21,* 80–85. doi:10.1097/GCO.0b013e32831d7f22

Lynch, H.T., Snyder, C.L., Lynch, J.F., Riley, B.D., & Rubinstein, W.S. (2003). Hereditary breast-ovarian cancer at the bedside: Role of the medical oncologist. *Journal of Clinical Oncology, 21,* 740–753. doi:10.1200/JCO.2003.05.096

Mahon, S.M. (2006). Impact of direct-to-consumer advertising on healthcare providers and consumers. *Clinical Journal of Oncology Nursing, 10,* 417–420. doi:10.1188/06.CJON.417-420

Mahon, S.M. (2009). Cancer genomics: Advocating for competent care for families. *Clinical Journal of Oncology Nursing, 13,* 373–376. doi:10.1188/09.CJON.373-376

Mahoney, M.C., Bevers, T., Linos, E., & Willett, W.C. (2008). Opportunities and strategies for breast cancer prevention through risk reduction. *CA: A Cancer Journal for Clinicians, 58,* 347–371. doi:10.3322/CA.2008.0016

Mahue-Giangreco, M., Ursin, G., Sullivan-Halley, J., & Bernstein, L. (2003). Induced abortion, miscarriage, and breast cancer risk of young women. *Cancer Epidemiology, Biomarkers and Prevention, 12,* 209–214.

Marchbanks, P.A., McDonald, J.A., Wilson, H.G., Folger, S.G., Mandel, M.G., Daling, J.R., ... Weiss, L.K. (2002). Oral contraceptives and the risk of breast cancer. *New England Journal of Medicine, 346,* 2025–2032. doi:10.1056/NEJMoa013202

Metcalfe, A., Haydon, J., Bennett, C., & Farndon, P. (2008). Midwives' view of the importance of genetics and their confidence with genetic activities in clinical practice: Implications for the delivery of genetics education. *Journal of Clinical Nursing, 17,* 519–530. doi:10.1111/j.1365-2702.2007.01884.x

Morimoto, L.M., White, E., Chen, Z., Chlebowski, R.T., Hays, J., Kuller, L., ... McTiernan, A. (2002). Obesity, body size, and risk of postmenopausal breast cancer: The Women's Health Initiative (United States). *Cancer Causes and Control, 13,* 741–751. doi:10.1023/A:1020239211145

National Cancer Institute. (2005). Summary report: Early reproductive events and breast cancer workshop. *Issues in Law and Medicine, 21,* 161–165.

National Comprehensive Cancer Network. (2010). *NCCN Clinical Practice Guidelines in Oncology™: Genetic/familial high-risk assessment: Breast and ovarian* [v.1.2010]. Retrieved from http://www.nccn.org/professionals/physician_gls/PDF/genetics_screening.pdf

Newcomer, L.M., Newcomb, P.A., Trentham-Dietz, A., Longnecker, M.P., & Greenberg, E.R. (2003). Oral contraceptive use and risk of breast cancer by histologic type. *International Journal of Cancer, 106,* 961–964. doi:10.1002/ijc.11307

O'Doherty, K., & Suthers, G.K. (2007). Risky communication: Pitfalls in counseling about risk, and how to avoid them. *Journal of Genetic Counseling, 16,* 409–417. doi:10.1007/s10897-006-9077-9

Oncology Nursing Society. (2006, March). *Breast cancer screening* [Position statement]. Pittsburgh, PA: Author.

Oncology Nursing Society. (2009a, March). *Cancer predisposition genetic testing and risk assessment counseling* [Position statement]. Pittsburgh, PA: Author.

Oncology Nursing Society. (2009b, March). *The role of the oncology nurse in cancer genetic counseling* [Position statement]. Pittsburgh, PA: Author.

Oncology Nursing Society. (2010, March). *Direct-to-consumer marketing of genetic and genomic tests* [Position statement]. Pittsburgh, PA: Author.

Orgéas, C.C., Sanner, K., Hall, P., Conner, P., Holte, J., Nilsson, S.J., ... Czene, K. (2009). Breast cancer incidence after hormonal infertility treatment in Sweden: A cohort study. *American Journal of Obstetrics and Gynecology, 200,* 72.e1–72.e7. doi:10.1016/j.ajog.2008.08.066

Pappo, I., Lerner-Geva, L., Halevy, A., Olmer, L., Friedler, S., Raziel, A., ... Ron-El, R. (2008). The possible association between IVF and breast cancer incidence. *Annals of Surgical Oncology, 15,* 1048–1055. doi:10.1245/s10434-007-9800-2

Peters, E. (2008). Numeracy and the perception and communication of risk. *Annals of the New York Academy of Sciences, 1128,* 1–7. doi:10.1196/annals.1399.001

Petrucelli, N., Daly, M.B., Culver, J.O.B., & Feldman, G.L. (2007, June 19). BRCA1 and BRCA2 hereditary breast/ovarian cancer. Retrieved from http://www.ncbi.nlm.nih.gov/bookshelf/br.fcgi?book=gene&part=brca1#brca1.Chapter_Notes

Pierce, J.P. (2009). Diet and breast cancer prognosis: Making sense of the Women's Healthy Eating and Living and Women's Intervention Nutrition Study. *Current Opinion in Obstetrics and Gynecology, 21,* 86–91. doi:10.1097/GCO.0b013e32831da7f2

Pinkowish, M.D. (2009). Many women treated with chest radiotherapy for childhood cancers are not getting mammograms as recommended by guidelines. *CA: A Cancer Journal for Clinicians, 59,* 141–142. doi:10.3322/caac.20019

Sandler, G.R., Wasserman, L., Fullerton, J.T., & Romero, M. (2004). Supporting patients through genetic screening for cancer risk. *Medsurg Nursing, 13,* 233–246.

Saslow, D., Boetes, C., Burke, W., Harms, S., Leach, M.O., Lehman, C.D., ... Russell, C.A. (2007). American Cancer Society guidelines for breast screening with MRI as an adjunct to mammography. *CA: A Cancer Journal for Clinicians, 57,* 75–89. doi:10.3322/canjclin.57.2.75

Shattuck-Eidens, D., Oliphant, A., McClure, M., McBride, C., Gupte, J., Rubano, T., ... Thomas, A. (1997). BRCA1 sequence analysis in women at high risk for susceptibility mutations. Risk factor analysis and implications for genetic testing. *JAMA, 278,* 1242–1250.

Singletary, S.E. (2003). Rating the risk factors for breast cancer. *Annals of Surgery, 237,* 474–482. doi:10.1097/01.SLA.0000059969.64262.87

Smith-Warner, S.A., Spiegelman, D., Yaun, S.S., Adami, H.O., Beeson, W.L., van den Brandt, P.A., ... Hunter, D.J. (2001). Intake of fruits and vegetables and risk of breast cancer: A pooled analysis of cohort studies. *JAMA, 285,* 769–776. doi:10.1001/jama.285.6.769

Sprague, B.L., Trentham-Dietz, A., Terry, M.B., Nichols, H.B., Bersch, A.J., & Buist, D.S.M. (2008). Fertility drug use and mammographic breast density in a mammography screening cohort of premenopausal women. *Cancer Epidemiology, Biomarkers and Prevention, 17,* 3128–3133. doi:10.1158/1055-9965.EPI-08-0503

Stopfer, J.E. (2000). Genetic counseling and clinical cancer genetics services. *Seminars in Surgical Oncology, 18,* 347–357. doi:10.1002/(SICI)1098-2388(200006)18:4<347::AID-SSU10>3.0.CO;2-D

Struewing, J.P., Hartge, P., Wacholder, S., Baker, S.M., Berlin, M., McAdams, M., ... Tucker, M.A. (1997). The risk of cancer associated with specific mutations of BRCA1 and BRCA2 among Ashkenazi Jews. *New England Journal of Medicine, 336,* 1401–1408. doi:10.1056/NEJM199705153362001

Stuebe, A.M., Willett, W.C., Xue, F., & Michels, K.B. (2009). Lactation and incidence of premenopausal breast cancer: A longitudinal study. *Archives of Internal Medicine, 169,* 1364–1371. doi:10.1001/archinternmed.2009.231

Taylor, A.J., & Taylor, R.E. (2009). Surveillance for breast cancer after childhood cancer. *JAMA, 301,* 435–436. doi:10.1001/jama.2009.9

Travis, L.B., Hill, D.A., Dores, G.M., Gospodarowicz, M., van Leeuwen, F.E., Holowaty, E., ... Gilbert, E. (2003). Breast cancer following radiotherapy and chemotherapy among young women with Hodgkin disease. *JAMA, 290,* 465–475. doi:10.1001/jama.290.4.465

Trepanier, A., Ahrens, M., McKinnon, W., Peters, J., Stopfer, J., Grumet, S.C., ... Vockley, C.W. (2004). Genetic cancer risk assessment and counseling: Recommendations of the National Society of Genetic Counselors. *Journal of Genetic Counseling, 13,* 83–114. doi:10.1023/B:JOGC.0000018821.48330.77

Tucker, W.T., & Ferson, S. (2008). Strategies for risk communication: Evolution, evidence, experience. *Annals of the New York Academy of Sciences, 1128,* ix–xii. doi:10.1196/annals.1399.000

Tyler, C.V., Jr., & Snyder, C.W. (2006). Cancer risk assessment: Examining the family physician's role. *Journal of the American Board of Family Medicine, 19,* 468–477.

Veronesi, U., Cascinelli, N., Mariani, L., Greco, M., Saccozzi, R., Luini, A., ... Marubini, E. (2002). Twenty-year follow-up of a randomized study comparing breast-conserving surgery with radical mastectomy for early breast cancer. *New England Journal of Medicine, 347,* 1227–1232. doi:10.1056/NEJMoa020989

Vogel, V.G. (2008). Epidemiology, genetics, and risk evaluation of postmenopausal women at risk of breast cancer. *Menopause, 15,* 782–789. doi:10.1097/gme.0b013e3181788d88

Wang, X.T. (2008). Risk communication and risky choice in context: Ambiguity and ambivalence hypothesis. *Annals of the New York Academy of Sciences, 1128,* 78–89. doi:10.1196/annals.1399.009

Zikmund-Fisher, B.J., Fagerlin, A., Roberts, T.R., Derry, H.A., & Ubel, P.A. (2008). Alternate methods of framing information about medication side effects: Incremental risk versus total risk of occurrence. *Journal of Health Communication, 13,* 107–124. doi:10.1080/10810730701854011

# CHAPTER 3

# Prevention and Detection

Suzanne M. Mahon, RN, DNSc, AOCN®, APNG

## Introduction

Although breast cancer remains a major public health problem, the pool of long-term survivors is ever increasing and the mortality rate from breast cancer continues to fall. Much of this success can be attributed to improved cancer screening, especially the widespread use of mammography. The routine use of screening mammography and the specialty use of other diagnostic modalities, including ultrasound and, more recently, magnetic resonance imaging (MRI), enable healthcare providers to identify early, nonpalpable cancers, replacing later-stage disease with a potentially curable diagnosis. Research continues to identify means to prevent breast cancer. Nurses play a major role in providing risk assessment services, implementing screening and prevention recommendations, ensuring appropriate follow-up, and providing comprehensive patient education. In order to provide these services and patient education, nurses must understand the principles of cancer prevention and early detection.

## Levels of Cancer Prevention and Early Detection

Primary cancer prevention encompasses a healthy lifestyle and includes all measures to avoid carcinogen exposure and promote health. The focus of primary prevention is to prevent a cancer from ever developing or to delay the development of a malignancy. For individuals with a particularly high risk of developing cancer (such as those with a known genetic predisposition), primary prevention may include the use of chemoprevention agents or prophylactic surgery to prevent or significantly reduce the risk of developing a malignancy.

Secondary prevention refers to the early detection and treatment of subclinical, asymptomatic, or early disease in peo-

ple without obvious signs or symptoms of cancer. Secondary cancer prevention includes identifying people at risk for developing malignancy and implementing appropriate screening recommendations based on the risk assessment. Screening may include physical examinations, self-examinations, radiologic procedures, laboratory tests, or other examinations. Examples of secondary breast cancer prevention include the use of a clinical breast examination (CBE) or mammography to detect a nonpalpable breast cancer. Screening tests seek to decrease the morbidity and mortality associated with cancer. Following a positive screening test, further diagnostic testing is required to determine if a malignancy exists.

Tertiary cancer prevention includes monitoring for and preventing recurrence of the originally diagnosed cancer and screening for second primary cancers and long-term effects of treatment in cancer survivors. This form of prevention is aimed at detecting complications and second cancers in long-term survivors when treatment is most likely to be effective and ultimately improve their quality of life.

## Primary Prevention

### Lifestyle Modifications

Primary prevention strategies have the potential to reduce breast cancer incidence in high-risk women. All women should be instructed to reduce known modifiable risk factors as much as possible (Colditz, 2005). This includes avoiding weight gain and obesity, engaging in regular physical activity, and minimizing alcohol intake. Because a large percentage of women in the United States are overweight or obese, strategies to maintain a healthy body weight are important to reduce the risk of both developing and dying from breast cancer. Growing evidence supports a modest protective effect of

*The author would like to acknowledge Dianne D. Chapman, ND, APRN, BC, for her work on this chapter in the first edition of this book.*

physical activity on breast cancer (Cummings et al., 2009). Most studies have found a reduced risk in women who exercise vigorously for 45–60 minutes on five or more days per week (American Cancer Society, 2009a, 2010b). The potential prevention may be due to the effects of physical activity on body mass, hormones, and energy.

Reducing alcohol intake may be a useful primary prevention strategy for decreasing breast cancer risk (Lof & Weiderpass, 2009). The increased risk for breast cancer is dose dependent and exists regardless of the type of alcoholic beverage consumed. For this reason, limiting or eliminating alcohol use may be an effective breast cancer prevention measure (Cummings et al., 2009).

## Chemoprevention

The use of drugs to reduce the risk of disease is referred to as *chemoprevention*. It is a form of primary cancer prevention. Increasing evidence suggests that, in women known to be at increased risk for breast cancer, the drugs tamoxifen and raloxifene reduce this risk (Mahoney, Bevers, Linos, & Willet, 2008; Nelson et al., 2009).

Tamoxifen has been used for more than three decades as an effective treatment for some breast cancers. The National Surgical Adjuvant Breast and Bowel Project (NSABP) P-1 trial confirmed that tamoxifen could be used for chemoprevention in the primary prevention of breast cancer (Fisher et al., 1998). This large randomized trial of more than 13,000 women first demonstrated that tamoxifen can also be used to reduce the risk of invasive and in situ breast cancer in women at high risk for developing the disease; however, the reduction in risk was limited to estrogen receptor (ER)–positive disease. After an average of seven years of follow-up, breast cancer risk was decreased by 42% in the group that received tamoxifen, with 25 cases of breast cancer diagnosed per 1,000 women in the group compared to 43 cases per 1,000 in the group who did not receive tamoxifen. Tamoxifen is approved by the U.S. Food and Drug Administration (FDA) to reduce the risk of invasive breast cancer for women, either premenopausal or postmenopausal, who are at increased risk for breast cancer. Tamoxifen (20 mg/day), taken for five years, may reduce the risk of developing ER-positive invasive breast cancer for up to 10 years.

In addition, the NSABP B-24 trial identified tamoxifen as a secondary prevention strategy for patients with estrogen-positive ductal carcinoma in situ (DCIS) to prevent ipsilateral and contralateral breast cancer (Fisher et al., 1999; Gasco, Argusti, Bonanni, & Decensi, 2005). The NSABP has conducted numerous studies that evaluated the efficacy of tamoxifen alone or as an adjunct to chemotherapy for treating breast cancer (Fisher et al., 1981, 1986, 1989, 1990, 1997, 1999). The NSABP studies indicated not only that tamoxifen was an effective treatment for breast cancer but also that it reduced the expected number of breast cancers that would be diagnosed in the contralateral breast.

A protective effect also was observed in an international randomized prevention trial involving more than 7,000 women (Cuzick et al., 2007). After a median follow-up time of eight years, breast cancer risk was reduced by 26% in the women who received tamoxifen, with 124 cases diagnosed among 3,579 women in the tamoxifen group compared to 168 cases among 3,575 women in the group not receiving tamoxifen. These long-term follow-up results indicate that the reduction in risk persists after completion of the five-year treatment schedule (Shen, Costantino, & Qin, 2008).

Tamoxifen is a selective ER modulator that binds to the receptor and acts as an agonist and antagonist, depending on the organ. Tamoxifen is an antagonist in the breast, occupying the ER and blocking the effects of estrogen. Tamoxifen has an agonist effect in the bones, liver, and uterus by producing estrogen-like effects (Cuzick et al., 2007). Serious adverse events may result from tamoxifen use. Tamoxifen use in the prevention setting may increase the risk of ischemic stroke, particularly in women 50 years of age or older. Follow-up data indicate that the risk of serious adverse events, such as thromboembolism, decreases after active treatment. A meta-analysis found that the risk of thromboembolic events increased 1.9-fold with tamoxifen use; pulmonary emboli were the most common events (Cuzick et al., 2007). The risk of superficial thrombophlebitis was three-fold higher. Therefore, tamoxifen is not recommended for women with a prior history of thromboembolic events, stroke, or transient ischemic attack.

The risk of uterine and endometrial cancer is estimated to nearly double with tamoxifen use, especially in women 50 years of age and older (Cuzick et al., 2007). In most cases, the uterine cancers were successfully treated stage 1 adenocarcinomas. The American Society of Clinical Oncology guideline (Visvanathan et al., 2009) recommends that women receiving tamoxifen have a baseline gynecologic examination before starting tamoxifen and annual follow-up continuing after treatment ends, with a timely, thorough workup for abnormal vaginal bleeding. Routine endometrial biopsy is not needed in the absence of abnormal vaginal bleeding. Women with abnormalities on endometrial biopsy performed because of abnormal vaginal bleeding may consider stopping tamoxifen use, in consultation with their gynecologist, oncologist, or primary care physician.

Vaginal discharge and hot flashes are commonly reported adverse effects associated with tamoxifen use. However, some trials reported that the gynecologic and vasomotor symptoms were greatest during active treatment and did not increase after treatment. Women in the tamoxifen arms also reported leg cramps and bladder control problems. Clinicians should inform women that such symptoms may arise with tamoxifen use. Tamoxifen may increase the incidence of cataracts, particularly in older women (Cuzick et al., 2007). Reported effects of tamoxifen on cognition are inconsistent and inconclusive. The risks and benefits associated with tamoxifen use should be carefully considered during the decision-making process.

Raloxifene is FDA approved for treating and preventing osteoporosis in women who are postmenopausal and for reducing the risk of invasive breast cancer in women who are postmenopausal and at increased risk for breast cancer. The Study of Tamoxifen and Raloxifene (STAR) trial compared the effectiveness of tamoxifen and raloxifene and found that raloxifene reduced the risk of invasive breast cancer to the same degree as tamoxifen, but it did not have the same protective effect against in situ cancer (DCIS or lobular carcinoma in situ) (Vogel et al., 2006). As with tamoxifen, the benefit appears to be limited to reducing the risk of developing an ER-positive breast cancer (Grady et al., 2008). Raloxifene appears to have a lower risk for certain side effects, such as endometrial cancer and blood clots in the legs or lungs, compared to tamoxifen (Vogel et al., 2006).

A reduction in risk was observed across the trials, primarily for ER-positive invasive breast cancer (Vogel et al., 2006). Raloxifene has equal efficacy to tamoxifen in reducing breast cancer risk for women who are postmenopausal. Raloxifene did not reduce noninvasive breast cancer as much as tamoxifen, but this finding was not statistically significant.

Raloxifene (60 mg/day), taken for five years, may be offered as an option to reduce the risk of ER-positive invasive breast cancer for women who are postmenopausal and at increased risk for breast cancer and for women who are postmenopausal with osteoporosis, in whom breast cancer risk reduction is a secondary benefit. The optimal duration of raloxifene use is not defined, but safety information for randomized trials is limited to eight years. The guideline recommends a duration of no longer than five years for primary breast cancer prevention. Women who are postmenopausal and for whom breast cancer risk reduction is a secondary outcome (to addressing osteoporosis) may take raloxifene for more than five years (Visvanathan et al., 2009).

Raloxifene is not recommended for breast cancer risk reduction in premenopausal women. Raloxifene does not have demonstrated activity against established breast cancer and should not be used to treat breast cancer or prevent its recurrence. It is not known to have an effect on overall or breast cancer–specific mortality, but a reduction in the number of diagnoses of breast cancer should be considered an important health outcome in and of itself, even in the absence of an ultimate reduction in breast cancer mortality (Visvanathan et al., 2009). For women with osteoporosis who are at risk for breast cancer, breast cancer risk reduction is an additional potential benefit. Fracture does not appear to be a risk of raloxifene, so women with a prior history of fractures or osteoporosis should not be excluded from considering raloxifene.

Like tamoxifen, raloxifene is not recommended for women with a prior history of deep venous thrombosis, pulmonary embolus, stroke, or transient ischemic attack. In the three trials comparing raloxifene to placebo, thrombotic events increased with raloxifene, but in two trials, the increase was not statistically significant. Reported adverse effects included venous thromboembolism, vasomotor symptoms, gynecologic symptoms, musculoskeletal problems, dyspareunia, hot flashes, leg cramps, bladder control problems, and peripheral edema (Cuzick et al., 2007). The risks and benefits associated with raloxifene use should be carefully considered during the decision-making process.

A woman at increased risk for breast cancer should discuss taking tamoxifen or raloxifene with her doctor. It is estimated that more than two million U.S. women could benefit from chemoprevention with these drugs (Freedman et al., 2003). All women taking tamoxifen and raloxifene should be cautioned about the signs and symptoms of these possible complications and report any symptoms that appear, including (a) pain, warmth, or swelling of the calf or thigh, (b) sudden loss of extremity or facial function or sensation, and (c) chest pain, pressure, or dyspnea. Women on tamoxifen should be instructed to report vaginal bleeding after menopause or excessive or unusual bleeding between menses. They should also have annual Pap tests and evaluations for any vaginal bleeding irregularities, which may include transvaginal ultrasound to evaluate the thickness of the endometrial lining or an endometrial biopsy to assess for hyperplasia or malignant pathology (Visvanathan et al., 2009). Risk factors for developing a thromboembolic event are increased in those who have had surgery within the past three months, a body mass index above 25 kg/m$^2$, a history of past or current smoking, hypertension, total cholesterol equal to or above 250, and a family history of heart disease (Cuzick et al., 2007). A patient presenting with leg swelling, warmth, or pain usually is evaluated for a thrombosis with a low-invasive imaging study such as ultrasonography. A ventilation/perfusion scan assesses pulmonary ventilation and perfusion and is useful for diagnosing a suspected pulmonary embolism. A patient with a suspected stroke should have a cardiology workup with chemistries, enzymes, and electrocardiogram, as well as imaging studies such as computed tomography, MRI, diffusion-weighted imaging to identify ischemia, and magnetic resonance perfusion study to determine the diagnosis and potential prognosis for recovery (Frizzell, 2005).

Based on the STAR trial comparing raloxifene and tamoxifen, raloxifene appears to have a more favorable adverse effect profile (Visvanathan et al., 2009). Women who were postmenopausal and taking raloxifene had a lower risk of deep vein thrombosis, pulmonary embolism, benign uterine complaints, gynecologic symptoms, and cataracts. It is likely that both tamoxifen and raloxifene increase arterial vascular events to a similar degree, especially for older women and those with risk factors for these events. The overall quality of life was similar in the raloxifene and tamoxifen arms, but the incidence of dyspareunia, weight gain, hot flashes, and musculoskeletal complaints was higher with raloxifene use, whereas the incidence of vasomotor symptoms, bladder incontinence, gynecologic symptoms, and leg cramps was higher with tamoxifen use. Tamoxifen and raloxifene have a similar favorable effect on fracture incidence.

## Chemoprevention in Women With Hereditary Predisposition

An estimated 70% of breast cancer is sporadic, and another 15%–20% is familial, meaning one or two family members have breast cancer but there is no obvious pattern of autosomal dominant transmission (National Comprehensive Cancer Network [NCCN], 2010c). Among women, an estimated 5%–10% of breast cancers and 10%–15% of ovarian cancers are due to inherited mutations in the *BRCA1* and *BRCA2* genes (Guillem et al., 2006). These autosomal dominant genes, which are highly penetrant, predispose individuals to significant risk for developing breast and/or ovarian cancer. The loss of the wild-type allele on chromosomes 17q (*BRCA1*) and 13q (*BRCA2*) suggests that these genes function as tumor suppressor genes (NCCN, 2010c). *BRCA1* and *BRCA2* are caretaker genes, which help to maintain genomic stability by recognizing and repairing DNA damage as well as having a role in cell-cycle checkpoint control. Many studies have estimated the risk of developing cancer in those with *BRCA1/2* mutations. The risk for younger women developing breast cancer is estimated to be 33%–50% by age 50 (NCCN, 2010c). The lifetime risk is estimated to be 87% by age 70. The lifetime risk of ovarian cancer ranges from 16%–60%. Membership in some populations infers an increased risk for having a *BRCA1/2* mutation. Founder mutations have been noted in those of Ashkenazi Jewish, Dutch, and Icelandic descent. An estimated 1 in 40 Ashkenazi women carries one of three mutations (185delAG and 5382insc on *BRCA1* and 6174delT on *BRCA2*) (NCCN, 2010c).

*BRCA1* and *BRCA2* mutations are associated with autosomal dominant inheritance patterns that can be inherited from the father or mother, meaning that a first-degree relative of a person with a *BRCA* mutation has a 50% likelihood of also having the mutation. Prevention strategies for carriers of a mutation vary from increased surveillance and chemoprevention to prophylactic removal of the breast and ovaries. Currently, sufficient evidence shows that prophylactic surgeries offer the best risk reduction for breast and ovarian cancers (Hartmann, Degnim, & Schaid, 2004; NCCN, 2010c).

Chemoprevention is an option sometimes considered by women at risk for hereditary breast and ovarian cancer. Initially, it was believed to be helpful in only those with a *BRCA2* mutation, but more recent epidemiologic evidence suggests it may be an appropriate option for all women at risk for hereditary breast and ovarian cancer (Guillem et al., 2006). It typically is initiated 5–10 years before the youngest age at onset of breast cancer in the family and continued for five years. Women who take tamoxifen, especially premenopausal women, need careful counseling about pregnancy prevention, and all women need to be aware of its potential side effects, including the risk of embolism (Daly et al., 2006; Narod, 2006).

Prophylactic mastectomy can result in a 90%–95% reduction in breast cancer (Daly et al., 2006; Domchek et al., 2006;

Guillem et al., 2006). This may be an appropriate option for many women, especially those who have already been diagnosed with cancer, have undergone multiple breast biopsies, have abnormalities on CBE or mammography, or have difficult-to-examine breasts clinically or on mammography. Prophylactic mastectomy may lead to significant overall survival in mutation carriers diagnosed with cancer (NCCN, 2010c). It is an irreversible procedure that can be emotionally difficult for many women. In most cases, a prophylactic mastectomy includes total mastectomy without an axillary node dissection. Skin-sparing and nipple-sparing procedures are sometimes offered with informed consent stating that when more breast tissue is left, the effectiveness of the procedure may be decreased (Guillem et al., 2006). Women who undergo a prophylactic mastectomy can opt for immediate reconstruction with a flap or implant or choose to use prosthetics. This is a difficult decision for a woman and usually requires much support and education. Some women find the online resources from Facing Our Risk of Cancer Empowered (known as FORCE, www.facingourrisk.org) to be especially helpful. This can allow some communication with women who have made this choice and can serve as a source of peer support.

Prophylactic bilateral salpingo-oophorectomy (BSO) may be a very prudent choice in women with known genetic susceptibility, especially because the effectiveness of screening for ovarian cancer is limited (Daly et al., 2006). It also has been shown to be a cost-effective measure in this population (Anderson et al., 2006). A BSO also may be associated with as much as a 90% reduction in risk for ovarian cancer and a 50% reduction in the risk for breast cancer (Guillem et al., 2006). The ideal age seems to be between 35 and 40 if childbearing is complete. Approximately 2%–6% of mutation-positive women in this age group will have occult ovarian cancers at the time of prophylaxis (Finch et al., 2006). This primary prevention strategy should be considered after a careful discussion of the potential benefits of a reduced risk of breast and ovarian cancer with the consequences of an early menopause associated with increased vasomotor symptoms and potential bone loss (Schmeler et al., 2006). Women at substantial risk for cervical and uterine problems and malignancies may want to consider a total abdominal hysterectomy (Domchek & Weber, 2006).

## Evaluating the Strengths and Limitations of Screening Modalities

In addition to conveying information about cancer risk, nurses must communicate information to patients about the accuracy of screening tests. It is not enough to simply recommend a screening test. Patients need to understand what the possibilities are regarding a true-positive or true-negative test result.

## Accuracy of Screening Tests

The accuracy of screening tests is described using a number of terms. A true-positive test (TP) is a abnormal test for cancer in an individual who actually has cancer. A true-negative test (TN) is a normal or negative screen for cancer in an individual who is subsequently found not to have cancer within a defined period after the last test. A false-negative test (FN) is a normal test for cancer in an individual who actually has cancer. A false-positive test (FP) is an abnormal test result for cancer screening in an individual who actually does not have cancer. An understanding of true and false test results is necessary to calculate information about sensitivity and specificity.

The *sensitivity* of a screening test is its ability to detect those individuals who have cancer. It is calculated by taking the number of TPs and dividing it by the total number of cancer cases (TP + FN). The *specificity* of a test is its ability to identify those individuals who actually do not have cancer. It is calculated by dividing the TN by the sum of the TN and FP cases. A high FP rate can result in unnecessary follow-up testing and anxiety in people who have a positive screen.

The *positive predictive value* is a measure of the validity of a positive test. It is the proportion of positive tests that are TP cases. The predictive value of a test depends on the disease prevalence. As the prevalence of a cancer increases in the population, the positive predictive value of the screening tests increases, even though its sensitivity and specificity remain unchanged. The *negative predictive value* is a measure of the validity of a negative test. It refers to the proportion of negative tests that are TNs.

The ideal screening test has a high specificity and sensitivity for detecting the cancer in its earliest stages. This is accomplished by having a high positive and negative predictability. Other factors that influence the screening test include the healthcare providers who are administering the screening examination and the quality of the radiology procedures.

*Acceptability* is the extent to which those for whom the test is recommended and designed agree to be tested. Components of acceptability include availability, safety, and expense/cost-effectiveness. The target disease should be a common form of cancer with high associated morbidity or mortality. The disease should have a preclinical stage before symptoms are evident, and effective treatment, capable of reducing morbidity and mortality, should be available if the disease is detected early.

## Improving the Accuracy of Screening

Healthcare providers can take several steps to improve the accuracy of screening tests. In terms of breast cancer screening, attaining certification, following professional guidelines, and following federal guidelines are critical steps. Guidelines are now in place for mammography centers that provide cancer screening services to ensure a minimum acceptable standard is met.

A mammography facility should be FDA certified. In an effort to standardize mammography facilities, the Mammography Quality Standards Act was implemented in 1992 to create performance standards for facility personnel and equipment. Surveys are conducted on a regular basis to ensure that the standards are being upheld, including properly functioning equipment, licensed/certified personnel, and documentation of continuing education. A listing of accredited facilities is available at www.fda.gov/cdrh/mammography/certified.html. Certification from relevant agencies should be publicly displayed.

The person conducting the examination or interpreting the radiologic test results profoundly affects the effectiveness of the cancer screening test. For example, some healthcare professionals are clearly better at performing CBEs than others and are more likely to detect a subtle breast change. Monitoring the quality of clinical examinations is important. Monitoring and improving the quality of physical examinations in the clinical setting is far more challenging but is nevertheless important to improve the sensitivity and specificity of the examination. Similarly, radiologists who interpret mammograms need to do so on a regular basis to maintain and develop their skills (Taplin et al., 2008).

Screening quality also may be improved by developing standardized instructions for patient preparation. This may not only improve patient compliance but also may help in obtaining the best possible screen.

Providers need to be continually updated on the newest guidelines and techniques for cancer screening. Such training should include a staff competency evaluation. New equipment is constantly being developed to enhance screening and diagnostic procedures. Agencies that provide screening services need to not just review such equipment but also develop policies on how they will test and possibly eventually adapt such equipment to their specific needs.

Once the healthcare provider identifies and communicates cancer risks and screening recommendations to the patient, the patient must decide which screening tests she desires. If a patient declines a recommended screening test, the patient should sign a waiver on a consent form acknowledging she was informed of the recommendation and is declining the recommended screening at that time. Information about cancer screening recommendations can be reinforced in a post-visit letter that summarizes the discussion of risk, informs the patient of the screening test results, reiterates any recommended follow-up, and summarizes the recommendations for cancer prevention and early detection.

A screening protocol or recommendation defines how cancer screening tests should be used. For example, ACS recommends that women of average risk initiate mammography at age 40 (ACS, 2010a). Such recommendations can vary among organizations and practitioners. A recommendation generally describes the target population to be served, the screening recommendation to be applied, and the interval at which the test should be undertaken.

A screening test aims to ensure that as few people as possible with the disease get through undetected (high sensitivity) and as few as possible without the disease are subject to further diagnostic tests (high specificity). Given high sensitivity and specificity, the likelihood that a positive screening test will give a correct result (positive predictive value) strongly depends on the prevalence of the disease within the population. If the prevalence of the disease is very low, even the best screening test will not be an effective public health program. Because the prevalence of breast cancer is estimated to be high (more than 2.5 million women are alive with a history of breast cancer [ACS, 2009a]), screening is reasonable. The perfect screening test for breast cancer does not exist. For this reason, tests often are combined to compensate for the limitations of any one test.

Most would agree that it makes sense to screen for and detect breast cancer in its earliest stages. Theoretically, treatment should be the least complicated and least toxic at this point, and the chance for long-term disease-free survival should be the greatest. Nurses often are confronted with questions about breast cancer prevention, screening modalities, and the early detection of cancer. They need to be able to instruct patients and families on the principles of screening, the rationale for the different recommendations put forth by national agencies, and controversies in screening.

Cancer screening is aimed at asymptomatic individuals with the goal of finding disease when it is most easily treated. It is important for patients to understand that screening is not prevention; the cancer must be measurable and present to be detected on a screening examination. True cancer prevention is aimed at keeping the cancer from ever developing. Screening tests seek to decrease both the morbidity and the mortality associated with cancer because theoretically, at an early stage, cancer is most effectively and easily treated. This is the traditional definition of cancer screening. Some also consider screening for genetic or molecular markers that put an individual at high risk for developing cancer to be a form of cancer screening. This is a rapidly emerging and targeted means to better quantify risk and offer primary prevention measures (some of which are drastic, such as prophylactic surgery).

Short-term outcomes may include measures of the number of people who are screened or who undergo genetic testing, the number of people with abnormal screens who have further diagnostic testing, the number of cancers detected, or the cost per cancer detected and risks associated with screening. Often, healthcare providers are most focused on the short-term benefits of screening, when larger strides in decreasing the morbidity and mortality associated with cancer could ultimately be achieved with a focus on more long-term goals and an emphasis on primary prevention behaviors, especially in relation to alcohol usage, obesity, poor dietary habits, and sedentary lifestyle (Schottenfeld & Beebe-Dimmer, 2006). Long-term outcomes may include site-specific cancers detected in the screened population, total costs, and the stage distribution of detected cancers (Tyler & Snyder, 2006). Knowledge of outcome measures is important for nurses who provide risk assessments and cancer screening services. Nurses need to be able to give detailed information about the risks and benefits that can arise during the screening process.

Screening guidelines change over time. ACS, for example, has been publishing guidelines for the early detection of cancer for more than 20 years (ACS, 2010a). Although the specific guidelines have changed over the years, the focus of the guidelines has changed very little. Healthcare providers are still expected to use the guidelines to select the best screening tests for an individual and to modify the guidelines in certain cases, such as if an individual has a particularly high risk for developing a specific malignancy.

Clinicians must remember that screening protocols are merely guidelines. They are not practice standards to be used blindly with every individual. Risk assessment is required in order to apply many of the guidelines. The goal of the ACS standards is the detection of malignancy. The U.S. Preventive Services Task Force (USPSTF) uses very strict criteria for assessing evidence of effectiveness. Cost-effectiveness of the screening recommendations is an important consideration for this group, for example. When providing information on cancer screening recommendations, nurses need to inform individuals why a certain recommendation is being made in their case.

Nurses often will make recommendations for various screening or detection measures, especially in people who carry a higher risk of developing a particular cancer based on their family history and genetic background. Nurses need to be able to accurately explain the risks and benefits of these screening tools to their patients. This requires an understanding of the measures of validity of a screening test. Specific recommendations for a screening test often vary among organizations such as ACS, USPSTF, or the National Cancer Institute. The specific criteria that each organization uses to make recommendations may vary, which is why the recommendations are not universal and can prove very confusing to the general public. There are, however, generally agreed-upon requirements and characteristics of acceptable screening tests. When presenting screening recommendations to individuals, it is important to include the rationale, strengths, and limitations of each test and to present this information in light of the individual's own risk for developing cancer. Often, individuals with a genetic susceptibility need recommendations that are more rigorous than those for individuals with average risk.

First, nurses need to review the scientific basis for each guideline. Each agency that promulgates a guideline should make this information available. An excellent place to obtain information about the scientific basis and the review process for a guideline is from the individual agency that generates the guideline or at the National Guideline Clearinghouse (www.guideline.gov). For some guidelines, the data support implementation only to a certain age, such as mammography. The ACS guidelines do not give an age at which to stop mammography but encourage clinicians to consider the overall health of the woman when recommending the screening (ACS, 2009a).

Second, nurses play a key role in interpreting these data to patients (Karliner et al., 2007; Lin et al., 2007). Nurses need to explain why a particular set of guidelines is being used for an individual patient. They need to remind each patient that these recommendations are guidelines, and some modifications may be made based on personal risk factor assessment and findings on a clinical examination. With some people who are in failing health, it is appropriate to discuss stopping cancer screening, although few of the guidelines provide specific direction in this area. Clearly, the benefits, risks, and potential limitations of each screening test need to be discussed individually and tailored according to the risk factor assessment.

Cancer risk communication influences patients' decisions to undergo cancer screening examinations. When a healthcare provider recommends a particular screening examination, the likelihood is increased that the individual will actually go on to have the recommended screening (Lin et al., 2007). Healthcare providers can make qualified recommendations for screening based on the myriad of guidelines available only if they understand the biases of various guidelines and have completed an accurate assessment of risk. In addition, decisions to undergo screening are influenced by the perceived benefit from undergoing the screening procedure. Such a decision must be balanced with a discussion of the risks associated with screening. Providing individuals with information about the sensitivity and specificity of a screening procedure is, indeed, challenging.

Figure 3-1 describes barriers to consider. The importance of targeting interventions that are culturally sensitive cannot be overestimated. People choose to engage in cancer screening interventions. If an intervention is not culturally sensitive or makes an individual uncomfortable, an opportunity for screening or increasing cancer awareness may be missed (ACS, 2009a, 2009b, 2009c, 2010b).

If the intended benefits of screening are to be realized, individuals need to have a clear understanding of the implications of the tests both before they are screened and after they receive the results. The potential benefits of screening are lost if individuals are never informed of the test results or the meaning of those results. Providing patients with information about screening results generates another opportunity to reinforce the information included in the risk factor assessment. After screening tests are completed, risk may be more apparent, and screening recommendations may need to be revised.

The cancer risk assessment begins the educational process related to cancer prevention and early detection. Without an

---

**Figure 3-1. Barriers to Engaging in Breast Cancer Screening**

**System Barriers**
- Conflicting recommendations create confusion about recommendations.
- Facilities may be geographically inaccessible or have inconvenient hours.
- Healthcare providers may be confused about the variety of recommendations from different agencies.
- Healthcare providers may not focus on wellness.
- Healthcare providers may not recommend screening.
- Risk assessment may not be conducted or may not be accurate to recommend appropriate screening.

**Patient Barriers**
- The woman underestimates the magnitude of her risk.
- The woman does not understand the potential benefits of screening.
- The woman lacks insurance or ability to pay for screening.
- The woman cannot access transportation to get to screening.
- The woman has other complications that prevent access to screening, including lack of availability during off-work hours or difficulty obtaining child care.
- Mammography or breast examination might be considered embarrassing.
- Mammography or a breast examination might be culturally unacceptable.
- The woman may speak another language.
- The woman may not have spousal, partner, or social support to complete screening.

*Note.* Based on information from American Cancer Society, 2009a, 2009b, 2009c, 2010a, 2010b; National Comprehensive Cancer Network, 2010c.

---

accurate and comprehensive risk assessment, it is impossible to provide the individual with appropriate and reasonable recommendations for primary and secondary cancer prevention. The risk factor assessment provides the oncology nurse with an opportunity to teach individuals about the epidemiology, risk factors, and signs and symptoms associated with various cancers. It transmits the framework individuals need to understand the importance of and rationale for primary and secondary cancer prevention strategies, as well as information about signs and symptoms that merit further evaluation.

## Patient Education

Empowering patients with enough information in understandable terms so that they can make an informed choice about cancer screening is the ultimate goal of cancer risk counseling. When a healthcare provider simply recommends a screening test or tries to scare a patient into undergoing a screening or genetic test by telling a poignant or compelling story, the patient may select or fail to select a screening test for the wrong reasons. Thus, it is important that providers offer balanced and accurate information. The downside of conveying a risk assessment such that the individual has enough information to make an informed decision is that it is extremely labor intensive for the healthcare provider.

Oncology nurses have a major responsibility to teach the public about cancer detection and screening. Individuals need to realize that cancer screening differs from diagnostic examinations for cancer. They also need to recognize that cancer screening is not perfect and, even when conducted properly, will still fail to detect some malignancies because of the limitations associated with different screening tests.

Research continues to suggest that the single most important factor in whether an individual has ever had a screening test, or has recently had a screening test, is a recommendation from the healthcare provider (ACS, 2010a). When nurses recommend screening to an individual, there is a far greater chance that the individual will actually go on to have appropriate screening. This recommendation can easily come in the form of patient education about cancer prevention and early detection.

Every cancer screening program should include a significant patient education component. Care needs to be taken in gathering appropriate and useful materials for this purpose. These materials may include brochures from cancer-related organizations or developed specifically for an agency's population. Posters can provide additional education and can be displayed in waiting and examination areas. Bulletin boards are a relatively simple means to provide brief public education specific to a population or topic. They have the advantage of being relatively easy to produce and change. Flip charts can be used for individual education; these can be either purchased or developed specifically for the group being served. Other educational aids might include anatomy charts and models or computer-assisted education.

When providing patients with information on cancer prevention and early detection, it is important to use educational materials that focus on wellness. More and more of these resources are becoming available. It is inappropriate to provide materials that focus on disease and treatment. In fact, some people find them distressing. The message of education and materials should be that early detection is associated with decreased morbidity and mortality and improved quality of life. Written patient education materials with a focus on nutrition, participation in chemoprevention trials, self-examination technique, and screening tests including mammography are available through the National Cancer Institute and ACS.

How long a person can retain information after counseling about cancer risk factors is unclear. Cancer screening programs and genetic counseling programs need to consider how information will be retained so that risk assessments can be updated, recommendations for screening modified if needed, and regular routine screening completed.

## Secondary Breast Cancer Prevention

Secondary cancer prevention (breast cancer screening and early detection) seeks to detect cancers in the earliest possible stage. The goal of secondary prevention is to detect cancer when treatment is most likely to be effective and is associated with the least morbidity. In breast cancer, secondary cancer prevention includes breast examinations and imaging modalities, especially mammography. An overview of the recommendations from a number of agencies is shown in Table 3-1. The proper use of screening and genetic testing can potentially decrease the morbidity and mortality associated with breast cancer. Screening is appropriate for asymptomatic women. Symptomatic women (see Figure 3-2) should be referred directly to a diagnostic evaluation, which might include an ultrasound, additional mammographic views, MRI, and biopsy.

## Clinical Breast Examination

Mammography and CBE often are recommended in tandem to properly screen average-risk women older than 40 years of age. Mammography has a variable false-negative rate between 10% and 30% (ACS, 2009a). For this reason, CBE is considered an important adjunct procedure to detect any breast abnormalities not noted on mammography. A minority of cancers are not seen on mammography because of increased density of breast tissue, the nature of certain types of breast cancer (invasive lobular), or inexplicable reasons. An experienced breast specialist may be able to discern suspicious breast changes that often are very subtle underlying areas of thickening, mild skin changes that might include dimpling or puckering, or a slight difference in the parenchymal texture of one breast when compared to the other. It also may be useful for detecting interval breast cancers between mammographic examinations (Smith, Cokkinides, Brooks, Saslow, & Brawley, 2010). Although CBE may indeed play an integral part in screening for breast cancer, no study has compared CBE alone versus no screening (NCCN, 2010b).

ACS (2010a) recommends that women undergo CBE every three years between the ages of 20 and 39 and then annually after age 40. The recommendation is that the examination should take place during periodic wellness health examinations. When CBE is performed, it is an opportunity for the healthcare provider to review and update the woman's family history, discuss the importance of early breast cancer detection, and answer any questions she may have about her own risk, new technologies, or other matters related to breast disease (Smith et al., 2010). During these discussions and examinations, healthcare professionals have the opportunity to and should emphasize the importance of awareness and recognition of breast changes and of contacting their physician promptly if changes are perceived. They also should emphasize the importance of awareness of a family history of breast

### Table 3-1. Comparison of Breast Cancer Screening Recommendations

| Guideline Component | ACS | ACOG | NCCN | USPSTF |
|---|---|---|---|---|
| Date released | 1997 (revised 2003; addendum released March 2007) | April 2003 (reaffirmed 2006) | 2008 (revised 2010) | 1997 (revised 2003; addendum released November 2009) |
| Age to start mammography | 40 | 40 | 40 | 50 |
| Interval to perform mammography | Annually | Annually | Annually | Biennial screening mammography for women aged 50–74 years |
| Age to stop mammography | As long as a woman is in reasonably good health and would be a candidate for treatment, she should continue to be screened with mammography. | Not stated | If there are severe comorbid conditions and a woman would not undergo intervention for findings, screening should be stopped. | Current evidence is insufficient to assess the additional benefits and harms of screening mammography in women 75 years or older. |
| Age to start clinical breast examination (CBE) | 20 | 20 | 20 | Insufficient data to assess the additional benefits and harms of CBE |
| Interval to perform CBE | At least every 3 years until age 40. Annually beginning at age 40. | Annually | Every 1–3 years until age 40. Annually beginning at age 40. | Not recommended |
| Breast self-examination (BSE) | Beginning in their 20s, women should be told about the benefits and limitations of BSE and reporting symptoms promptly. Women who choose to do BSE should receive instruction and have their technique reviewed. It is acceptable for women to choose not to do BSE or to do BSE irregularly. | Counsel women that BSE has the potential to detect palpable breast cancer and can be performed if the woman desires. There is no reason to recommend against BSE. | Encourage breast awareness. | Recommends against teaching BSE. |
| Breast magnetic resonance imaging | Recommended for<br>• Women with a known *BRCA* mutation<br>• Women with a first-degree relative of *BRCA* carrier, but untested<br>• Women with a lifetime risk of 20%–25% or greater on a model that is largely dependent on family history | No recommendation for or against | Recommended for women with a lifetime risk of > 20% | Current evidence is insufficient to assess the additional benefits and harms of either digital mammography or magnetic resonance imaging instead of film mammography as screening modalities for breast cancer. |
| References | ACS, 2009a; Saslow et al., 2007 | ACOG, 2003 | NCCN, 2010a, 2010b | USPSTF, 2009 |

ACOG—American Congress of Obstetricians and Gynecologists; ACS—American Cancer Society; NCCN—National Comprehensive Cancer Network; USPSTF—U.S. Preventive Services Task Force

and ovarian cancers in first- and second-degree relatives on both the maternal and paternal sides of the family. An opportunity to update the family history should take place during encounters for other preventive care or screening.

The clinical usefulness of CBE and breast self-examination (BSE) is driven by the skill of the examiner. The more thorough the steps, the more likely a small or subtle change will be detected. The reported sensitivity is 35%–47% (Barton & Elmore, 2009). CBE offers an excellent opportunity for patient education and return demonstration of BSE technique in motivated women. Figures 3-3 through 3-12 demonstrate the steps of CBE.

## Breast Self-Examination

Physicians, nurses, and professional organizations have routinely recommended BSE has as an adjunct tool to facilitate the early detection of breast cancer for many years (ACS, 2010a). However, very few studies have been done to substantiate its effectiveness (i.e., decrease in mortality) or to evaluate its associated financial and emotional costs (Smith et al., 2010). Although many organizations no longer recommend monthly BSE, ACS recommends that women should be informed about the potential benefits, limitations, and harm (principally the possibility of a false-positive result) associated with BSE. Women then may choose to perform BSE regularly, occasionally, or not at all (ACS, 2009a). If a woman chooses to perform periodic BSE, she should receive instructions in the

---

**Figure 3-2. Signs and Symptoms of Breast Cancer**

- Lump or mass in the breast
- Swelling in all or part of the breast
- Skin irritation or dimpling
- Breast pain
- Nipple pain
- Nipple inversion in a previously everted nipple
- Nipple eversion in a previously inverted nipple
- Redness, scaliness, or thickening of the nipple or breast skin
- Nipple discharge other than breast milk

*Note.* Based on information from American Cancer Society, 2009a.

---

**Figure 3-3. Clinical Breast Examination—Arms Relaxed**

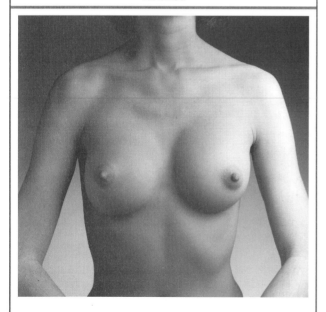

The clinical breast examination begins with the arms relaxed at the side and the woman undressed to the waist.

*Note.* Photo by Photogroup. Used courtesy of the National Cancer Institute.

---

**Figure 3-4. Clinical Breast Examination—Arms Squeezing at Waist**

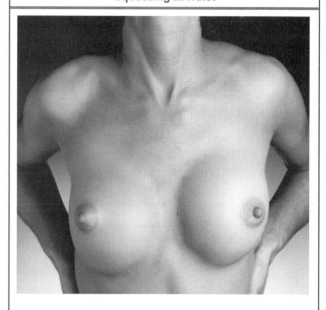

Next, have the woman squeeze her hands at her waist, and observe for dimpling or puckering or other changes.

*Note.* Photo by Photogroup. Used courtesy of the National Cancer Institute.

---

**Figure 3-5. Clinical Breast Examination—Arms Above Head**

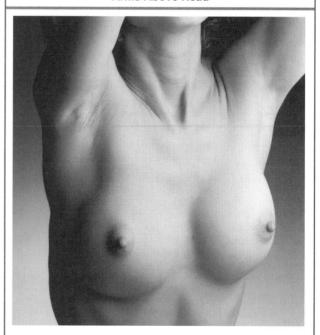

Have the patient raise her hands above the head to observe for dimpling, puckering, or other breast changes.

*Note.* Photo by Photogroup. Used courtesy of the National Cancer Institute.

## Figure 3-6. Clinical Breast Examination— Leaning Forward

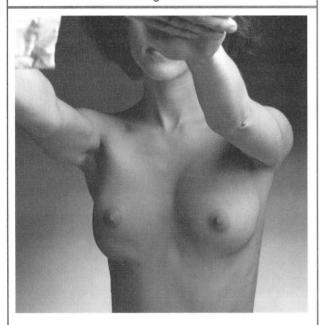

Have the woman lean forward, and observe for dimpling, puckering, retraction, or other breast changes.

*Note.* Photo by Photogroup. Used courtesy of the National Cancer Institute.

## Figure 3-8. Clinical Breast Examination— Sweep the Breast

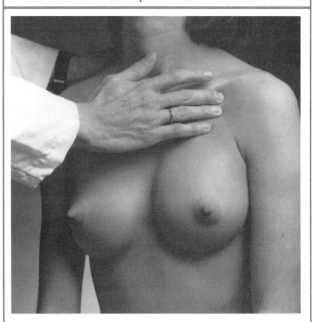

Sweep the hand over the breast beginning at the clavicle to palpate any lumps or irregularities.

*Note.* Photo by Photogroup. Used courtesy of the National Cancer Institute.

## Figure 3-7. Clinical Breast Examination—Palpation of Supraclavicular and Infraclavicular Lymph Nodes

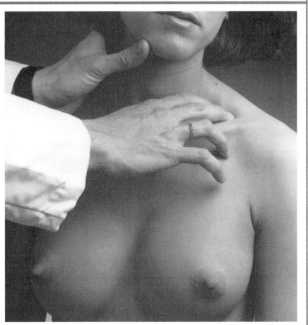

Palpate the supraclavicular and infraclavicular lymph nodes for abnormalities.

*Note.* Photo by Photogroup. Used courtesy of the National Cancer Institute.

## Figure 3-9. Clinical Breast Examination—Palpate for Axillary Lymph Nodes

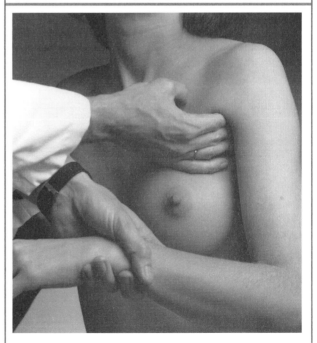

Palpate for axillary lymph node abnormalities.

*Note.* Photo by Photogroup. Used courtesy of the National Cancer Institute.

### Figure 3-10. Clinical Breast Examination—Palpate for Masses

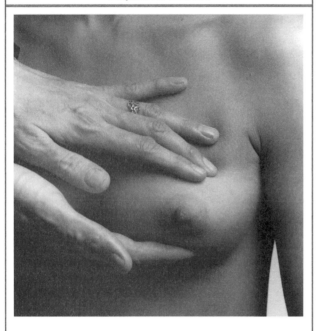

Support the breast under one hand, and palpate for masses. Note any nipple discharge.

*Note.* Photo by Photogroup. Used courtesy of the National Cancer Institute.

### Figure 3-11. Clinical Breast Examination—Breast Palpation in Supine Position

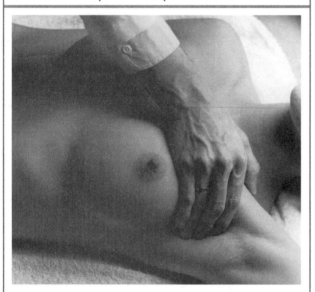

Place a towel or small pillow under the side to be examined while the patient is lying down. This spreads out the breast tissue. Examine the breast systematically in circles or strips, pressing deep, deeper, and still deeper until the entire breast is covered.

*Note.* Photo by Photogroup. Used courtesy of the National Cancer Institute.

### Figure 3-12. Clinical Breast Examination—Palpate Behind the Nipple

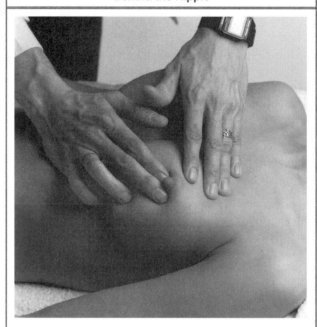

Press the nipple down. There should not be any resistance behind the nipple.

*Note.* Photo by Photogroup. Used courtesy of the National Cancer Institute.

technique and periodically have her technique reviewed. Ideally this is done during the CBE and follows the same steps in Figures 3-3 through 3-12, except the woman examines herself. The underlying rationale for increased breast awareness is that women who have increased awareness or who practice BSE may find lumps earlier than women who do not perform BSE and that the lumps are smaller and more easily treated, thereby decreasing mortality.

Despite the recommendation, women will still choose to perform monthly BSE if they feel it is helpful or if their healthcare practitioner actively encourages them to do so. One of the biggest benefits of BSE is that it allows women to be proactive in their breast health. Women in the United States are very aware of the prevalence of breast cancer and often are willing to take steps to enhance early detection. The ACS guidelines include BSE as an option starting at age 20. Between ages 20 and 40, women should have a CBE every one to three years. Women older than age 40 are urged to have an annual CBE and mammogram and to report any breast changes promptly (ACS, 2010a).

In addition, women who choose BSE should know the proper technique and timing of the examination. Nurses often initiate and reinforce this teaching when patients come in for a routine examination or when an appointment is made to address a perceived breast problem. The best time for menstruating women to perform BSE is right after their period ends, and menopausal women should choose a particular day of the month (such as when bills are paid, when the bank statement arrives, etc.) to remind them to do BSE. The current practice of BSE is a two-step activity. First, after a bath or shower, the breasts are visually examined, turning from side to side in front of a mirror with arms down, arms pressing on the hips, and arms raised over the head. These different positions alter the tension on the pectoralis muscle below the breast to best identify any puckering or change in the breast contour. The woman also notes any difference in the skin color or texture and any nipple changes (e.g., new evidence of inversion or protrusion, scaly or crusty appearance). At this point, the woman should palpate the supraclavicular, infra-clavicular, and axillary lymph nodes for any changes. The remainder of the palpation examination is best performed lying down, as this allows the breast tissue to spread out evenly over the chest wall. The woman should be instructed to use the flat pads of the first three fingers for the examination and to place a pillow or towel under the shoulder and use the opposite hand of the side to be examined. The entire breast is examined from the bra line to the collar bone and from the breastbone to the outer portion of the breast. After moving the pillow or towel to the other shoulder, the woman examines the other breast in the same manner. The pattern can be circular or up and down, according to preference. Women who practice BSE regularly have a sense of the normal architecture of their breasts and are more aware of subtle changes that may occur.

## Screening Mammography

Mammography is used for two separate indications. The first indication is as a routine screening procedure for women who have no known problems and are adhering to health promotion guidelines recommended by their healthcare provider. The second indication for mammography is when the woman or healthcare provider notes an abnormality during monthly BSE or a routine examination. The mammogram then becomes a diagnostic imaging tool to investigate the area in question. A perfect screening tool would be one that has no risk of side effects that may potentially cause harm and has 100% sensitivity and specificity; that is, it would detect all abnormalities and identify only those that need further investigation, thereby eliminating false positives and false negatives. A perfect tool is probably unattainable, though. More effective screening tools for early detection are always under investigation, but mammography remains the "gold standard" at this time (ACS, 2009a). This has led to controversy in screening guidelines (see Table 3-1).

Screening mammography is a low-dose x-ray examination of the breast that is performed on women with no complaints or symptoms of breast cancer (see Figure 3-13). The goal of screening mammography is to detect a breast tumor when it is still too small to be felt by a physician or the patient. Re-

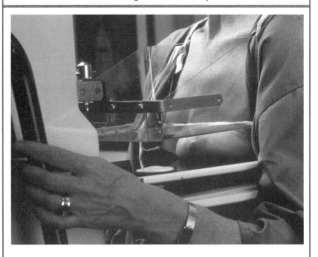

**Figure 3-13. Conventional Mammography Equipment Demonstrating Breast Compression**

Shown is a breast being compressed to get the optimum mammographic image.

*Note.* Photo by Bill Branson. Used courtesy of the National Cancer Institute.

search has shown that the early detection of small breast cancers by screening mammography greatly improves a woman's chances for successful treatment (ACS, 2010a). For example, if breast cancer is detected on mammography and treated while it is still confined to the breast ducts (DCIS), the cure rate approaches 100% (Karssemeijer et al., 2009).

A screening mammogram is ordered annually usually beginning at age 40 in women with average risk who are asymptomatic. Medicare and other commercial insurance companies cover annual screening mammography. Medicare has certain parameters regarding annual mammography. The yearly examination must be scheduled after one calendar year has elapsed, or Medicare will not cover the cost. The films are taken by a technologist, and cases are batched to be read by the radiologist at a later time. The standard screening mammogram consists of two views of each breast, four in all. One view is a cranial-caudal view that provides an image from top to bottom. The second view not only images the breast but also includes a portion of the pectoralis muscle in order to assess the axillary lymph nodes. This view, the medial-lateral-oblique, is accomplished through a diagonal view of the breast on an angle from the armpit to the lower inner aspect of the breast (American College of Radiology [ACR], 2003). The primary purpose of a screening mammogram is to identify any new changes in the breast. If a change is detected, a diagnostic mammogram will be recommended to determine whether the change is real or artifactual. Although most cases in which patients are called back for more films result in benign findings, the process takes a significant emotional toll on patients because they often will worry about the potential diagnosis of breast cancer. This anxiety is exacerbated by the fact that most additional studies cannot be performed immediately, and it is not uncommon to wait a week for the additional workup.

Most guidelines for breast cancer screening do not specify an upper age for stopping screening. For example, ACS (2010b) recommends yearly mammograms beginning at age 40 and continuing as long as the woman is in good health. Few studies have described women's decision-making patterns to stop mammography, but it appears some women and their healthcare providers, recognizing that the expected benefit of early detection declines with remaining life expectancy, consciously decide to discontinue screening following a serious health event (Mandelblatt et al., 2005). Although most women discontinue screening following serious health events, many do not (Howard, Huang, & Adams, 2009).

During mammography, the technologist will position the patient and image each breast separately. One at a time, each breast is carefully positioned on a special plate and then gently compressed with a paddle (often made of clear acrylic glass [Plexiglas®, Altuglas International] or another plastic) (see Figure 3-13). This compression flattens the breast so that the maximum amount of tissue can be imaged and examined. Correct positioning of the breast during mammography is extremely important. If the entire breast is not in the x-ray field, or if something is blocking the x-ray field (such as a piece of jewelry or the shoulder or opposite breast), the diagnosis can be compromised. It also is easier to apply proper compression when the breast is positioned correctly. It is important that the patient be fully informed about each step of the mammogram procedure to ensure that she can fully participate and cooperate in the examination. During the actual x-ray exposure, patients must remain absolutely still and hold their breath to eliminate image blurring caused by patient motion and breathing. Breast compression may cause some discomfort, but it only lasts for a brief time during the mammography procedure. Patients should feel firm pressure related to the compression but no significant pain. During the mammography examination, breast compression should only be applied for a few seconds for each view. Breast compression is necessary during mammography to flatten the breast so less tissue overlap occurs for better visualization of anatomy and potential abnormalities. For example, inadequate compression can lead to poor imaging of microcalcifications, tiny calcium deposits that often are an early sign of breast cancer (NCCN, 2010b). The compression also reduces overlapping normal shadows, which can appear as suspicious regions on the film. Other reasons for compression include that it allows for the use of a lower x-ray dose because a thinner amount of breast tissue is being imaged; it immobilizes the breast to eliminate image blurring caused by motion; and it reduces x-ray scatter, which also leads to image degradation. It is important for women to understand what the compression does and why it is necessary; nurses should include this in patient education.

At some facilities, mammography technologists may place adhesive markers to the breast skin prior to taking images of the breast. The purpose of the adhesive markers is twofold: first, to identify areas with moles, blemishes, or scars so that they are not mistaken for abnormalities, and second, to identify areas that may be of concern (e.g., if a lump was felt during physical examination).

Screening mammography is a relatively low-cost procedure. The average cost for screening mammography in the United States is about $125–$150 (Smith et al., 2010). Medicare was amended to cover mammography in 1991. Depending on a woman's health coverage program, screening mammography may incur little or no out-of-pocket cost.

Mammography will detect about 80%–90% of breast cancers in women without symptoms (ACS, 2009a). It is somewhat more accurate in postmenopausal women than in premenopausal women because their breasts tend to be less dense. Reported overall sensitivity of mammography is estimated to be 75% (ACS, 2009a). The sensitivity of mammography can vary from 60% to 90% for women with dense tissue. Younger women often have denser breasts, but breast density can remain throughout life, potentially obscuring nonpalpable abnormalities (see Figures 3-14 and 3-15).

The most commonly used method for assessing and reporting breast density in mammography is ACR's Breast Imaging Reporting and Data System (BI-RADS®) describing four different categories: (a) entirely fat, (b) scattered fibroglandular densities, (c) heterogeneously dense, and (d) extremely dense (ACR, 2003). The BI-RADS classifications are routinely used as a part of a radiologist's mammographic assessment, and the information is typically available in the report to the woman. This system has been adopted in Europe and provides standardization for classification of a breast mass. BI-RADS rates the density of breast tissue; the presence of a mass; the shape and border appearance of the mass; the presence, type, and distribution of calcifications (macro or micro); and architectural distortion. It also rates associated findings that further clarify a mass or calcifications, such as axillary adenopathy, skin or nipple retraction, and skin thickening. The presence or absence of abnormal findings is calculated and given a number that ranges from zero (incomplete evaluation, needs more imaging) to six (known cancer) (ACR, 2003). A summary of the categories and recommendations can be found in Table 3-2. This information needs to be communicated to the woman and the referring provider (see Figure 3-16). A growing body of research is developing models that incorporate breast density to estimate one's risk of developing breast cancer (Tice et al., 2008). Women who have a BI-RADS breast density classification of heterogeneously dense or extremely dense should also be informed that the sensitivity of a mammogram may be reduced.

**Figure 3-14. Mammogram Image of Dense and Fatty Breasts**

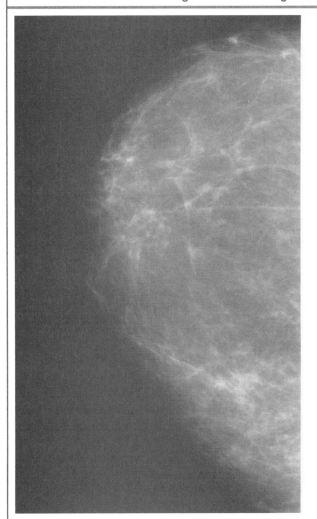 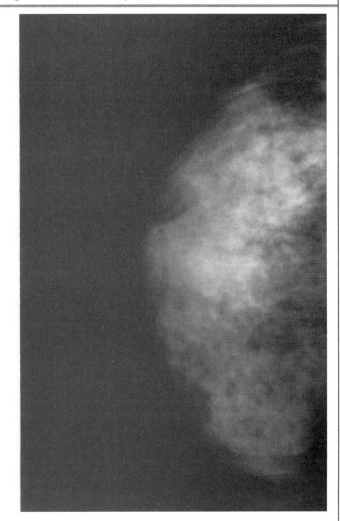

Shown is a side-by-side of two normal mammograms showing the difference between a dense breast (left) and a fatty breast (right). The dense breast is that of a 39-year-old woman; the fatty breast is that of a 59-year-old woman. Abnormal lesions are easier to detect and diagnose in a fatty breast, making mammography more accurate.

*Note.* Image by Dr. Kathy Cho, NIH Radiology. Used courtesy of the National Cancer Institute.

The benefits of mammography include a reduction in the risk of dying of breast cancer, and if breast cancer is detected early, there is a possibility of less aggressive surgery and less aggressive or less toxic adjuvant therapy (ACS, 2010a). Women also should be told about the limitations and potential harms of mammography. The harms of mammography include radiation risk, short- and long-term anxiety associated with false-positive results, biopsy for benign lesions, and the possibility that some breast cancers detected on mammography are nonaggressive and thus overtreated. The risk of a radiation-induced cancer from low-dose mammography is so low that although theoretically possible, it would be very difficult to systematically measure (Smith et al., 2010). The most common and more directly measurable harm associated with

mammography includes the inconvenience from additional imaging resulting from false positives, benign biopsy for abnormal findings, and short- and long-term anxiety resulting from false-positive results. For most women, the anxiety is of limited duration and without long-term or lasting effects. Clear communication about imaging results is associated with reduced anxiety (ACS, 2009a). Women must understand that mammography will not detect all breast cancers and that some breast cancers detected with mammography may still have a poor prognosis. Some women avoid mammography because of radiation exposure concerns, ultimately delaying early detection if a problem exists (Smith et al., 2010).

Women may avoid mammography because they underestimate the importance of the examination or have had prior bad

### Figure 3-15. Mammogram Showing Small Lesion

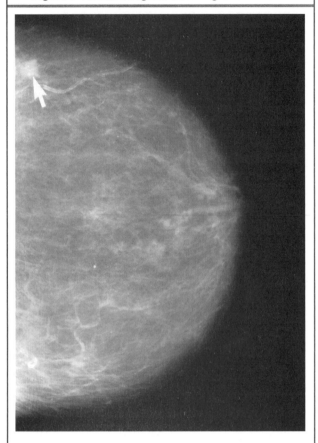

Shown on mammogram is a small cancerous lesion, as well as calcific deposits in veins.

*Note.* Image courtesy of the National Cancer Institute.

rable" to film mammography in terms of detecting breast cancer (Vernacchia & Pena, 2009). Digital mammography systems cost approximately 1.5–4 times as much as standard film mammography systems. Although procedural time saved by using digital mammography over standard film mammography justifies part of the cost for facilities that perform several thousand mammograms each year, it is not completely clear whether the high cost of digital mammography is justifiable in terms of its benefits in detecting breast cancer (Hendrick et al., 2010). Digital mammography may lead to a small in-

### Table 3-2. BI-RADS™ Assessment Categories for Mammography*

| Category | Interpretation | Risk Information |
|---|---|---|
| 0 | Need additional imaging | – |
| 1 | Negative mammogram | Continue annual screening mammography (for women 40 and older). |
| 2 | Benign finding such as a cyst or fibroadenoma | Continue annual screening mammography (for women 40 and older). |
| 3 | Probably benign finding—Short interval follow-up suggested. | Probably benign finding; less than 2% chance of cancer. Usually receives a six-month follow-up mammogram; most level 3 abnormalities do not undergo biopsy. |
| 4 | Suspicious abnormality—Biopsy should be considered. | Most abnormalities are benign but may require biopsy because this category can be malignant in 25%–50% of cases. |
| 5 | Highly suggestive of malignancy—Appropriate action should be taken. | Typically biopsy is performed, and if results are benign, the abnormality usually receives re-biopsy because the first biopsy may not have sampled the correct area. The percentage of category 5 abnormalities that will be cancer is approximately 95%. |
| 6 | Known biopsy-proven malignancy | Definitive treatment will be needed. Malignancy has been proved by biopsy obtained during an imaging study. |

*The American College of Radiology established the Breast Imaging Reporting and Data System (BI-RADS™) to guide the breast cancer diagnostic routine. Radiologists sometimes refer to each BI-RADS category as a "level."

*Note.* Based on information from American College of Radiology, 2003.

experiences with mammography. Nurses have an important role in teaching women about what to expect during mammography. Suggested teaching points are shown in Figure 3-17.

In standard mammography, images are recorded on film using an x-ray cassette. The film is viewed by the radiologist using a light box and then stored in a jacket in the facility's archives. With digital mammography, the breast image is captured using a special electronic x-ray detector, which converts the image into a digital picture for review on a computer monitor. The digital mammogram is then stored on a computer. With digital mammography, the magnification, orientation, brightness, and contrast of the image can be altered after the examination is completed to help the radiologist see certain areas more clearly.

Several studies have demonstrated that digital mammography is at least as accurate as standard mammography and in many instances may be more accurate (ACS, 2009a). To date, studies of digital mammography and standard film mammography have shown that digital mammography is "compa-

---

**Figure 3-16. Information Typically Found in a Mammogram Report**

- **Patient information:** Usually appears at the top of the report and includes the patient's name and age and the reason for the mammogram (e.g., annual screening mammogram, referred by physician to evaluate new right breast lump).
- **Clinical history:** The patient's medical and family history of breast cancer or other breast conditions are noted.
- **Procedure(s):** May explain what types of mammogram views were taken. Typical views for screening mammograms include the cranial-caudal (CC) and the medial-lateral-oblique (MLO) views. Typical views for a diagnostic mammogram that might be described include CC, MLO, and supplemental views tailored to the specific problem. These can include spot compression views, magnification views, and any other images obtained.
- **Findings:** May describe what was found from the mammogram. Size, location, and characteristics of breast abnormalities may be noted. Primary signs of breast cancer may include spiculated masses or clustered pleomorphic microcalcifications. Secondary signs of breast cancer may include asymmetrical tissue density, skin thickening or retraction, or focal distortion of tissue. Some radiologists also may include comments about breast density and distribution of the breast tissue.
- **Impression:** The radiologist's overall assessment of the findings. Usually includes a classification of the mammogram using the Breast Imaging Reporting and Data System (BI-RADS™) developed by the American College of Radiology.
- **Recommendation:** Some radiologists may give specific instructions on what actions should be taken next. For example, the radiologist could recommend no action necessary, a six-month follow-up mammogram, other diagnostic maneuvers, or biopsy.

*Note.* Based on information from American College of Radiology, 2003.

---

crease in the number of small DCIS cancers detected (Karssemeijer et al., 2009).

From the patient's perspective, a digital mammogram is the same as a standard film-based mammogram in that breast compression and radiation are necessary to create clear images of the breast. The time needed to position the patient is the same for each method. However, conventional film mammography requires several minutes to develop the film, whereas digital mammography provides the image on the computer monitor in less than a minute after the exposure/data acquisition. Thus, digital mammography provides a shorter examination for the woman and may possibly allow mammography facilities to conduct more mammograms in a day. During a facility's conversion from film to digital mammography, there may be a higher rate of callbacks, and women should be informed of this possible outcome (Sala et al., 2009). Digital mammography also can be manipulated to correct for under- or overexposure after the examination is completed, thus eliminating the need for some women to undergo repeat mammograms before leaving the facility. Potential benefits of digital mammography include improved contrast between dense and non-dense breast tissue, faster image acquisition, shorter examination time, easier image storage, possible manipulation of breast images for more accurate detection of breast cancer, the ability to correct under- or overexposure of films without having to repeat mammograms, and electronic transmittal of images over telephone lines or a network for remote consultation with other physicians.

Results of the Digital Mammographic Imaging Screening Trial demonstrated that digital mammography may be more accurate than standard film mammography at detecting breast cancer in some women. According to the study results, digital and standard film mammography had similar accuracy rates for many women. However, digital mammography was significantly better at screening women in any of the following categories: (a) women younger than age 50, regardless of what level of breast tissue density, (b) women who are pre- or perimenopausal, and (c) women known to have heterogeneously or very dense breasts (Pisano et al., 2005).

Computer-aided detection (CAD) technology is a recent advance in the field of breast imaging. The CAD technology basically works like a second pair of eyes, reviewing a patient's mammogram film after the radiologist has already made

---

**Figure 3-17. Patient Education Regarding Mammography**

- To help minimize discomfort during mammography, the woman should schedule a mammogram to take place one week after menses begin, when breasts are the least tender.
- If possible, she should bring previous mammogram reports if using a new facility or bring a list of where and when previous mammograms have been completed to facilitate obtaining previous films or images for comparison.
- On the day of the examination, she should not wear talcum powder, deodorant, lotion, or perfume under the arms or on the breasts. These substances can cause artifacts on mammogram images, making the images harder to interpret. For example, aluminum particles in some powders and deodorants can mimic microcalcifications on the mammogram image.
- The patient should wear a two-piece outfit so that she only has to remove her top and bra for the examination. A blouse that buttons in the front is optimal because it can be easily removed, whereas pullover tops are less convenient.
- Any jewelry worn (especially earrings or necklaces) should be easily and quickly removable, especially if the patient will undergo a procedure that requires her to lie face down.
- Any breast symptoms or problems that a woman is experiencing should be described to the technologist performing the examination. She also should be prepared to discuss with the mammography technologist any pertinent history: prior surgeries, hormone use, and family or personal history of breast cancer. Prior to mammography, she should discuss with her clinician any new findings or problems in her breasts.
- The patient should be instructed that she should learn the results of the mammogram from the physician or the mammography center within 10 days. The woman should not assume that the mammogram is negative if she does not hear from the clinic.

---

an initial interpretation. If the computer software detects any breast abnormalities or "regions of interest" on the mammogram film, it marks them. The radiologist can then go back and review the mammogram film again to determine whether the marked areas are suspicious and require further examination (with additional imaging tests or biopsy). With the CAD technology, the radiologist still makes the final interpretation of the mammogram. Based on clinical studies, researchers have estimated that for every 100,000 breast cancers currently detected with screening mammograms, the CAD technology could result in the detection of an additional 20,500 breast cancers (The et al., 2009).

Every mammography facility should be ACR accredited, and a copy of the certificate of accreditation should be readily visible at the mammography center. This ensures that quality-care standards are in place (see Figure 3-18).

## Detection Issues in Special Populations

Because breast cancer accounts for approximately 28% of all new female cancers (ACS, 2010a), more efforts are needed to ensure that all women have access to screening. The uninsured and underinsured routinely encounter barriers to basic health care. Some cultural groups may have misconceptions about the efficacy of breast cancer screening and do not

---

### Figure 3-18. Minimal Standards for Mammography

The following regulations are required of every mammography facility in the United States:

- Physicians who interpret mammograms, radiologic technologists who perform mammography, and medical physicists who survey mammography equipment must have adequate training and experience.
- Each mammography facility must have an effective quality-control program and maintain thorough records.
- Each facility must submit typical mammography images to the U.S. Food and Drug Administration (FDA) for review. The FDA will evaluate the quality and amount of radiation used to obtain the images (radiation levels are required to be low).
- Each mammography facility must develop systems for following up on mammograms that reveal abnormalities and for obtaining biopsy results.
- Each mammography facility must undergo yearly inspections by FDA- or state-certified inspectors.
- Mammography facilities are required to provide patients with written results of their mammograms in easy-to-understand language within 30 days of the mammogram.
- Patients also may obtain their original mammogram (not a copy) from the facility so that they may compare the results with previous mammograms.
- For cases in which an abnormality is detected on the patient's mammogram, the facility is required to notify the patient and her physician (if appropriate) and recommend a suitable course of action.

*Note.* Based on information from American College of Radiology, 2003.

---

adhere to recommendations or access clinical examinations and mammography. Improving primary, secondary, and tertiary prevention methods is not the only solution to reducing incidence and death rates; improving access to clinical examinations and mammography for all cultural groups is necessary as well.

## Uninsured and Underinsured Populations

Disparities clearly exist in cancer prevention and early detection utilization. Research continues to demonstrate that a direct consequence of lack of insurance or underinsurance is lower screening rates and limited access to primary care for prompt evaluation of symptoms (Ward et al., 2008). This means that this population is much more likely than those with private insurance to be diagnosed at later stages of tumor development, when treatment is less likely to be effective and is associated with increased morbidity, mortality, and economic costs (Méndez, Evans, & Stone, 2009). For example, 75% of women ages 40–64 who had private insurance had received a mammogram in the past two years, compared to 56% of women with Medicaid and 38% of women without insurance. Similarly, 8% of women with private insurance had a stage III or IV breast cancer at diagnosis, whereas 18% of uninsured women and 19% of women with Medicaid had stage III or IV breast cancer at diagnosis (ACS, 2009a). Even a co-pay of $12.50 results in fewer women being screened (approximately 8.8%) and has been identified as a barrier to mammography utilization (ACS, 2009a).

Even when programs such as the National Breast and Cervical Cancer Early Detection Program (NBCCEDP), administered by the Centers for Disease Control and Prevention (CDC), are available to these groups, promoting access to these programs remains a significant challenge. This program, which began in 1990 and is now available in all 50 states, the District of Columbia, four U.S. territories, and 13 American Indian/Alaska Native tribal organizations, was developed to enable low-income, uninsured, and underinsured women to gain access to breast and cervical cancer screening and diagnostic services when needed. Sadly, in 2006, only 15% of eligible women received a screening mammogram (ACS, 2010b). An estimated 8%–11% of U.S. women of screening age are eligible to receive NBCCEDP services (CDC, 2010). Eligibility for the program is determined by established guidelines for women living at or below 250% of the federal poverty level. Services for breast health include CBE, mammography, diagnostic testing for women whose screening outcome is abnormal, surgical consultation, and referrals to treatment. Since 1991, the NBCCEDP has served more than 3 million women, provided more than 7.2 million screening examinations, and diagnosed 30,963 breast cancers (CDC, 2010). At age 65, women become eligible for Medicare, which provides coverage for breast cancer screening, including annual mammography.

## Minority Groups

Disparities among racial groups exist in the utilization of screening mammography. These disparities stem from many factors, including misconceptions or a lack of knowledge, low-income status, unemployment, and lack of insurance. Women who have not finished high school have lower rates for mammography screening than high school graduates (ACS, 2010b). The mammography screening rate for low-income women is 24% lower than that for higher-income women (Bigby & Holmes, 2005). Mammography utilization rates and screening rates for African Americans are comparable to those for Caucasian women. However, non-White women are less likely to follow up on abnormal mammography results. Hispanic, American Indian, and Alaska Native women have lower rates of mammography screening than Caucasian women (Bigby & Holmes, 2005).

Studies have documented unequal receipt of prompt, high-quality treatment for African American women compared to White women (ACS, 2009a, 2009b). In 2005, the proportion of African American women aged 40 and older who reported receiving a mammogram within the past two years was 64.9% (ACS, 2009b). Only 49.9% of African American women reported having a mammogram within the past year.

Hispanic women also are more likely to be diagnosed with larger breast tumors than non-Hispanic White women. Differences in mammography utilization and delayed follow-up of abnormal screening results probably contribute to this difference. Differences in access to care and treatment likely contribute to this disparity (ACS, 2009c). In 2005, 59.6% of Hispanic women aged 40 and older had a mammogram within the past two years, compared to 68.1% of non-Hispanic Whites. Among Hispanic subgroups (ACS, 2009c), Central and South American and Cuban women show a higher prevalence of breast cancer screening (63.9% and 72.7%, respectively) than Mexican women (54.5%), who are the least likely to have had a recent mammogram. Despite increases in the prevalence of screening, breast cancer is detected at an advanced stage more often in Hispanics than in non-Hispanic Whites (ACS, 2009c). This difference has been largely attributed to lower frequency of and longer intervals between mammograms and lack of timely follow-up of suspicious mammograms.

Efforts need to be made to provide culturally sensitive care and increase participation in screening programs and to ensure that women with abnormalities in screening examinations receive prompt and appropriate care (Albano et al., 2007). Screening programs should consider the environment where the screening is being delivered, the economic status of the population being served, their comfort with technology, religious and worldviews/beliefs, language and health literacy, social structure and support of family and friends, and beliefs and values (Kagawa-Singer, Dadia, Yu, & Surbone, 2010). Intervention programs such as navigator programs that fol-

low patients throughout treatment in order to enhance communication among the surgeon, oncologist, and patient have been shown to reduce disparities in breast cancer morbidity and mortality (ACS, 2009a).

## Young Women

Breast cancer is rare in young women (approximately 1,230 annual cases in women younger than 30 [ACS, 2009a]), and diagnostic methods often are applied inappropriately and inconsistently when a lump or mass is found in the breast (Jatoi, Anderson, & Rosenberg, 2008). Developmentally, breast lumps are more common in this age group, and a clinician may have a low index of suspicion for breast cancer. Compounding these biases is the fact that breast cancer may be more difficult to diagnose in this age group because of normal hormonal fluctuations during the menstrual cycle that result in a nodular presentation commonly referred to as fibrocystic change. Because mammography often is not useful in young, dense breasts, ultrasound, clinical examination, and possibly a tissue sample should be performed to exclude the possibility of breast cancer (ACS, 2009a).

Screening recommendations for those at risk for hereditary breast and ovarian cancer are usually initiated at a much earlier age than in the general population. The decision of when to begin screening is based on family and personal history; screening often begins approximately 10 years before the youngest age at which a person was diagnosed with cancer in the family (Brandt, Bermejo, Sundquist, & Hemminki, 2010). This is because of the early age at cancer onset seen in this population. Women from these families should be educated about the signs and symptoms of breast cancer (lump, thickening, change in breast skin or color, nipple direction, or nipple discharge) and ovarian cancer (vague abdominal pain or gastrointestinal symptoms, weight loss or bloating). Training in BSE may offer women some sense of control and should begin at age 18. Mammography typically is initiated at age 25. Women need to be clearly instructed on the limitations of mammography in the younger age groups because of the density of the breast tissue.

Conventional screening for women with a high lifetime risk of developing breast cancer often is inadequate because of the increased breast density in young women, the frequency of atypical imaging presentations, and the rapid growth of hereditary breast cancer, resulting in a higher rate of interval cancer (Kuhl et al., 2005). Screening recommendations differ for women with a known mutation in *BRCA1* or *BRCA2* and include mammography, ultrasound, and MRI of the breast with imaging every six months (NCCN, 2010c). MRI has been shown to be more diagnostic than mammography in young women because it is not affected by breast density. Mutation carriers have an 87% lifetime risk of developing breast cancer, and annual screening may not provide adequate scrutiny for these high-risk women. This screening strategy ensures that an imaging study is performed every six months with the goal of detecting breast cancer as early as possible.

## Women With Disabilities

Mammography and breast cancer screening for people with disabilities is fraught with physical and sociologic barriers. Women with disabilities are living longer, and preventive measures should be available for health maintenance. Women with disabilities are less likely than those without disabilities to receive a physician recommendation for screening mammography, and this is particularly the case among older women and those with multiple disabilities (Yankaskas et al., 2010). The lower rates of mammography usage among the disabled may result from the difficulties of the actual screening process, especially for those with mobility limitations, as a mammogram requires that the patient stand (Wei, Findley, & Sambamoorthi, 2006). Women with disabilities, especially intellectual disabilities, may experience more fear and anxiety about cancer screening than the general population. Self-examination also may be compromised by spasm, pain, lack of strength, and immobility.

Positioning patients for mammography is challenging for patients who are in a wheelchair or those who are unable to stand for prolonged periods. Also, women who have spinal cord injuries or muscular disease often are unable to be positioned for adequate imaging. Patients must be able to remain still, raise their arms, and rotate their shoulders as well as bend at the waist to optimize imaging. Very few health facilities are designed to provide necessary preventive health delivery for women with disabilities. The facility must have access for wheelchairs in every room, examination tables that can be raised and lowered, hydraulic lifts, and a staff trained in disability awareness and sensitivity, as well as the proper procedures for transferring and positioning (Wei et al., 2006).

Barriers such as appropriate information, transport, and assistance also may prevent women with disabilities from getting to the facility. Once there, communication difficulties, physical limitations, psychological barriers, and staff attitudes become barriers to a successful outcome. Education for health personnel as well as adaptation of the mammographic technique to suit the physical limitations of women with disabilities are critical to increasing participation and ensuring successful outcomes. Importantly, there is a need to identify women for whom having a mammogram is not an option and for whom alternative breast screening methods should be provided (Poulos, Balandin, Llewellyn, & Dew, 2006).

## Older Adults

Increasing age is a significant risk factor for developing breast cancer. During 2002–2006, 95% of new cases and 97% of breast cancer deaths occurred in women age 40 and older (ACS, 2009a). During that same time, the median age at breast cancer diagnosis was 61 years. This means that 50% of women who developed breast cancer were age 61 or younger at the time of diagnosis. The lifetime risk for a 70-year-old woman of average risk for developing breast cancer is 1 in 14 for women ages 60–79, and an estimated 35% of women are older than 70 at the time of diagnosis. Recent surveillance figures indicate that 50.2% of women older than 65 had a mammogram within the past year (ACS, 2009a). ACS guidelines recommend that women receive yearly screening mammography if they are in good health and would be a candidate for treatment if diagnosed (ACS, 2010a). A great deal of debate exists regarding the age at which screening mammography should be discontinued. It is a well-known fact that early detection prolongs survival, and age remains the greatest risk factor for the development of breast cancer. Factors that support screening for older adults include the increased incidence in the population, the ease of determining mammographic abnormalities in fatty-replaced breast tissue, and retrospective studies that indicate probable benefit. NCCN (2010b) and ACS (2010a) do not advocate a distinct age cutoff but recommend considering comorbidities and life expectancy. Women who have health issues that would preclude chemotherapy, hormone replacement, and surgery for breast cancer, such as severe heart disease, sedentary or bedridden lifestyle, pulmonary disease, or other organ disease that would make life expectancy less than five years, would be candidates for ceasing mammography. It is unreasonable to perform screening tests if the person has a medical condition that makes treatment inadvisable.

## Tertiary Prevention

Tertiary cancer prevention includes the ongoing surveillance and early detection of second primary malignancies and other treatment-related complications in cancer survivors. Tertiary prevention is an emerging role for oncology nurses, especially with regard to women being treated for breast cancer. The care and rehabilitation of women with breast cancer should include strategies to promote the early detection of second primary cancers, as well as strategies to reduce the risk factors for second malignancies and other long-term complications, such as osteoporosis or lymphedema.

Although women are living longer after an initial diagnosis of cancer, environmental and lifestyle risk factors, treatment modalities, and the underlying genetic basis of breast cancer predispose many breast cancer survivors to developing second primary malignancies. Long-term side effects from chemotherapy that require assessment and early management include cardiotoxicity, neuropathy, ototoxicity, and renal failure. Other survivors experience complications related to surgery or radiotherapy, including paresthesias and lymphedema (see Chapter 9). Survivors also are at risk for psychosocial problems that stem from the effects of the diagnosis or treatment (see Chapter 10). Healthcare professionals need to address each of these potential problems with a plan for assessment of the risk, prevention, detection, and early intervention.

A second primary cancer is defined as the occurrence of a new cancer that is biologically independent of the original primary cancer (López et al., 2009). Second cancers may occur because of a genetic predisposition to the second cancer. Treatment with chemotherapeutic agents, especially alkylating agents, is another etiologic source. These agents have been associated with an increased risk of developing hematologic malignancies. Treatment with radiation therapy also has been associated with second primary cancers. Still other second cancers probably occur as a result of random chance. An understanding of the etiology, risk factors, and subsequent development of a second cancer ultimately should result in improved screening and surveillance for survivors.

The observation of multiple primary cancers was first reported in 1889 (Neugut, Meadows, & Robinson, 1999). Initial criteria for classifying multiple primary cancers were first reported in the 1930s. Despite these published reports, little attention has been directed toward screening for second primary cancers. No large, prospective, randomized trials have evaluated the efficacy of monitoring patients closely to detect second cancers (López et al., 2009).

Only recently has attention been focused on the medical and psychosocial needs of long-term survivors of malignancy. The National Cancer Institute established the Office of Cancer Survivorship in 1996. A major focus of this office is the dissemination of information on the risks for developing second primary cancers. As people with cancer live longer after the initial diagnosis and experience high levels of functioning after treatment, it is becoming increasingly important to provide preventive therapies and screening for the late consequences of the first diagnosis.

Currently, the population of cancer survivors living longer periods of time after their initial cancer diagnosis is ever growing. Recent estimates, according to ACS (2009a), suggest that more than 2.5 million women are living with a history of breast cancer. This is largely a result of improved earlier detection of malignancy and the development of more effective therapies. These improvements in treatment have created a new population of patients. The needs of these patients are unique, and healthcare providers are challenged to identify risks, detect problems early, and provide care for these patients. Tertiary prevention is aimed at this population.

The exact etiology of a second primary cancer is not always clear. Many of these cancers are thought to be treatment related. Others are related to environmental exposures. It has been recognized for some time that an individual who had cancer in one paired organ is at increased risk for developing a second cancer in the contralateral unaffected organ, especially in the case of breast cancer. The underlying premise is that whatever predisposed a person to develop the first cancer would also predispose the patient to develop the sec-

ond cancer in the contralateral organ. Women with breast cancer have an elevated risk of developing a second primary cancer. There is a strong relationship between younger age at diagnosis of the primary breast cancer and risk of subsequent cancer. Women diagnosed with early-onset breast cancer (before age 40) have almost a 3-fold increased risk of any subsequent cancer, with a 4.5-fold increased risk of subsequent breast cancer (ACS, 2009a). Genetic predisposition, notably mutations in *BRCA1* and *BRCA2* genes, contributes to the excess risk of subsequent cancer among women with early-onset breast cancer. For those women with a known mutation in *BRCA1* or *BRCA2*, the cumulative risk is estimated to be 87% for breast cancer and 60% for ovarian cancer (NCCN, 2010c). Women who are younger at the diagnosis of their first primary breast cancer tend to have a shorter interval between malignancies. These women should be counseled about the potential benefits of prophylactic mastectomy and oophorectomy (Rebbeck, Kauff, & Domchek, 2009). Prophylactic oophorectomy may be associated with an 85% reduction in the risk of ovarian cancer and 50% reduction in the risk of developing breast cancer. Prophylactic mastectomy may reduce the risk of breast cancer by more than 95%.

It is only recently that there has been both public and professional awareness that the very treatment that eradicated their first cancer often places cancer survivors at risk for a subsequent second primary cancer. This is particularly true of radiation therapy, chemotherapy, and hormonal therapy. The use of combined therapies probably has a synergistic effect and further increases the risk (López et al., 2009).

To date, most of the second primary cancers associated with radiotherapy for childhood cancers have been bone and soft tissue sarcomas and carcinomas of the thyroid gland, breast, and skin (López et al., 2009). Factors that influence the development of second malignancies include the total dose and number of fractions, the source of energy, combinations of chemotherapeutic agents, and age at exposure (i.e., younger age increases the risk) (ACS, 2010a). These second cancers can occur years to decades after the initial therapy. The organ at risk depends on the site where the radiation was delivered and how well the surrounding tissue was protected by shielding (Taylor & Taylor, 2009). Risk may be increased in women who have received radiotherapy because of scatter radiation exposure; however, the magnitude of the risk is unknown. Although the data were limited, results of a trial of radiation therapy after lumpectomy as compared to mastectomy showed no increase in the risk of second malignancies in the contralateral breast in women receiving radiation therapy (López et al., 2009).

Chemotherapeutic agents also have been associated with second primary cancers, especially hematologic malignancies. These have been reported with alkylating agents, vinca alkaloids, antimetabolites, and antitumor antibiotics (Sánchez et al., 2008). Alkylating agents in particular have been associated with leukemias, myelodysplastic syndrome, sarcomas, and bladder cancer. These malignancies can occur within several years of treatment. The leukemias that occur as a consequence of treatment tend to be extremely resistant to chemotherapy when compared to de novo leukemia (Sánchez et al., 2008).

Tamoxifen frequently is used in the treatment of estrogen-dependent breast cancer. Although most clinicians use tamoxifen for only five years, the risk of endometrial cancer is increased in these women (NCCN, 2010b). The risk is higher in those with other risk factors for the development of endometrial cancer.

Women who have been successfully treated for one breast cancer need to be informed about the risk of a second breast cancer and have appropriate screening. In general, this includes annual mammography, biannual CBE, regular self-examination, and prompt management of any change in the breast examination. For women with a diagnosis of breast cancer who still have a uterus (especially those taking tamoxifen), an annual gynecologic examination is indicated. Women should be instructed regarding the early symptoms of endometrial cancer, which require prompt reporting to a healthcare provider. These include abnormal spotting, bleeding, or discharge, especially in postmenopausal women (ACS, 2010a).

The early detection of ovarian cancer presents a significant challenge to healthcare providers. At present, no evidence exists to suggest that ultrasound, pelvic examination, or CA-125 testing decreases the morbidity and mortality associated with ovarian cancer (NCCN, 2010c). Women need to be instructed on the limitations of these screening examinations and informed that ovarian cancer has few early signs or symptoms. For those with a known mutation in *BRCA1* or *BRCA2*, a prophylactic oophorectomy may be a prudent prevention strategy.

## Psychosocial Concerns

Anxiety and fear about cancer recurrence are documented concerns in long-term survivors of cancer. Little is known about how much survivors realize they are at risk for a second primary cancer and how fearful they are of developing one. This problem has received little attention. Every cancer survivor has a different risk of developing a second primary cancer. Clearly, efforts are needed to better understand patients' perceptions and anxiety related to this risk.

Information about a second risk for cancer should be communicated in a nonthreatening way. Survivors need to understand that their prognosis is actually excellent when concern shifts to screening for second cancers. Healthcare providers should articulate that screening and prevention recommendations are being given to detect cancers early and further increase long-term survival and quality of life. Just as assessment of risk for second malignancies should occur in long-term follow-up, so should assessment of overall adjustment and quality of life. For patients having difficulty adjusting to long-term survival, further intervention with a health professional with expertise in psychosocial management sometimes may be indicated.

## Implications for Nurses

Healthcare providers who work with long-term survivors of cancer are well suited to provide the comprehensive risk assessments and education that patients need regarding development of a second cancer. The process of selecting appropriate screening strategies begins with an individual risk assessment. Each cancer survivor should be considered individually. Risk factors should be documented and interpreted for the patient. The risk factor assessment should guide the selection of appropriate screening strategies.

Specific screening guidelines for second primary malignancies are vague. Currently, screening for second cancers is similar to screening for first cancers, such as following the guidelines for screening in asymptomatic people published by ACS (2010a) and a variety of other groups. These guidelines need to be tailored to the individual risks of the cancer survivor.

Cancer survivors also need to be educated about the signs and symptoms of second malignancies that should be reported. This education helps to make patients better advocates for themselves and more involved in their care. Furthermore, appropriate self-examination technique should be discussed with long-term cancer survivors. Healthcare providers should offer to teach women proper BSE practices during the professional examination. This enables women to best learn self-examination and better appreciate their own anatomic landmarks. Women who have had breast surgery should be taught how to examine the affected breast and what constitutes a normal and abnormal finding.

In addition, all survivors probably can benefit from knowledge of how to properly examine their skin. Many survivors have received photosensitizing chemotherapy and need to know how to protect their skin from further damage and how to examine for changes that might signal an early skin cancer.

Regular follow-up appointments provide an opportunity for continuity of care and to assess patients' long-term adjustment to the cancer diagnosis. Efforts should be made to help survivors to become active participants in their long-term follow-up. This is an opportunity to teach not only survivors about healthy lifestyles and the importance of cancer screening but also their family members. After treatment is completed, the stress level of patients and families is often lower, and they may be more receptive to this teaching.

Despite the potential benefits of long-term follow-up, as many as 60% of survivors report no regular medical follow-up visits (Wilkins & Woodgate, 2008). Ethnicity also plays an important role in predicting secondary prevention practices. When all preventive services, including cancer screening, are considered, research shows that African American survivors receive fewer services compared to survivors of other ethnicities (Mayer et al., 2007).

Tertiary prevention for cancer survivors can be approached in several ways (Snyder et al., 2009). Tertiary prevention care should consider surveillance for recurrence, screening for second cancers, identification of and interventions for consequences of cancer and its treatment, instruction and implementation of health promotion strategies, and a plan for coordination between oncology specialists and primary care providers. Cancer survivors should continue to work with their healthcare providers to receive age- and gender-appropriate screening for many types of cancers (Wilkins & Woodgate, 2008). These typically follow recommendations such as the ACS (2010a) recommendations for cancer prevention and early detection (Ng & Travis, 2008).

A number of models exist for providing long-term care (McCabe & Jacobs, 2008). A disease-specific model for long-term survivors focuses on the early identification of problems such as lymphedema, fatigue, psychological distress, and weight gain and promotes an organized set of services to assess and address these problems. The comprehensive survivorship clinic model typically offers a consultative service, where the survivor is referred to the survivorship staff for a one-time visit while ongoing care continues to be provided by the original treatment team. A multidisciplinary team develops a treatment summary and follow-up care plan for the survivor, which includes surveillance for late complications as well as health promotion recommendations. Another model is the nurse practitioner–led clinic, where an advanced practice nurse in collaborative practice with the treatment team provides continuing regular care to manage the survivor at a predetermined time after the completion of therapy.

## Diagnostic Evaluation

For women with a symptom of breast cancer or an abnormality detected on a screening examination, a diagnostic evaluation is indicated. This might include additional radiographic studies and, in some cases, a biopsy. Women need support and education as they undergo a diagnostic evaluation; for most, it is extremely anxiety provoking.

### Diagnostic Mammography

About 5%–10% of women have their mammogram interpreted as abnormal or inconclusive until further tests are done. Women with implants also may be candidates for diagnostic mammography (NCCN, 2010b). Other women who may be candidates for diagnostic mammography include women with a history of breast cancer, women with breast change, or women at high risk for developing breast cancer (e.g., *BRCA1* or *BRCA2* carriers). In most instances, additional tests (imaging studies and/or biopsy) lead to a final interpretation of normal breast tissue or a benign finding.

The goal of diagnostic mammography is to pinpoint the exact size and location of breast abnormality and to image the surrounding tissue and lymph nodes. A diagnostic mammogram is performed in real time; that is, the radiologist looks at each view and determines whether additional views are needed to better evaluate a specific questionable area. The radiologist then meets with the woman immediately after the films are completed and discusses the results.

In many cases, diagnostic mammography will help show that the abnormality is highly likely to be benign. Typically, when this occurs, the radiologist may recommend that the woman return at a later date for a follow-up mammogram, usually in six months. However, if an abnormality seen with diagnostic mammography is suspicious, additional breast imaging (with examinations such as ultrasound or biopsy) may be ordered. Biopsy is the only definitive way to determine whether a woman has breast cancer.

### Ultrasound

Ultrasound imaging is a noninvasive test that involves exposing the breast to high-frequency sound waves to produce pictures of the inside of the body. Ultrasound examinations do not use radiation. Because ultrasound images are captured in real time, they can show the structure and movement of the body's internal organs, as well as blood flowing through blood vessels.

In an ultrasound examination, a transducer is passed over the breast that both sends the sound waves and records the echoing waves. When the transducer is pressed against the skin, it directs small pulses of inaudible, high-frequency sound waves into the body. As the sound waves bounce off internal organs, fluids, and tissues, the microphone in the transducer records tiny changes in the sound's pitch and direction. These signature waves are instantly measured and displayed by a computer, which in turn creates a real-time picture on the monitor. The primary use of breast ultrasound is to help diagnose breast abnormalities during a physical examination and to further assess abnormalities detected on mammography. Ultrasound imaging can help to determine whether an abnormality is solid (which may be either benign or malignant) or fluid-filled (usually a benign cyst requiring no further evaluation) (NCCN, 2010b). When an ultrasound examination reveals a suspicious breast abnormality, a physician may choose to perform an ultrasound-guided biopsy. With current high-resolution ultrasound, specific observations can accurately characterize most cystic masses, thereby facilitating management decisions (Huff, 2009).

Benefits of ultrasound include that it is noninvasive and is usually painless. In general, it is widely available, easy to use, and less expensive than other imaging methods. Ultrasound imaging does not use any ionizing radiation but often provides a clear picture of soft tissues, which do not show up well on x-ray images. Ultrasound may help detect and classify a breast lesion that cannot be interpreted adequately through mammography alone.

No known risks are associated with ultrasound, but it does not replace annual mammography and careful CBE because many cancers are not visible with ultrasound. Many calcifications seen with mammography cannot be seen with ultrasound. Some early breast cancers show up only as calcifications on mammography imaging.

## Magnetic Resonance Imaging

A breast MRI, also known as magnetic resonance mammography, can be an excellent but expensive diagnostic tool for finding extremely small breast cancers or recurrences, occult breast cancers, and suspicious abnormalities in high-risk women with dense breasts and for delineating the level of suspicion for multiple questionable breast abnormalities found on a mammogram. It also is often used to assess implant rupture and may be helpful in the staging of newly diagnosed breast cancers (NCCN, 2010b). MRI has a high sensitivity rate (95%–100%), but this modality has limitations (i.e., its ability to identify microcalcifications is not always reliable, benign lesions may produce false-positive results and unnecessary biopsies) (Houssami & Hayes, 2009).

Premenopausal women experience significant changes in breast volume, breast parenchyma pattern, and water content during the menstrual cycle. Conducting the MRI study at the appropriate point in the cycle minimizes the possibility of false-positive results. Therefore, women need to time the study with their menstrual cycle, between the sixth and sixteenth day (Ellis, 2009), which often postpones the test for weeks. Also, a woman may not be a candidate for MRI because of claustrophobia or implanted medical devices. At this time, MRI does not have adequate specificity (37%–97%) to be a useful screening tool (Lehman et al., 2007), and insurance companies are reluctant to pay for MRI without documentation of specific medical necessity.

MRI uses magnetic fields instead of radiation to produce very detailed, cross-sectional images of the body. MRI examinations for breast imaging typically use a contrast material (usually gadolinium diethylenetriamine penta-acetic acid [commonly known as DTPA]), which enhances the ability of the MRI to capture detailed images of breast tissue. NCCN recommends that breast MRI examinations should be performed and interpreted by an expert breast imaging team working in concert with the multidisciplinary treatment team (Lehman & Smith, 2009). Breast MRI examinations require a dedicated breast coil and breast imaging radiologists familiar with the optimal timing sequences and other technical details for image interpretation. The imaging center should have the ability to perform MRI-guided needle sampling or wire localization of MRI-detected findings (Lehman et al., 2007). Otherwise, the scan must be repeated at another facility at the time of the biopsy. Women need to be informed that MRI

is also more expensive than mammography and often is not covered by insurance companies, except in high-risk women or for diagnostic purposes.

In a review of 11 prospective comparative studies, the addition of annual contrast-enhanced MRI of the breast to mammography demonstrated more than 90% sensitivity, more than twice that of mammography alone (Warner, 2008). False-positive rates were higher with the addition of MRI, but specificity improved on successive rounds of screening. Although survival data are not yet available, the stage distribution of these tumors predicts a significant reduction in breast cancer mortality rate compared with that of screening without MRI. Further research is necessary to define the optimal screening schedule for different subgroups.

Although MRI may eventually prove to be cost-effective and advantageous for women at elevated risk because of other combinations of risk factors, at this time recommendations for annual screening mammography and MRI are directed strictly for women known or estimated to be high-risk mutation carriers (lifetime risk estimated to be 20% or greater) or for women with a history of high-dose radiation therapy at a young age (NCCN, 2010b). ACS (2010a) and NCCN (2010b) have concluded that evidence is insufficient to recommend for or against MRI screening in women with a 15%–20% lifetime risk as defined by these same family history–based risk estimation models, or women with a history of DCIS or lobular carcinoma in situ, a history of biopsy-proven proliferative lesions, a prior history of breast cancer, or extremely dense breasts. MRI is not recommended for women at average risk, although investigations are under way to determine whether it should be considered for other higher-risk groups (Lehman, DeMartini, Anderson, & Edge, 2009; Saslow et al., 2007).

Some recommend against the routine use of preoperative MRI in women with established, early-stage breast cancer (Houssami & Hayes, 2009). The ACS position is that it should be discouraged until (and if) high levels of evidence demonstrate that preoperative MRI either improves surgical care, reduces the number of required surgeries, or reduces local recurrence and death due to breast cancer (ACS, 2009a).

## Breast Biopsy

A new abnormality that has been identified either through mammography or by palpation often will need tissue sampling. This can be accomplished using various tools and decision strategies. The biopsy spectrum ranges from minimally invasive to more invasive, and the type of biopsy selected often depends on the suspicion and location of the finding (NCCN, 2010b).

The importance of appropriate and adequate biopsy technique and sampling should not be underestimated. The distinction between benign and malignant lesions requires tissue examination. This is usually accomplished with a tissue sample obtained by biopsy. Lesions that are suspicious by imaging and those that are suspicious clinically can be sampled by biopsy. Biopsy techniques in the diagnosis of breast conditions include fine-needle aspiration (FNA), core needle biopsy (CNB), and open surgical biopsy. Both FNA and CNB usually are same-day procedures completed in the physician's office or imaging department. FNA does not provide a tissue sample that is conclusive for a diagnosis of invasive versus in situ carcinoma and may not provide adequate tissue for the identification of markers such as ER, progesterone receptor, and HER2. In contrast, CNB specimens usually yield a specimen that makes those assessments possible (Burstein, Harris, & Morrow, 2008). CNB tissue sampling is accomplished by the insertion of a hollow, large-core needle through the skin. One or more samples may be taken. CNB can be done with or without imaging and may be combined with vacuum suction (Bruening et al., 2010).

Palpable or clinically suspicious lesions may be biopsied with or without image guidance. For lesions with no clinical findings, biopsy can be performed in combination with imaging including MRI, ultrasound, or mammography. For example, FNA and needle biopsy can be ultrasound guided. Biopsy also can be MRI guided or completed in combination with mammography in a procedure known as a stereotactic biopsy.

## Fine-Needle Aspiration

FNA often is used when there is a palpable finding most consistent with a cyst. Breast cysts typically feel rubbery and are mobile. The healthcare provider uses a small-gauge needle (approximately 22 gauge) with a 10–20 ml syringe to pierce the mass and withdraw the fluid. Cystic contents usually are yellow to muddy colored, and the fluid can vary from thin to very turbid. If the patient has a history of benign cyst aspirations, the provider may not send the contents to cytology each time, provided that the fluid is consistent with prior aspirations. However, the patient should always have a return appointment in one to two months to confirm that the cyst has not refilled. If the area has refilled, a CNB may be recommended (NCCN, 2010b).

If the lump cannot be felt, ultrasound may be used to help the physician guide the needle into the breast and to the lesion. No incision is made, and a very small bandage is put over the site where the needle entered. FNA is the easiest and fastest method of obtaining a breast biopsy and is very effective for women who have fluid-filled cysts. However, the pathologic evaluation can be incomplete because the tissue sample is very small. When FNA is used alone, about 10% of breast cancers may be missed. The effectiveness of this procedure depends on the skill of the surgeon or radiologist who performs it (O'Flynn, Wilson, & Michell, 2010).

## Core Needle Biopsy

Core biopsy provides a more definitive diagnosis than FNA, and many providers choose this method because a core

of tissue yields a larger number of cells to examine, thereby reducing false-negative rates. Core biopsies for palpable masses are easily performed in the office. A larger gauge needle (14 gauge) is inserted into a spring-loaded device. After the area is anesthetized with a local anesthetic, the healthcare provider pulls the trigger on the device that directs the needle into the mass. One or multiple core samples can be obtained. The patient should be cautioned that a loud "pop" will be heard and not to be startled. The core or cores then go to pathology.

## Stereotactic Biopsy

Radiology-assisted biopsies are most frequently done for nonpalpable abnormalities. The radiologist will recommend the approach, either stereotactic or ultrasound guided, that will best target the area in question. Stereotactic biopsy is performed using a specially designed table. This table is equipped with an opening through which the breast is suspended (see Figure 3-20). The mammographic equipment is located beneath the table in line with the breast. The breast is compressed, and the radiologist or surgeon targets the area by obtaining a pair of images at 15° angles to calculate the exact coordinates (Kepple et al., 2004). The biopsy area then is localized with a 1 cm × 1 cm grid. The needle apparatus (14 gauge or 8- or 11-gauge vacuum-assisted device) is lined up with the grid to ensure that the correct area is targeted (Kepple et al., 2004). After the area is anesthetized using a local anesthetic, several core samples are obtained and sent to pathology. More than one area of the breast may be sampled. Stereotactic biopsies are recommended for abnormalities of moderate suspicion. They can be highly accurate in obtaining tissue of suspicious areas. In a meta-analysis of 83 studies of stereotactic- and ultrasonography-guided CNB, the pro-

**Figure 3-20. Stereotactic Biopsy Performed in the Prone Position**

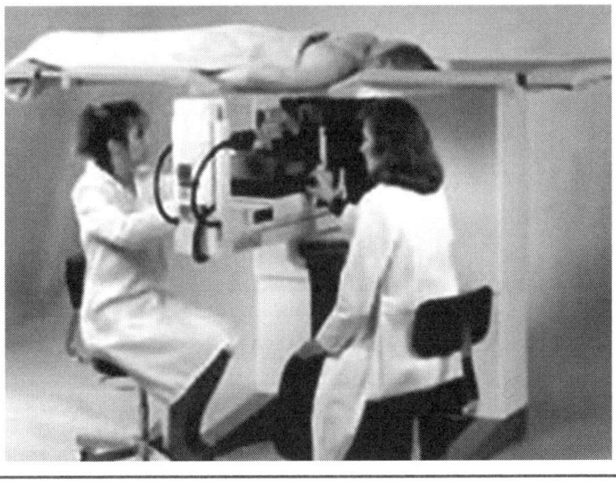

*Note.* Image courtesy of www.imaginis.com. Used with permission.

cedures seem to be almost as accurate as open surgical biopsy and with lower complication rates (Bruening et al., 2010).

Sedation is not required for this procedure. Once the patient is in the procedure area, local anesthesia is administered. Recovery generally is quick and uncomplicated. Most patients are able to resume normal activity almost immediately afterward. Pain is minimal and usually can be managed with an over-the-counter pain reliever.

The radiologist may leave a small titanium clip at the biopsy site following a stereotactic biopsy. A woman with a large tumor may elect to have neoadjuvant chemotherapy to shrink the tumor and improve the cosmetic outcome for later surgery. In some instances, the tumor disappears, and the target site is lost if breast preservation has been planned. The clip assists the radiologist in targeting the area of the tumor so that an adequate surgical excision can take place. A clip also may be left when calcifications are being targeted for a large-gauge needle biopsy or a wire-localized biopsy. If the pathology indicates a cancer, the area can be reexcised using the clip as a guide. The standard of care is to take a post-biopsy clip placement film to ensure the proper location (NCCN, 2010b). A serious complication of using a clip is migration of the clip immediately or at a later time. A new mammogram and a careful assessment of the clip placement must be made prior to evaluating any patient for surgery.

## Wire-Localized Biopsy

A wire-localized biopsy uses breast imaging to target an area in preparation for surgical removal (NCCN, 2010b). A radiologist who recommends an image-guided biopsy is assured that the wire tip can be accurately placed through or alongside the lesion. A hookwire most often is used as the guide because the hook helps to keep the wire in place. Wire placement for nonpalpable lesions can be accomplished through a stereotactic method or using ultrasonography. Multiple wires can be placed either for multiple lesions or to delineate the borders of a large mass. After placement is confirmed through ultrasound or mammography, the patient is sent to the operating room with the placement films. The surgeon uses the films and guide wire to remove the target area. Once the mass is removed, the specimen is sent to mammography, where a film is taken to confirm that the area in question has been completely excised.

## Excisional Biopsy

Before the advances in breast imaging and needle biopsy techniques, open surgical biopsy was used for diagnosis of breast cancer. The preferred standard of current practice, however, is that CNB should be the initial diagnostic approach (NCCN, 2010b). Diagnosis by needle biopsy results in fewer complications, decreased incidence of reexcision, decreased total number of breast surgeries, and decreased cost. Initial

needle biopsy also allows for a discussion of surgical options with the patient before a breast incision is made and facilitates a surgical plan that allows axillary node procedures to be completed in the same surgical visit as the breast surgery (Bruening et al., 2010; Burstein et al., 2008; Friese, Neville, Edge, Hassett, & Earle, 2009; Pocock, Taback, Klein, Joseph, & El-Tamer, 2009). Open surgical biopsy as a diagnostic tool should be reserved for those cases in which needle biopsy cannot be used (deep chest wall lesions, for example), cases in which inadequate samples were obtained by needle biopsy, or cases in which imaging or needle biopsy cannot provide a diagnosis but physical findings warrant a biopsy (NCCN, 2010b; Roses & Giuliano, 2005).

Indications also exist for open surgical biopsy following CNB. These indications include atypical ductal hyperplasia, atypical lobular hyperplasia or lobular carcinoma in situ, radial scar, and papillary lesions. In these situations, excision of the area with an open surgical technique is recommended to adequately assess for the presence of in situ or invasive disease and to provide adequate tissue for accurate tumor classification (Burstein et al., 2008; Roses & Giuliano, 2005). In cases in which the area of excision can only be identified by imaging, wire localization precedes the surgical biopsy.

The area is numbed with a local anesthetic, and a sedative usually is administered. A small incision of about 1–2 inches is made as close to the lump as possible. The surgeon removes a piece of tissue or, if it is small, the entire lump, and the incision is sutured. Often the surgeon will ink the edges of the specimen with different colors to indicate the orientation and provide histopathologic information if the lesion is malignant. This type of biopsy usually is done on an outpatient basis.

After the decision to do the biopsy has been made, the physician should inquire whether the patient is taking anticoagulants, including aspirin. It is common for anticoagulants to be discontinued several days prior to a scheduled operation to avoid abnormal bleeding during the procedure.

Following the procedure, the patient goes to the recovery room and is monitored by the nursing staff. Recovery from a biopsy done under local anesthesia generally is rapid. Postoperative pain usually is minimal and resolves within a few days. However, pain medication may be prescribed. Patients may return to work the day after biopsy, if their job is not physically demanding. For one to two weeks after the procedure, patients should avoid heavy lifting. The incision should completely heal within one month, and the stitches dissolve or are removed a week to 10 days later at the doctor's office.

Many patients are concerned about the cosmetic appearance of their breast following biopsy. The incision leaves a small scar that fades in time. The location of the lesion, its size, and the amount of surrounding tissue removed determines whether the breast changes in appearance. For example, if a very large lump was removed, the scar may be large and may leave an indentation in the breast. Few complications are associated with biopsy. Infection can occur, and the incision site should be watched for redness, swelling, or fluid leakage, which should be reported to the physician immediately. Nurses should instruct patients to keep the biopsy site clean and dry and to call the healthcare provider if any signs of bleeding or infection develop. Depending on how the incision was closed, the patient also will need information about dressing changes and showering. Steri-Strip™ (3M Health Care) adhesive skin closures often are used to close the biopsy wound. Typically, patients should not bathe until these strips fall off. The recommendation for showering or bathing may differ among surgeons, and specific instructions need to be communicated to patients.

Many surgeons prefer that a woman wear a bra continuously for the first week to provide additional support and protection for the biopsy site. Nurses providing postoperative education should check on the preferences of each particular surgeon. Occasionally a seroma may develop, but it will reabsorb in a few weeks.

## Conclusion

Prevention and early diagnosis strategies have changed dramatically in the past decade. Mammography has evolved into a recommended and accepted study for the early detection of breast cancer. That has been evident through the decrease in breast cancer mortality despite slight increases in incidence. MRI of the breast has proved to be an important screening and diagnostic tool for women with an occult breast cancer because of tissue density and other factors, as well as *BRCA* mutation carriers who choose close surveillance over prophylactic mastectomy. Other more sensitive tools will continue to be developed in the future, and genetic testing will expand to include many other cancers. Nurses may understandably feel challenged by new technology and genetic advances because patients will expect them to be familiar with the intricacies and rationale for new imaging studies and to provide education regarding their cancer risk based on personal and family history. This task will not be easy, as nurses often do not have time to attend outside educational programs, but educational alternatives may include taking online courses and scheduling in-services within the institution.

## References

Albano, J.D., Ward, E., Jemal, A., Anderson, R., Cokkinides, V.E., Murray, T., ... Thun, M.J. (2007). Cancer mortality in the United States by education level and race. *Journal of the National Cancer Institute, 99,* 1384–1394. doi:10.1093/jnci/djm127

American Cancer Society. (2009a). *Breast cancer facts and figures 2009–2010.* Atlanta, GA: Author.

American Cancer Society. (2009b). *Cancer facts and figures for African Americans 2009–2010.* Atlanta, GA: Author.

American Cancer Society. (2009c). *Cancer facts and figures for Hispanics/Latinos 2009–2011.* Atlanta, GA: Author.

American Cancer Society. (2010a). *Cancer facts and figures 2010.* Atlanta, GA: Author.

American Cancer Society. (2010b). *Cancer prevention and early detection facts and figures 2010.* Atlanta, GA: Author.

American College of Obstetricians and Gynecologists. (2003). *Breast cancer screening* (ACOG Practice Bulletin No. 42). Washington, DC: Author.

American College of Radiology. (2003). *Breast Imaging Reporting and Data System (BI-RADS®) atlas.* Reston, VA: Author.

Anderson, K., Jacobson, J.S., Heitjan, D.F., Zivin, J.G., Hershman, D., Neugut, A.I., & Grann, V.R. (2006). Cost-effectiveness of preventive strategies for women with a *BRCA1* or a *BRCA2* mutation. *Annals of Internal Medicine, 144,* 397–406.

Barton, M.B., & Elmore, J.G. (2009). Pointing the way to informed medical decision making: Test characteristics of clinical breast examination. *Journal of the National Cancer Institute, 101,* 1223–1224. doi:10.1093/jnci/djp279

Bigby, J., & Holmes, M.D. (2005). Disparities across the breast cancer continuum. *Cancer Causes and Control, 16,* 35–44. doi:10.1007/s10552-004-1263-1

Brandt, A., Bermejo, J.L., Sundquist, J., & Hemminki, K. (2010). Breast cancer risk in women who fulfill high-risk criteria: At what age should surveillance start? *Breast Cancer Research and Treatment, 121,* 133–141. doi:10.1007/s10549-009-0486-y

Bruening, W., Fontanarosa, J., Tipton, K., Treadwell, J.R., Launders, J., & Schoelles, K. (2010). Systematic review: Comparative effectiveness of core-needle and open surgical biopsy to diagnose breast lesions. *Annals of Internal Medicine, 152,* 238–246. doi:10.1059/0003-4819-152-1-201001050-00190

Burstein, H.J., Harris, J.R., & Morrow, M. (2008). Malignant tumors of the breast. In V.T. DeVita Jr., S. Hellman, & S.A. Rosenberg (Eds.), *Cancer: Principles and practice of oncology* (8th ed., pp. 1606–1654). Philadelphia, PA: Lippincott Williams & Wilkins.

Centers for Disease Control and Prevention. (2010). National Breast and Cervical Cancer Early Detection Program national aggregate data. Retrieved from http://www.cdc.gov/cancer/nbccedp/data/summaries/national_aggregate.htm#breast

Colditz, G.A. (2005). Epidemiology and prevention of breast cancer. *Cancer Epidemiology, Biomarkers and Prevention, 14,* 768–772. doi:10.1158/1055-9965.EPI-04-0157

Cummings, S.R., Tice, J.A., Bauer, S., Browner, W.S., Cuzick, J., Ziv, E., ... Kerlikowske, K. (2009). Prevention of breast cancer in postmenopausal women: Approaches to estimating and reducing risk. *Journal of the National Cancer Institute, 101,* 384–398. doi:10.1093/jnci/djp018

Cuzick, J., Forbes, J.F., Sestak, I., Cawthorn, S., Hamed, H., Holli, K., & Howell, A. (2007). Long-term results of tamoxifen prophylaxis for breast cancer—96-month follow-up of the randomized IBIS-I trial. *Journal of the National Cancer Institute, 99,* 272–282. doi:10.1093/jnci/djk049

Daly, M.B., Axilbund, J.E., Bryant, E., Buys, S., Eng, C., Friedman, S., ... Weitzel, J.N. (2006). Genetic/familial high-risk assessment: Breast and ovarian clinical practice guidelines. *Journal of the National Comprehensive Cancer Network, 4,* 156–176.

Domchek, S.M., Friebel, T.M., Neuhausen, S.L., Wagner, T., Evans, G., Isaacs, C., ... Rebbeck, T.R. (2006). Mortality after bilateral salpingo-oophorectomy in BRCA1 and BRCA2 mutation carriers: A prospective cohort study. *Lancet Oncology, 7,* 223–229. doi:10.1016/S1470-2045(06)70585-X

Domchek, S.M., & Weber, B.L. (2006). Clinical management of *BRCA1* and *BRCA2* mutation carriers. *Oncogene, 25,* 5825–5831. doi:10.1038/sj.onc.1209881

Ellis, R.L. (2009). Optimal timing of breast MRI examinations for premenopausal women who do not have a normal menstrual cycle. *American Journal of Roentgenology, 193,* 1738–1740. doi:10.2214/AJR.09.2657

Finch, A., Shaw, P., Rosen, B., Murphy, J., Narod, S.A., & Colgan, T.J. (2006). Clinical and pathologic findings of prophylactic salpingo-oophorectomies in 159 BRCA1 and BRCA2 carriers. *Gynecologic Oncology, 100,* 58–64. doi:10.1016/j.ygyno.2005.06.065

Fisher, B., Costantino, J.P., Wickerham, D.L., Redmond, C.K., Kavanah, M., Cronin, W.M., ... Wolmark, N. (1998). Tamoxifen for prevention of breast cancer: Report of the National Surgical Adjuvant Breast and Bowel Project P-1 Study. *Journal of the National Cancer Institute, 90,* 1371–1388.

Fisher, B., Dignam, J., Wolmark, N., DeCillis, A., Emir, B., Wickerham, D.L., ... Margolese, R.G. (1997). Tamoxifen and chemotherapy for lymph node-negative, estrogen receptor-positive breast cancer. *Journal of the National Cancer Institute, 19,* 1673–1682.

Fisher, B., Dignam, J., Wolmark, N., Wickerham, D.L., Fisher, E.R., Mamounas, E., ... Oishi, R.H. (1999). Tamoxifen in treatment of intraductal breast cancer: National Surgical Adjuvant Breast and Bowel Project B-24 randomised controlled trial. *Lancet, 353,* 1993–2000. doi:10.1016/S0140-6736(99)05036-9

Fisher, B., Redmond, C., Brown, A., Fisher, E.R., Wolmark, N., Bowman, D., ... Legault-Poisson, S. (1986). Adjuvant chemotherapy with and without tamoxifen in the treatment of primary breast cancer: 5-year results from the National Surgical Adjuvant Breast and Bowel Project Trial. *Journal of Clinical Oncology, 4,* 459–471.

Fisher, B., Redmond, C., Brown, A., Wolmark, N., Wittliff, J., Fisher, E.R., ... Shibata, H. (1981). Treatment of primary breast cancer with chemotherapy and tamoxifen. *New England Journal of Medicine, 305,* 1–6. doi:10.1056/NEJM198107023050101

Fisher, B., Redmond, C., Legault-Poisson, S., Dimitrov, N.V., Brown, A.M., Wickerham, D.L., ... Glass, A.G. (1990). Postoperative chemotherapy and tamoxifen compared with tamoxifen alone in the treatment of positive-node breast cancer patients aged 50 years and older with tumors responsive to tamoxifen: Results from the National Surgical Adjuvant Breast and Bowel Project B-16. *Journal of Clinical Oncology, 8,* 1005–1018.

Fisher, B., Redmond, C., Wickerham, D.L., Wolmark, N., Bowman, D., Couture, J., ... Robidoux, A. (1989). Systemic therapy in patients with node-negative breast cancer. A commentary based on two National Surgical Adjuvant Breast and Bowel Project (NSABP) clinical trials. *Annals of Internal Medicine, 111,* 703–712.

Freedman, A.N., Graubard, B.I., Rao, S.R., McCaskill-Stevens, W., Ballard-Barbash, R., & Gail, M.H. (2003). Estimates of the number of US women who could benefit from tamoxifen for breast cancer chemoprevention. *Journal of the National Cancer Institute, 95,* 526–532. doi:10.1093/jnci/95.7.526

Friese, C.R., Neville, B.A., Edge, S.B., Hassett, M.J., & Earle, C.C. (2009). Breast biopsy patterns and outcomes in Surveillance, Epidemiology, and End Results–Medicare data. *Cancer, 115,* 716–724. doi:10.1002/cncr.24085

Frizzell, J.P. (2005). Acute stroke: Pathophysiology, diagnosis, and treatment. *AACN Clinical Issues, 16,* 421–440.

Gasco, M., Argusti, A., Bonanni, B., & Decensi, A. (2005). SERMs in chemoprevention of breast cancer. *European Journal of Cancer, 41,* 1980–1989. doi:10.1016/j.ejca.2005.04.017

Grady, D., Cauley, J.A., Geiger, M.J., Kornitzer, M., Mosca, L., Collins, P., ... Barrett-Connor, E. (2008). Reduced incidence of invasive breast cancer with raloxifene among women at increased coronary risk. *Journal of the National Cancer Institute, 100,* 854–861. doi:10.1093/jnci/djn153

Guillem, J.C., Wood, W.C., Moley, J.F., Berchuck, A., Karlan, B.Y., Mutch, D.G., ... Offit, K. (2006). ASCO/SSO review of current role of risk-reducing surgery in common hereditary syndromes.

*Journal of Clinical Oncology, 24,* 4642–4660. doi:10.1200/JCO.2005.04.5260

Hartmann, L.C., Degnim, A., & Schaid, D.J. (2004). Prophylactic mastectomy for BRCA1/2 carriers: Progress and more questions. *Journal of Clinical Oncology, 22,* 981–983. doi:10.1200/JCO.2004.01.925

Hendrick, E.R., Pisano, E.D., Averbukh, A., Moran, C., Berns, E.A., Yaffe, M.J., ... Gatsonis, C. (2010). Comparison of acquisition parameters and breast dose in digital mammography and screen-film mammography in the American College of Radiology Imaging Network digital mammographic imaging screening trial. *American Journal of Roentgenology, 194,* 362–369. doi:10.2214/AJR.08.2114

Houssami, N., & Hayes, D.F. (2009). Review of preoperative magnetic resonance imaging (MRI) in breast cancer: Should MRI be performed on all women with newly diagnosed, early stage breast cancer? *CA: A Cancer Journal for Clinicians, 59,* 290–302. doi:10.3322/caac.20028

Howard, D.H., Huang, Y.L., & Adams, E.K. (2009). Discontinuation of screening mammography after serious health events. *Archives of Internal Medicine, 169,* 2162–2163. doi:10.1001/archinternmed.2009.396

Huff, J.G. (2009). The sonographic findings and differing clinical implications of simple, complicated, and complex breast cysts. *Journal of the National Comprehensive Cancer Network, 7,* 1101–1105.

Jatoi, I., Anderson, W.F., & Rosenberg, P.S. (2008). Qualitative age-interactions in breast cancer: A tale of two diseases? *American Journal of Clinical Oncology, 31,* 504–506. doi:10.1097/COC.0b013e3181844d1c

Kagawa-Singer, M., Dadia, A.V., Yu, M.C., & Surbone, A. (2010). Cancer, culture, and health disparities: Time to chart a new course? *CA: A Cancer Journal for Clinicians, 60,* 12–39. doi:10.3322/caac.20051

Karliner, L.S., Napoles-Springer, A., Kerlikowske, K., Haas, J.S., Gregorich, S.E., & Kaplan, C.P. (2007). Missed opportunities: family history and behavioral risk factors in breast cancer risk assessment among a multiethnic group of women. *Journal of General Internal Medicine, 22,* 308–314. doi:10.1007/s11606-006-0087-y

Karssemeijer, N., Bluekens, A.M., Beijerinck, D., Deurenberg, J.J., Beekman, M., Visser, R., ... Broeders, M.J. (2009). Breast cancer screening results 5 years after introduction of digital mammography in a population-based screening program. *Radiology, 253,* 353–358. doi:10.1148/radiol.2532090225

Kepple, J., Van Zee, K.J., Dowlatshahi, K., Henry-Tillman, R.S., Israel, P.Z., & Klimberg, V.S. (2004). Minimally invasive breast surgery. *Journal of the American College of Surgeons, 199,* 961–975. doi:10.1016/j.jamcollsurg.2004.07.032

Kuhl, C.K., Schrading, S., Leutner, C.C., Morakkabati-Spitz, N., Wardelmann, E., Fimmers, R., ... Schild, H.H. (2005). Mammography, breast ultrasound, and magnetic resonance imaging for surveillance of women at high familial risk for breast cancer. *Journal of Clinical Oncology, 23,* 8469–8476. doi:10.1200/JCO.2004.00.4960

Lehman, C.D., Gatsonis, C., Kuhl, C.K., Hendrick, R.E., Pisano, E.D., Hanna, L., ... Schnall, M.D. (2007). MRI evaluation of the contralateral breast in women with recently diagnosed breast cancer. *New England Journal of Medicine, 356,* 1295–1303. doi:10.1056/NEJMoa065447

Lehman, C.D., DeMartini, W., Anderson, B.O., & Edge, S.B. (2009). Indications for breast MRI in the patient with newly diagnosed breast cancer. *Journal of the National Comprehensive Cancer Network, 7,* 193–201.

Lehman, C.D., & Smith, R.A. (2009). The role of MRI in breast cancer screening. *Journal of the National Comprehensive Cancer Network, 7,* 1109–1115

Lin, C.J., Block, B., Nowalk, M.P., Woods, M., Ricci, E.M., Morgen-
lander, K.H., & Heron, D.E. (2007). Breast cancer risk assessment
in socioeconomically disadvantaged urban communities. *Journal
of the National Medical Association, 99*, 752–756.

Lof, M., & Weiderpass, E. (2009). Impact of diet on breast cancer
risk. *Current Opinion in Obstetrics and Gynecology, 21*, 80–85.
doi:10.1097/GCO.0b013e32831d7f22

López, M.L., Lana, A., Díaz, S., Folgueras, M.V., Sánchez, L., Co-
mendador, M.A., … Cueto, A. (2009). Multiple primary cancer:
An increasing health problem. Strategies for prevention in cancer survivors. *European Journal of Cancer Care, 18*, 598–605.
doi:10.1111/j.1365-2354.2008.00974.x

Mahoney, M.C., Bevers, T., Linos, E., & Willett, W.C. (2008). Opportunities and strategies for breast cancer prevention through
risk reduction. *CA: A Cancer Journal for Clinicians, 58*, 347–
371. doi:10.3322/CA.2008.0016

Mandelblatt, J.S., Schechter, C.B., Yabroff, K.R., Lawrence, W., Dignam, J., Extermann, M., … Balducci, L. (2005). Toward optimal
screening strategies for older women: Costs, benefits, and harms of
breast cancer screening by age, biology, and health status. *Journal
of General Internal Medicine, 20*, 487–496. doi:10.1111/j.1525-
1497.2005.0116.x

Mayer, D.K., Terrin, N.C., Menon, U., Kreps, G.L., McCance, K., Par-
sons, S.K., & Mooney, K.H. (2007). Screening practices in cancer
survivors. *Journal of Cancer Survivorship, 1*, 17–26. doi:10.1007/
s11764-007-0007-0

McCabe, M.S., & Jacobs, L. (2008). Survivorship care: Models
and programs. *Seminars in Oncology Nursing, 24*, 202–207.
doi:10.1016/j.soncn.2008.05.008

Méndez, J.E., Evans, M., & Stone, M.D. (2009). Promoters and barriers to mammography screening in multiethnic inner city patients.
*American Journal of Surgery, 198*, 526–528. doi:10.1016/j.amjsurg
.2009.07.002

Narod, S.A. (2006). Modifiers of risk of hereditary breast cancer.
*Oncogene, 25*, 5832–5836. doi:10.1038/sj.onc.1209870

National Comprehensive Cancer Network. (2010a, August 7). *NCCN
Clinical Practice Guidelines in Oncology™: Breast cancer risk reduction* [v.2.2010]. Retrieved from http://www.nccn.org/professionals/
physician_gls/PDF/breast_risk.pdf

National Comprehensive Cancer Network. (2010b, November 19).
*NCCN Clinical Practice Guidelines in Oncology™: Breast cancer
screening and diagnosis* [v.1.2011]. Retrieved from http://www.
nccn.org/professionals/physician_gls/PDF/breast-screening.pdf

National Comprehensive Cancer Network. (2010c, October 21).
*NCCN Clinical Practice Guidelines in Oncology™: Genetic/fa-
milial high-risk assessment: Breast and ovarian* [v.1.2010]. Retrieved from http://www.nccn.org/professionals/physician_gls/
PDF/genetics_screening.pdf

Nelson, H.D., Fu, R., Griffin, J.C., Nygren, P., Smith, M.E., & Hum-
phrey, L. (2009). Systematic review: Comparative effectiveness of
medications to reduce risk for primary breast cancer. *Annals of Internal Medicine, 151*, 703–715, W-226–W-235. doi:10.1059/0003-
4819-151-10-200911170-00147

Neugut, A.I., Meadows, A.T., & Robinson, E. (1999). Introduction.
In A.I. Neugut, A.T. Meadows, & E. Robinson (Eds.), *Multiple
primary cancers* (pp. 3–11). Philadelphia, PA: Lippincott Williams & Wilkins.

Ng, A.K., & Travis, L.B. (2008). Subsequent malignant neoplasms
in cancer survivors. *Cancer Journal, 14*, 429–434. doi:10.1097/
PPO.0b013e31818d8779

O'Flynn, E.A., Wilson, A.R., & Michell, M.J. (2010). Image-guided breast biopsy: State-of-the-art. *Clinical Radiology, 65*, 259–
270. doi:10.1016/j.crad.2010.01.008

Pisano, E.D., Gatsonis, C., Hendrick, E., Yaffe, M., Baum, J.K., Acha-
ryya, S., … Rebner, M. (2005). Diagnostic performance of dig-

ital versus film mammography for breast-cancer screening. *New
England Journal of Medicine, 353*, 1773–1783. doi:10.1056/
NEJMoa052911

Pocock, B., Taback, B., Klein, L., Joseph, K.A., & El-Tamer, M.
(2009). Preoperative needle biopsy as a potential quality measure
in breast cancer surgery. *Annals of Surgical Oncology, 16*, 1108–
1111. doi:10.1245/s10434-008-0188-4

Poulos, A.E., Balandin, S., Llewellyn, G., & Dew, A.H. (2006). Wom-
en with cerebral palsy and breast cancer screening by mammography. *Archives of Physical Medicine and Rehabilitation, 87*, 304–
307. doi:10.1016/j.apmr.2005.09.020

Rebbeck, T.R., Kauff, N.D., & Domchek, S.M. (2009). Meta-analysis
of risk reduction estimates associated with risk-reducing salpingo-
oophorectomy in *BRCA1* or *BRCA2* mutation carriers. *Journal of
the National Cancer Institute, 101*, 80–87. doi:10.1093/jnci/djn442

Roses, D.F., & Giuliano, A.E. (2005). Surgery for breast cancer. In
D.F. Roses (Ed.), *Breast cancer* (2nd ed., pp. 401–452). Philadelphia, PA: Elsevier Churchill Livingstone.

Sala, M., Comas, M., Macià, F., Martinez, J., Casamitjana, M., &
Castells, X. (2009). Implementation of digital mammography in
a population-based breast cancer screening program: Effect of
screening round on recall rate and cancer detection. *Radiology,
252*, 31–39. doi:10.1148/radiol.2521080696

Sánchez, L., Lana, A., Hidalgo, A., Rodríguez, J.M., Del Valle, M.O.,
Cueto, A., … López, M.L. (2008). Risk factors for second primary tumours in breast cancer survivors. *European Journal of Cancer Prevention, 17*, 406–413. doi:10.1097/CEJ.0b013e3282f75ee5

Saslow, D., Boetes, C., Burke, W., Harms, S., Leach, M.O., Lehman, C., … Russell, C.A. (2007). American Cancer Society guidelines for breast screening with MRI as an adjunct to mammography. *CA: A Cancer Journal for Clinicians, 57*, 75–89. doi:10.3322/
canjclin.57.2.75

Schmeler, K.M., Sun, C.C., Bodurka, D.C., White, K.G., Soliman,
P.T., Uyei, A.R., … Lu, K.H. (2006). Prophylactic bilateral salpingo-oophorectomy compared with surveillance in women with
BRCA mutations. *Obstetrics and Gynecology, 108*, 515–520.
doi:10.1097/01.AOG.0000228959.30577.13

Schottenfeld, D., & Beebe-Dimmer, J. (2006). Alleviating the burden of cancer: A perspective on advances, challenges, and future
directions. *Cancer Epidemiology, Biomarkers and Prevention, 15*,
2049–2055. doi:10.1158/1055-9965.EPI-06-0603

Shen, Y., Costantino, J.P., & Qin, J. (2008). Tamoxifen chemoprevention treatment and time to first diagnosis of estrogen receptor-negative breast cancer. *Journal of the National Cancer Institute, 100*, 1448–1453. doi:10.1093/jnci/djn320

Smith, R.A., Cokkinides, V., Brooks, D., Saslow, D., & Brawley, O.W.
(2010). Cancer screening in the United States, 2010: A review of
current American Cancer Society guidelines and issues in cancer screening. *CA: A Cancer Journal for Clinicians, 60*, 99–119.
doi:10.3322/caac.20063

Snyder, C.F., Frick, K.D., Peairs, K.S., Kantsiper, M.E., Herbert,
R.J., Blackford, A.L., … Earle, C.C. (2009). Comparing care for
breast cancer survivors to non-cancer controls: A five-year longitudinal study. *Journal of General Internal Medicine, 24*, 469–
474. doi:10.1007/s11606-009-0903-2

Taplin, S., Abraham, L., Barlow, W.E., Fenton, J.J., Berns, A.E., Car-
ney, P.A., … Elmore, J.G. (2008). Mammography facility characteristics associated with interpretive accuracy of screening mammography. *Journal of the National Cancer Institute, 100*, 876–
887. doi:10.1093/jnci/djn172

Taylor, A.J., & Taylor, R.E. (2009). Surveillance for breast cancer after childhood cancer. *JAMA, 301*, 435–436. doi:10.1001/
jama.2009.9

The, J.S., Schilling, K.J., Hoffmeister, J.W., Friedmann, E., McGin-
nis, R., & Holcomb, R.G. (2009). The detection of breast can-

cer with full-field digital mammography and computer-aided detection. *American Journal of Roentgenology, 192*, 337–340. doi:10.2214/AJR.07.3884

Tice, J.A., Cummings, S.R., Smith-Bindman, R., Ichikawa, L., Barlow, W.E., & Kerlikowske, K. (2008). Using clinical factors and mammographic breast density to estimate breast cancer risk: Development and validation of a new predictive model. *Annals of Internal Medicine, 148*, 337–347.

Tyler, C.V., Jr., & Snyder, C.W. (2006). Cancer risk assessment: Examining the family physician's role. *Journal of the American Board of Family Medicine, 19*, 468–477.

U.S. Preventive Services Task Force. (2009). Screening for breast cancer: U.S. Preventive Services Task Force recommendation statement. *Annals of Internal Medicine, 151*, 716–726, W-236. doi:10.1059/0003-4819-151-10-200911170-00008

Vernacchia, F.S., & Pena, Z.G. (2009). Digital mammography: Its impact on recall rates and cancer detection rates in a small community-based radiology practice. *American Journal of Roentgenology, 193*, 582–585. doi:10.2214/AJR.08.1720

Visvanathan, K., Chlebowski, R.T., Hurley, P., Col, N.F., Ropka, M., Collyar, D., ... Lippman, S.M. (2009). American Society of Clinical Oncology clinical practice guideline update on the use of pharmacologic interventions including tamoxifen, raloxifene, and aromatase inhibition for breast cancer risk reduction. *Journal of Clinical Oncology, 27*, 3235–3258. doi:10.1200/JCO.2008.20.5179

Vogel, V.G., Costantino, J.P., Wickerham, D.L., Cronin, W.M., Cecchini, R.S., Atkins, J.N., ... Wolmark, N. (2006). Effects of tamoxifen vs raloxifene on the risk of developing invasive breast cancer and other disease outcomes: The NSABP Study of Tamoxifen and Raloxifene (STAR) P-2 Trial. *JAMA, 295*, 2727–2741. doi:10.1001/jama.295.23.joc60074

Ward, E., Halpern, M., Schrag, N., Cokkinides, V., DeSantis, C., Bandi, P., ... Jemal, A. (2008). Association of insurance with cancer care utilization and outcomes. *CA: A Cancer Journal for Clinicians, 58*, 9–31. doi:10.3322/CA.2007.0011

Warner, E. (2008). The role of magnetic resonance imaging in screening women at high risk of breast cancer. *Topics in Magnetic Resonance Imaging, 19*, 163–169. doi:10.1097/RMR.0b013e31818bc994

Wei, W., Findley, P.A., & Sambamoorthi, U. (2006). Disability and receipt of clinical preventive services among women. *Women's Health Issues, 16*, 286–296. doi:10.1016/j.whi.2006.09.002

Wilkins, K.L., & Woodgate, R.L. (2008). Preventing second cancers in cancer survivors [Online exclusive]. *Oncology Nursing Forum, 35*, E12–E22. doi:10.1188/08.ONF.E12-E22

Yankaskas, B.C., Dickens, P., Bowling, J.M., Jarman, M.P., Luken, K., Salisbury, K., ... Lorenz, C.E. (2010). Barriers to adherence to screening mammography among women with disabilities. *American Journal of Public Health, 100*, 947–953. doi:10.2105/AJPH.2008.150318

# CHAPTER 4

# Pathophysiology and Staging

Susan G. Yackzan, APRN, MSN, AOCN®

## Introduction

The development of breast cancer is a complex process brought about by accumulating abnormalities in cells and in the supporting microenvironment. These aberrations may be the result of inherited or environmental factors. They are multiple and varied, may number in the hundreds or thousands, and result in diverse breast cancer presentation and classification. Significant national and international scientific efforts have resulted in a vastly increased knowledge base regarding the pathophysiology of breast cancer with the hope of a more complete understanding and increased clinical application in the not-so-distant future (Conzen, Grushko, & Olopade, 2008; Korkola & Gray, 2010).

## Anatomy and Physiology of the Breast

Breasts, also known as mammary glands, function physiologically as apocrine glands in the production of milk. During fetal development, breasts develop on the ventral side of the embryo. By the fifth week of gestation, a milk line or streak develops as an ectodermal thickening and extends bilaterally from the axilla to the thigh (Rosen, 2009). Most of this line atrophies by the sixth or seventh week of gestation, leaving a small portion bilaterally in the pectoral region. By the tenth to sixteenth week, the nipple and areolas have formed in those areas, followed by the downgrowth of short ducts that branch internally from the nipples. By the end of fetal development, 15–25 mammary ducts are present (Phillips & Price, 2002).

From birth until the onset of puberty, breast development is largely quiescent. With the onset of puberty, gonadotropin-releasing hormones are secreted by the hypothalamus, causing the release of follicle-stimulating hormone (FSH) and luteinizing hormone from the pituitary. FSH stimulates the maturation of ovarian follicles, resulting in estrogen production. In the presence of other hormones, such as glucocorticoids, insulin, and growth hormone, estrogen stimulates the develop-

ment of periductal stroma, the deposition of fat, and further growth of the ductal system in breast tissue (Kass, Mancino, Rosenbloom, Klimberg, & Bland, 2009). Progesterone exposure, also in concert with other hormones, stimulates lobuloalveolar development. Breasts are mature but inactive after puberty. The final stage of breast development occurs with pregnancy and involves cellular proliferation and lobuloalveolar differentiation (Phillips & Price, 2002).

The adult breast is normally protuberant and circular, with a pigmented areola and nipple (see Figure 4-1). Elevated ductal openings called Montgomery tubercles normally are present on the areola. Bilaterally, the breasts lie

**Figure 4-1. Surface Anatomy of the Adult Breast**

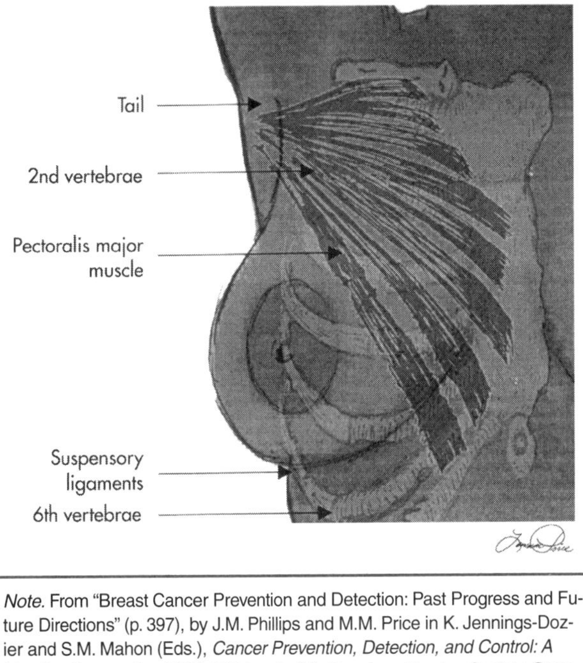

*Note.* From "Breast Cancer Prevention and Detection: Past Progress and Future Directions" (p. 397), by J.M. Phillips and M.M. Price in K. Jennings-Dozier and S.M. Mahon (Eds.), *Cancer Prevention, Detection, and Control: A Nursing Perspective*, 2002, Pittsburgh, PA: Oncology Nursing Society. Copyright 2002 by the Oncology Nursing Society. Reprinted with permission.

over the pectoral fascia, may extend from the second to the sixth vertebrae, and lie between the midaxillary line and the sternal edge (Phillips & Price, 2002). The Cooper accessory ligaments extend from the deep layers of the breast through the lobes and attach to the overlying skin, giving shape to the breast and anchoring the gland to the skin. Breast tissue extending toward the axilla is known as the tail of Spence.

Internally, the breast is made up of adipose, epithelial, and fibrous tissue (see Figure 4-2). From the nipple, each breast is organized into 15–25 lobes that are radially arranged and associated with ducts that join together so that only 5–10 ducts open on the surface of the nipple. Within the lobes of the breast, ducts branch out and end in the functional, secretory unit of the breast known as the terminal duct lobular unit (TDLU), where milk is produced (Phillips & Price, 2002; Rosen, 2009). Each TDLU is composed of alveoli or saccules that branch from the terminal ducts. Ducts are lined with squamous epithelium in the superficial portion, changing to a glandular, columnar, or cuboidal epithelium distal to the lactiferous sinus. From this squamocolumnar junction, the ductal system is lined with two types of epithelial cells, luminal cells that secrete milk and myoepithelial cells that eject the milk. Myoepithelial cells consist of both smooth muscle and epithelial cells and are found between the luminal cells and the basement membrane in the basal lamina or in what may be referred to as the basal layer. Changes in these myoepithelial cells may prove important in the process of carcinogenesis and invasion of malignant cells through the basement membrane (Adriance, Inman, Petersen, & Bissell, 2005; Rosen, 2009).

## Classification

The majority of primary breast cancers are adenocarcinomas, which traditionally are divided into subtypes based

---

### Figure 4-2. Internal Anatomy of the Adult Breast

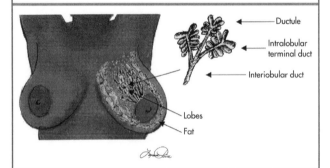

*Note.* From "Breast Cancer Prevention and Detection: Past Progress and Future Directions" (p. 397), by J.M. Phillips and M.M. Price in K. Jennings-Dozier and S.M. Mahon (Eds.), *Cancer Prevention, Detection, and Control: A Nursing Perspective,* 2002, Pittsburgh, PA: Oncology Nursing Society. Copyright 2002 by the Oncology Nursing Society. Reprinted with permission.

---

on growth patterns and microscopic findings. The two major subtypes are ductal and lobular carcinomas (Burstein, Harris, & Morrow, 2008). Breast carcinomas are further classified as either in situ (noninvasive) or invasive. Other types of cancer that occur in the breast include stromal tumors, lymphomas, and metastases from other sites.

## Breast Carcinomas

### Carcinoma in Situ

In situ breast carcinomas are defined by the presence of malignant epithelial cells within the ducts or lobules with no extension beyond the basement membrane. In situ carcinomas do not exhibit lymphvascular invasion. They are further described as ductal carcinoma in situ (DCIS) or lobular carcinoma in situ (LCIS) (Lester, 2005; Wood, Muss, Solin, & Olopade, 2005). The distinction between DCIS and LCIS is not based on the presence of cancer cells within distinct ducts or lobules. In fact, most breast carcinomas of both types occur in the TDLU. Differentiation is based on the type and growth pattern of cells (Sims, Clarke, Howell, & Howell, 2008). In situ carcinomas are expected to account for 21% of all breast cancer incidence in the United States in 2010 (Jemal, Siegel, Xu, & Ward, 2010). If left untreated and observed over 20 years, invasive carcinoma can be expected to occur in about 25%–35% of in situ carcinomas. This is a rate of about 1% per year (Lester, 2005).

**Ductal carcinoma in situ (intraductal or noninvasive ductal carcinoma):** DCIS most commonly presents as a nonpalpable lesion that is detected by mammography and often is found in association with microcalcifications. DCIS also may present as a density found on mammogram or as an incidental finding upon biopsy of other lesions. Before the advent of mammographic screening, DCIS accounted for less than 5% of all carcinomas (Lester, 2005).

As noted previously, DCIS is defined by the existence of malignant epithelial cells with no extension beyond the basement membrane. A wide range of pathologic findings may be seen with DCIS. DCIS may occur as a small, localized lesion or as a very extensive lesion that has spread throughout the ducts of the breast. DCIS may present as multifocal disease occurring in separate areas of the breast. Multifocal disease is found more frequently in association with DCIS lesions greater than 2–2.5 cm (Rosen, 2009). DCIS often is present as a component of invasive tumors and is thought to be a precursor lesion for invasive cancer.

DCIS has several subtypes. Subtypes were traditionally defined microscopically by cell morphology and include comedocarcinoma, cribriform, papillary, micropapillary, and solid (see Table 4-1). Other less common subtypes exist. Classification by cell type lacks prognostic value and is complicated by the fact that 30%–60% of DCIS lesions may include a mixture of more than one subtype

### Table 4-1. Subtypes of Ductal Carcinoma in Situ

| Subtype | Features |
|---|---|
| Comedocarcinoma | Solid growth; may fill lumen<br>Large, pleomorphic cells<br>High-grade nuclei<br>Central necrotic core (may be calcified)<br>Periductal fibrosis and inflammation commonly present<br>Myoepithelial layer may be affected |
| Cribriform | Cells that form fenestrations (sieve-like pattern)<br>Cells are smaller and more uniform compared to comedocarcinoma<br>General lack of necrosis |
| Papillary | Neoplastic cells arranged in fernlike pattern<br>Papillae project into the lumen of the duct.<br>Fibrovascular stromal architecture |
| Micropapillary | Features of papillary with smaller papillae<br>Papillae may coalesce and appear as bulbous protrusions or bridges across the ducts. |
| Solid | Cancer cells completely fill the ducts.<br>Small foci or necrosis or lack of necrosis<br>May be present with comedocarcinoma |

*Note.* Based on information from Lester, 2005; Povoski & Barsky, 2009; Rosen, 2009.

(Burstein et al., 2008). DCIS can be categorized as nuclear grade 1 (low), 2 (intermediate), or 3 (high). Prognostic indicators include the size of the lesion, margin status, and grade (Povoski & Barsky, 2009). Estrogen receptor (ER) and progesterone receptor (PR) status can be assessed on DCIS specimens, and more than 70% of DCIS lesions will be ER positive (Burstein et al., 2008). Other markers also can be assessed on some lesions, including HER2, p53, and E-cadherin.

**Lobular carcinoma in situ:** LCIS is typically an incidental finding and is not commonly associated with any clinical or mammographic abnormalities. LCIS is estimated to account for 1%–4% of all breast cancer cases and is found in 1%–2% of core biopsy specimens (Wood et al., 2005). In age distribution, LCIS tends to be more prominent than DCIS in younger, premenopausal women (Singh, 2006). It is more frequently multifocal and bilateral as compared to DCIS. The risk of subsequent cancer occurs with nearly equal frequency in both the ipsilateral and contralateral breast after a LCIS diagnosis. The majority of subsequent cancers are invasive ductal carcinomas (Lester, 2005; Wood et al., 2005).

Controversy exists as to whether LCIS is a precursor lesion or simply a marker of high risk for development of future carcinoma. Some lesions are associated with an almost 10-fold increased risk of invasive cancer, whereas others are associated with very little risk of invasive cancer. Evolving terminology alludes to this heterogeneous mix, with terms such as *atypical lobular hyperplasia* (ALH), which is used to describe similar but less well-developed lesions, and *lobular neoplasia*, which is used to describe both LCIS and ALH (Burstein et al., 2008; Povoski & Barsky, 2009).

LCIS appears histologically as a proliferation of noncohesive cells. LCIS lesions are almost uniformly ER/PR positive, lack E-cadherin expression, and usually are HER2 negative (Burstein et al., 2008; Lester, 2005; Rosen, 2009).

### Invasive (Infiltrating) Carcinomas

Microscopically, invasive or infiltrating carcinomas extend beyond the basement membrane. Extension may continue through the breast parenchyma and into lymphvascular spaces and may metastasize into regional lymph nodes or distant sites.

The majority of invasive breast carcinomas occur in the upper outer quadrant of the breast. When found mammographically as calcifications, invasive carcinomas usually are small, and lymph nodes typically are negative. A noted density is the most common mammographic finding for invasive carcinomas. Invasive carcinomas exhibiting this pattern usually are half the size of masses found first by palpation and have nodal metastases in less than 20% of the cases. In women not undergoing mammography, invasive carcinomas usually present as a palpable mass, and positive lymph nodes can be anticipated in 50% of those cases (Lester, 2005).

As with in situ carcinomas, the distinction between invasive ductal or lobular carcinoma does not actually designate a site of origin. Most carcinomas arise in the TDLU regardless of type (Burstein et al., 2008). Components of in situ carcinoma can be found in most invasive carcinomas and often share histologic patterns with the invasive component (Schnitt & Guidi, 2004).

Classification of invasive carcinomas traditionally is based on cytology, growth pattern of cells, secretion, architectural features, and biologic behavior (Jaffer, 2005). The classification of invasive (or infiltrating) ductal carcinomas (IDCs) includes cancers that do not exhibit significant identifying features of a specific subtype such as lobular, medullary, tubular, or mucinous. As such, the label *IDC* is not a subtype in itself. It is rather a term for a group of breast cancers that cannot be defined in other ways and is referred to as IDC of no special type (referred to as NST) or IDC not otherwise specified (referred to as NOS). The majority of breast carcinomas fall into this general category of IDC. Classification into a specific subtype requires defining histology in 90% of the tumor (Shapiro & Barsky, 2009). Table 4-2 outlines several of the subtypes of invasive breast carcinoma along with significant identifying features. In some cases, histology of tumors may be mixed.

**Invasive ductal carcinomas of no special type:** IDC usually presents as a palpable mass or abnormality found on mammogram and may rarely present as Paget disease of the nipple. Histopathology is variable within this category and may be variable within a single tumor (Shapiro & Barsky, 2009). Well-differentiated tumors are typically ER/PR positive and do not overexpress HER2. Poorly differentiated tumors may be ER/PR negative and HER2 positive. IDCs usually contain areas of associated DCIS. More aggressive DCIS tends to be associated with higher-grade IDC. Less aggressive DCIS tends to be associated with lower-grade IDC (Lester, 2005). Important prognostic features include tumor size, axillary node status, tumor grade, and lymph-vascular invasion.

Gene expression profiling may be useful in identifying subtypes of IDC and is an active area of study. Relevance for prognosis and clinical decision making must be defined. In addition, the usefulness of profiling will depend upon widely available and consistent testing techniques (Lester, 2005).

**Invasive lobular carcinoma:** Invasive lobular carcinomas (ILCs) make up the second largest proportion of invasive carcinomas. The usual presentation is a mammographic density or palpable mass. ILC also may present as a vague thickening and diffuse pattern on mammogram. An increased risk of multifocal disease in the ipsilateral breast has been associated with ILC, as has the presence of bilateral cancer (Lester, 2005; Wood et al., 2005).

The hallmark pathology of ILC is a pattern of infiltration characterized by uniform cells that appear to invade the stroma in a single-file or linear strand (Bleiweiss & Jaffer, 2005; Wood et al., 2005). This has traditionally been called the Indian file pattern. Mutation of E-cadherin has been correlated with ILC. A component of LCIS is present in most ILCs. Well-differentiated tumors usually are hormone receptor positive, and HER2 overexpression is rare. Poorly differentiated tumors are the opposite, often lacking hormone receptors and exhibiting HER2 positivity. The metastatic pattern for ILC is different than for other types of breast carcinoma and includes preferential sites such as the peritoneum, retroperitoneum, leptomeninges, gastrointestinal tract, ovaries, and uterus. ILC rarely metastasizes to the lungs and pleura (Lester, 2005).

Several variant forms exist within this category, and not all ILCs exhibit the single-file pattern. Variant ILCs usually contain classic ILC within the lesion and as a group may be more aggressive in behavior (Bleiweiss & Jaffer, 2005).

**Medullary carcinoma:** Accounting for approximately 5% of invasive cancers, medullary carcinomas usually present as a well-circumscribed mass. Occurrence is more common in younger women, and this type of breast carcinoma is more commonly associated with *BRCA1* mutation (Jaffer, 2005; Shapiro & Barsky, 2009). This tumor type may have a history of rapid, explosive growth (Lester, 2005). Microcalcifications usually are not found. Lymphadenopathy may be present but may be benign, reactive lymphadenopathy (Jaffer, 2005).

Characteristic features of medullary carcinomas include poorly differentiated cells growing in a sheet-like (syncytial) pattern and lymphoplasmacytic infiltrates. A component of DCIS is not uncommon. HER2 overexpression is not usually seen, and areas of necrosis may be present (Jaffer, 2005; Shapiro & Barsky, 2009).

Medullary carcinoma usually confers a more favorable prognosis than IDC of no special type. If many, but not all, of the important histopathologic features are present, these tumors may be classified as atypical medullary carcinomas (Wood et al., 2005). Atypical tumors may not predict the same favorable prognosis (Jaffer, 2005).

**Tubular carcinoma:** Historically, tubular carcinomas have accounted for a very small portion (1%–3%) of invasive breast carcinomas. The incidence of tubular carcinomas has increased in populations of women who undergo screening mammography. Tubular carcinomas represent up to 10%

### Table 4-2. Features of Subtypes of Breast Cancer

| Type | Prominent Features | Occurrence |
|---|---|---|
| Invasive ductal | Wide variation of characteristics<br>Consistency usually hard<br>Border usually irregular but may be distinct<br>Tan-white tumors | 65%–80% |
| Invasive lobular | Hallmark pattern of single-file cell infiltration (Indian file pattern)<br>Several variant forms<br>Consistency usually hard with irregular margins<br>Borders usually irregular<br>Atypical metastatic pattern<br>Tendency to be multifocal | 10%–15% |
| Medullary | Well-circumscribed mass; may be lobulated<br>Soft, fleshy tumor<br>Prominent lymphoplasmacytic infiltrates | 5% |
| Tubular | Histologically low-grade features<br>Consistency usually firm<br>Border usually irregular | 1%–3% |
| Mucinous (colloid) | Well-circumscribed mass<br>Usually soft, gelatinous tumor<br>Large, extracellular pools of mucin | 2% |

*Note.* Based on information from Bleiweiss & Jaffer, 2005; Jaffer, 2005; Lester, 2005; Rosen, 2009; Shapiro & Barsky, 2009; Singh, 2006; Wood et al., 2005.

of the tumors less than 1 cm in diameter at diagnosis (Lester, 2005). They are more common in postmenopausal women (Singh, 2006).

Tubular carcinomas are usually found mammographically as a spiculated (with spikes or needle-like points) density or abnormality. Microcalcifications may or may not be present (Jaffer, 2005; Shapiro & Barsky, 2009). Tubular carcinomas usually are small and often have an associated DCIS component. They usually are well differentiated and ER positive, do not overexpress HER2, lack significant chromosomal changes, and generally exhibit good prognostic features (Jaffer, 2005; Wood et al., 2005). Positive axillary nodes are found in less than 10% of tubular carcinoma cases (Lester, 2005).

**Mucinous carcinoma (colloid):** Mucinous carcinomas (also known as colloid cancers) usually occur in older women. Mucinous carcinomas often present as a palpable mass and usually are well-circumscribed masses that may have grown slowly over many years (Lester, 2005; Wood et al., 2005). The incidence of mucinous carcinoma is slightly higher in the *BRCA1*-positive population (Lester, 2005). The incidence of positive axillary nodes and distant metastases is lower with mucinous carcinoma than with IDC in general.

Mucinous carcinomas are characterized by the presence of large, extracellular pools of mucin in the tumor. They usually exhibit favorable prognostic features, including low to intermediate grade, positive ER/PR status, and negative HER2 status (Jaffer, 2005).

**Carcinoma of mixed histology:** Some invasive carcinomas may share features of both IDC and ILC (Bleiweiss & Jaffer, 2005). In some cases, components of both histologies are present in the same tumor and may contain a transitional zone between the two patterns. In other cases, tumor cells may exhibit the cytologic features of one type but invasive characteristics of the other. Still other tumors may exhibit cytologic and invasive characteristics of both tumor types simultaneously (Schnitt & Guidi, 2004).

**Other types:** Several other subtypes exist that together account for less than 1%–2% of all invasive breast carcinomas. Adenoid cystic carcinomas are associated with an excellent prognosis and are similar to adenoid cystic carcinomas arising in the salivary glands. Secretory carcinomas show predominant secretory activity and usually are low-grade tumors. Because cases had been recorded in children, this type of IDC was previously known as juvenile IDC. However, it also may be found in adults and thus has been renamed. Invasive cribriform carcinoma is a well-differentiated cancer associated with a favorable prognosis. Micropapillary invasive carcinomas are very rare and usually are found in older women. They exhibit a more aggressive behavior and may show lymphatic invasion and positive axillary nodes. Micropapillary carcinomas usually are ER positive and may be HER2 positive or negative. Metaplastic carcinomas (carcinoma with metaplasia) are highly variant tumors and may contain elements of epithelial and mesenchymal tissues. Metaplastic carcinomas may exhibit squamous differentiation. Elements of cartilage, bone, muscle, and spindle cells, among other cell types, have been reported in metaplastic carcinomas. Other subtypes include neuroendocrine tumors, apocrine carcinomas, lipid- and glycogen-rich carcinomas, and invasive carcinomas with osteoclast-like giant cells (Jaffer, 2005; Shapiro & Barsky, 2009; Wood et al., 2005).

## Inflammatory Breast Carcinoma

Inflammatory breast carcinoma (IBC) is a very aggressive type of breast cancer that accounts for 1%–5% of breast cancer cases. It is defined by the clinical characteristics of redness, warmth, edema (peau d'orange), breast enlargement, and tenderness, which are believed to be caused by tumor emboli in the dermal lymphatics. Onset of symptoms usually is quite rapid, and IBC is not associated with a particular histologic subtype. Biopsy-proven presence of cancer cells in the dermal lymphatics is indicative of IBC, although a diagnosis can be made on clinical presentation alone in the presence of a biopsy-proven breast cancer. A mass may or may not be palpable, and axillary nodes often are positive at the time of presentation (Burstein et al., 2008; Jaffer, 2005; Rosen, 2009).

## Paget Disease

Paget disease is a rare form of breast cancer, accounting for only 1%–3% of cases. The underlying pathology involves the presence of large round tumor cells (Paget cells) within the nipple epidermis. Clinical signs include nipple or areolar erythema, an eczema-like appearance, ulceration, crusting, irritation, and discharge. Nipple discharge, retraction, or inversion also may be present. A biopsy of the involved area is recommended for diagnosis (Burstein et al., 2008; Caliskan et al., 2008).

Paget disease may be associated with or without an underlying ductal carcinoma, either DCIS or invasive. If present, an associated cancer may be located in any part of the breast. The pathophysiology of Paget disease is not certain. Malignant cells may extend throughout the ductal system from an in situ lesion, may be transformed cells within the epidermis of the nipple, or may migrate from an invasive carcinoma in the breast (Burstein et al., 2008; Caliskan et al., 2008).

## Occult Breast Cancer

Rarely, in an estimated less than 1% of cases, breast carcinoma occurs as an occult presentation with positive axillary nodes or distant metastases without a detectable primary lesion. A thorough examination to locate the primary should include physical examination and imaging studies including mammography, ultrasound, breast magnetic resonance imaging, and positron-emission tomography. Diagnoses other than breast carcinoma must be excluded, including carcinomas of other sites (lung, pancreas, gastrointestinal tract, thyroid, ovaries, kidney), noncarcinomatous malignancy (melanoma, lymphoma, germ cell tumors), and nonmalignant causes (Estabrook & Giron, 2005; Wood et al., 2005). An appropriate biopsy technique yielding an adequate sample for study is essential to confirm the occult tumor as consistent with breast origin. Approximately 30% of occult carcinomas have no gross evidence of disease. In those cases, biopsy of multiple random sections of breast tissue may reveal pathology (Rosen, 2009). In rare cases, a tumor may remain occult, in which case a treatment plan is pursued despite the lack of identified primary. If not treated, 50% of patients can be expected to develop clinically evident breast disease (Burstein et al., 2008).

## Stromal Breast Tumors

Nonepithelial breast cancers arising from the breast stroma are far less common than epithelial cancers. Stromal tumors may range from benign to malignant tumors. Fibroadenomas are benign stromal tumors. Phyllodes tumors, historically known as cystosarcoma phyllodes, are usually low-grade, benign tumors that behave in a manner similar to fibroadenomas (Lester, 2005). Evidence has shown that phyllodes tumors may develop from fibroadenomas, perhaps in the manner of progressive carcinogenesis (Jaffer, 2005). The true malignant nature of phyllodes tumors is defined by the clinical course, however. The behavior of phyllodes tumors may be unpredictable, and both benign and malignant phyllodes tumors may recur. Phyllodes tumors that occur as high-grade/malignant lesions exhibit marked cellular atypia and mitotic activity, resembling sarcomas. Wide excision with tumor-free margins is the treatment of choice for both benign and malignant phyllodes tumors. Tumors that recur require reexcision with wider margins and possibly mastectomy and radiation therapy (Wood et al., 2005). Metastasis of phyllodes tumors occurs in a pattern consistent with sarcomas and has been reported up to 12 years after initial diagnosis. The most common sites of metastasis are the lung, pleura, and bone (Ellis, Sawyer, Rampaul, & Pineda, 2006).

Sarcomas of the breast are very rare, accounting for about 1% of all breast malignancies. They can be distinguished from malignant phyllodes tumors or metaplastic carcinomas by the absence of any epithelial components within the tumors. Sarcomas of the breast look like sarcomas in other body sites and can include angiosarcomas, fibrous histiocytomas, fibrosarcomas, rhabdomyosarcomas, liposarcomas, and leiomyosarcomas. Sarcomas usually present as a breast mass, often exhibiting rapid growth. The most common site of metastasis is

the lung. Spread to axillary lymph nodes is not common, as sarcomas spread via the hematogenous route (Estabrook & Giron, 2005; Jaffer, 2005). A slightly increased risk (0.3%–4%) of angiosarcomas after radiation therapy has been noted, most often occurring within 5–10 years after radiation therapy (Lester, 2005).

## Other Breast Cancers

Primary lymphomas of the breast are extremely rare. Presentation usually evolves as a painless breast mass, sometimes with a history of rapid enlargement. Masses usually are found in the upper outer quadrant of the breast and more frequently in the right breast. Presentation with multiple masses is possible. Bilateral presentation also is possible and appears to be associated with pregnant or postpartum patients and patients with Burkitt lymphoma. A very unusual presentation mimics the skin changes characteristic of IBC. Axillary nodes may be involved. B symptoms such as fever, night sweats, anorexia, weight loss, and weakness are uncommon but present in some cases, especially with high-grade histologies. All histologic types of lymphoma have been reported to occur in the breast, but most are diffuse, B-cell non-Hodgkin lymphoma (Jaffer, 2005; Morgan & Simpson, 2006; Rosen, 2009; Wood et al., 2005).

Metastasis to the breast from nonmammary sites is rare and almost never occurs in the absence of other metastases. Metastasis from nonmammary cancers accounts for approximately 1% of breast malignancies. Malignancies that can metastasize to the breast include melanoma, lung, kidney, stomach, ovarian, cervical, thyroid, gastric, renal cell, colorectal, thyroid, and head and neck cancers; and sarcoma, medulloblastoma, neuroblastoma, and mesothelioma (Jaffer, 2005; Rosen, 2009).

## Staging

Staging is the process of grouping patients based on the extent of their disease for the purpose of classification into prognostic groups and to inform treatment decisions. Clinical staging includes a complete physical examination, imaging studies, and pathologic examination of the breast or other tissues as needed to make a diagnosis. Pathologic staging includes the pathologic examination of biopsied, resected, or surgically explored primary tumor, lymph nodes, and metastatic sites in addition to the clinical staging data (Edge et al., 2010). Pathologic staging is particularly important in breast cancer because of the prognostic implications of tumor type, size, and extension. Breast cancer staging is incomplete without pathologic staging. The widely accepted staging system for breast cancer is the American Joint Committee on Cancer (AJCC) system and is outlined in Figure 4-3.

**Figure 4-3. American Joint Committee on Cancer Tumor, Node, Metastasis (TNM) Staging System for Breast Cancer**

**Primary Tumor (T)**

The T classification of the primary tumor is the same regardless of whether it is based on clinical or pathologic criteria, or both. Size should be measured to the nearest millimeter. If the tumor size is slightly less than or greater than a cutoff for a given T classification, it is recommended that the size be rounded to the millimeter reading that is closest to the cutoff. Designation should be made with the subscript "c" or "p" modifier to indicate whether the T classification was determined by clinical (physical examination or radiologic) or pathologic measurements, respectively. In general, pathologic determination should take precedence over clinical determination of T size.

| | |
|---|---|
| TX | Primary tumor cannot be assessed |
| T0 | No evidence of primary tumor |
| Tis | Carcinoma in situ |
| Tis (DCIS) | Ductal carcinoma in situ |
| Tis (LCIS) | Lobular carcinoma in situ |
| Tis (Paget's) | Paget disease of the nipple is NOT associated with invasive carcinoma and/or carcinoma in situ (DCIS and/or LCIS) in the underlying breast parenchyma. Carcinomas in the breast parenchyma associated with Paget disease are categorized based on the size and characteristics of the parenchymal disease, although the presence of Paget disease should still be noted. |
| T1 | Tumor $\leq$ 20 mm in greatest dimension |
| T1mi | Tumor $\leq$ 1 mm in greatest dimension |
| T1a | Tumor > 1 mm but $\leq$ 5 mm in greatest dimension |
| T1b | Tumor > 5 mm but $\leq$ 10 mm in greatest dimension |
| T1c | Tumor > 10 mm but $\leq$ 20 mm in greatest dimension |
| T2 | Tumor > 20 mm but $\leq$ 50 mm in greatest dimension |
| T3 | Tumor > 50 mm in greatest dimension |
| T4 | Tumor of any size with direct extension to the chest wall and/or to the skin (ulceration or skin nodules)* |

* Invasion of the dermis alone does not qualify as T4.

| | |
|---|---|
| T4a | Extension to the chest wall, not including only pectoralis muscle adherence/invasion |
| T4b | Ulceration and/or ipsilateral satellite nodules and/or edema (including peau d'orange) of the skin, which do not meet the criteria for inflammatory carcinoma |
| T4c | Both T4a and T4b |
| T4d | Inflammatory carcinoma** |

** Inflammatory carcinoma is restricted to cases with typical skin changes involving a third or more of the skin of the breast. While the histologic presence of invasive carcinoma invading dermal lymphatics is supportive of the diagnosis, it is not required, nor is dermal lymphatic invasion without typical clinical findings sufficient for a diagnosis of inflammatory breast cancer.

**Regional Lymph Nodes (N)**

*Clinical*

| | |
|---|---|
| NX | Regional lymph nodes cannot be assessed (e.g., previously removed) |
| N0 | No regional lymph node metastases |
| N1 | Metastases to movable ipsilateral level I, II axillary lymph node(s) |
| N2 | Metastases in ipsilateral level I, II axillary lymph nodes that are clinically fixed or matted; or in clinically detected* ipsilateral internal mammary nodes in the *absence* of clinically evident axillary lymph node metastases |

*(Continued on next page)*

## Figure 4-3. American Joint Committee on Cancer TNM Staging System for Breast Cancer *(Continued)*

| | |
|---|---|
| N2a | Metastases in ipsilateral level I, II axillary lymph nodes fixed to one another (matted) or to other structures |
| N2b | Metastases only in clinically detected* ipsilateral internal mammary nodes and in the *absence* of clinically evident level I, II axillary lymph node metastases |
| N3 | Metastases in ipsilateral infraclavicular (level III axillary) lymph node(s) with or without level I, II axillary lymph node involvement; or in clinically detected* ipsilateral internal mammary lymph node(s) with clinically evident level I, II axillary lymph node metastases; or metastases in ipsilateral supraclavicular lymph node(s) with or without axillary or internal mammary lymph node involvement |
| N3a | Metastases in ipsilateral infraclavicular lymph node(s) |
| N3b | Metastases in ipsilateral internal mammary lymph node(s) and axillary lymph node(s) |
| N3c | Metastases in ipsilateral supraclavicular lymph node(s) |

### Pathologic (pN)*

| | |
|---|---|
| pNX | Regional lymph nodes cannot be assessed (e.g., previously removed, or not removed for pathologic study) |
| pN0 | No regional lymph node metastasis identified histologically |

*Note:* Isolated tumor cell clusters (ITC) are defined as small clusters of cells not greater than 0.2 mm, or single tumor cells, or a cluster of fewer than 200 cells in a single histologic cross-section. ITCs may be detected by routine histology or by immunohistochemical (IHC) methods. Nodes containing only ITCs are excluded from the total positive node count for purposes of N classification but should be included in the total number of nodes evaluated.

| | |
|---|---|
| pN0(i–) | No regional lymph node metastases histologically, negative IHC |
| pN0(i+) | Malignant cells in regional lymph node(s) no greater than 0.2 mm (detected by hematoxylin and eosin stain (H&E) or IHC including ITC) |
| pN0(mol–) | No regional lymph node metastases histologically, negative molecular findings (RT-PCR)** |
| pN0(mol+) | Positive molecular findings (reverse transcriptase polymerase chain reaction [RT-PCR])**, but no regional lymph node metastases detected by histology or IHC |
| pN1 | Micrometastases; or metastases in 1–3 axillary lymph nodes; and/or in internal mammary nodes with metastases detected by sentinel lymph node biopsy but not clinically detected*** |
| pN1mi | Micrometastases (greater than 0.2 mm and/or more than 200 cells, but none greater than 2.0 mm) |
| pN1a | Metastases in 1–3 axillary lymph nodes, at least one metastasis greater than 2.0 mm |
| pN1b | Metastases in internal mammary nodes with micrometastases or macrometastases detected by sentinel lymph node biopsy but not clinically detected*** |
| pN1c | Metastases in 1–3 axillary lymph nodes and in internal mammary lymph nodes with micrometastases or macrometastases detected by sentinel lymph node biopsy but not clinically detected |
| pN2 | Metastases in 4–9 axillary lymph nodes; or in clinically detected**** internal mammary lymph nodes in the *absence* of axillary lymph node metastases |
| pN2a | Metastases in 4–9 axillary lymph nodes (at least one tumor deposit greater than 2.0 mm) |
| pN2b | Metastases in clinically detected**** internal mammary lymph nodes in the *absence* of axillary lymph node metastases |
| pN3 | Metastases in 10 or more axillary lymph nodes; or in infraclavicular (level III axillary) lymph nodes; or in clinically detected**** ipsilateral internal mammary lymph nodes in the *presence* of 1 or more positive level I, II axillary lymph nodes; or in more than 3 axillary lymph nodes and in internal mammary lymph nodes with micrometastases or macrometastases detected by sentinel lymph node biopsy but not clinically detected***; or in ipsilateral supraclavicular lymph nodes |
| pN3a | Metastases in 10 or more axillary lymph nodes (at least one tumor deposit greater than 2.0 mm); or metastases to the infraclavicular (level III axillary lymph) nodes |

*(Continued on next page)*

| Figure 4-3. American Joint Committee on Cancer TNM Staging System for Breast Cancer *(Continued)* | |
|---|---|
| pN3b | Metastases in clinically detected**** ipsilateral internal mammary lymph nodes in the *presence* of 1 or more positive axillary lymph nodes; or in more than 3 axillary lymph nodes and in internal mammary lymph nodes with micrometastases or macrometastases detected by sentinel lymph node biopsy but not clinically detected*** |
| pN3c | Metastases in ipsilateral supraclavicular lymph nodes |

\* Classification is based on axillary lymph node dissection with or without sentinel lymph node biopsy. Classification based solely on sentinel lymph node biopsy without subsequent axillary lymph node dissection is designated (sn) for "sentinel node," for example, pN0(sn).

\*\* RT-PCR: reverse transcriptase/polymerase chain reaction

\*\*\* "Not clinically detected" is defined as not detected by imaging studies (excluding lymphoscintigraphy) or not detected by clinical examination.

\*\*\*\* "Clinically detected" is defined as detected by imaging studies (excluding lymphoscintigraphy) or by clinical examination and having characteristics highly suspicious for malignancy or a presumed pathologic macrometastasis based on fine needle aspiration biopsy with cytologic examination.

**Distant Metastasis (M)**

| | |
|---|---|
| M0 | No clinical or radiographic evidence of distant metastases |
| cM0(i+) | No clinical or radiographic evidence of distant metastases, but deposits of molecularly or microscopically detected tumor cells in circulating blood, bone marrow or other non-regional nodal tissue that are no larger than 0.2 mm in a patient without symptoms or signs of metastases |
| M1 | Distant detectable metastases as determined by classic clinical and radiographic means and/or histologically proven larger than 0.2 mm |

*Note.* From *AJCC Cancer Staging Manual* (7th ed., pp. 358–360), by S.B. Edge, D.R. Byrd, C.C. Compton, A.G. Fritz, F.L. Greene, and A. Trotti III (Eds.), 2010, New York, NY: Springer, www.springer.com. Copyright 2010 by American Joint Committee on Cancer. Adapted with permission.

Tumor (T), node (N), and metastasis (M) form the basis of the AJCC staging system. Stage and prognostic grouping is outlined in Table 4-3. The assigned tumor size, or T, may be based on both clinical and pathologic staging. The measurement judged to be most accurate for the individual case should be used. T size should be measured for the invasive component of a tumor only. Nodal status focuses on the regional lymph nodes. Breast lymphatics drain by three routes: axillary, transpectoral, and internal mammary. For staging purposes, intramammary lymph nodes are coded as axillary. Supraclavicular nodes are classified as regional lymph nodes. Metastasis to any other lymph nodes, including cervical or contralateral internal mammary lymph nodes, is classified as distant (M1). Ipsilateral axillary, interpectoral and lymph nodes along the axillary vein are often classified as level I, II, or III. Level I or low axillary nodes are lateral to the lateral border of the pectoralis minor muscle. Level II or mid-axillary nodes lie between the medial and lateral borders of the pectoralis minor muscle and include interpectoral (Rotter) lymph nodes. Level III or apical axillary nodes are medial to the medial margin of the pectoralis minor muscle (Edge et al., 2010).

Histologic grade should be assigned for all invasive carcinomas (Edge et al., 2010). A pathologist completes the grading on routine sections that are assessed and scored. Scores are assigned based on three tumor features: degree of tubule formation, number of mitoses, and amount of nuclear pleomorphism (Santillan, Kiluk, & Cox, 2009). Each of the three features is reviewed and receives a score of one to three points according to severity (with one being favorable and three being more severe). Scores are summed to calculate a final total score, which can range from three to nine. Totals of three to five indicate a well-differentiated or low-grade tumor (grade 1), totals of six to seven indicate a moderately differentiated or intermediate-grade tumor (grade 2), and totals of eight to nine indicate a poorly differentiated or high-grade tumor (grade 3) (Edge et al., 2010).

## Prognostic and Predictive Factors

Prognostic factors are measurements taken at the time of surgery or diagnosis to estimate outcome (see Table 4-4). Many of these factors are assessed by evaluating biopsy or surgical specimens. The TNM staging system incorporates important prognostic factors such as invasive disease, nodal status, extension, and tumor size (Burstein et al., 2008; Santillan et al., 2009). Predictive factors are clinical or pathologic characteristics used to determine the likelihood of response to treatment (Lester, 2005; Sheldon, 2005). Some are well established, whereas others are still under investigation.

## Extent of Invasion

Pathologic examination of a tumor is necessary to determine the extent of invasion. In situ carcinoma by definition is confined and not metastatic. In the AJCC staging system, in

## Table 4-3. Breast Cancer Stage/Prognostic Groups

| Stage | T | N | M |
|---|---|---|---|
| 0 | Tis | N0 | M0 |
| IA | T1* | N0 | M0 |
| IB | T0 | N1mi | M0 |
| | T1* | N1mi | M0 |
| IIA | T0 | N1** | M0 |
| | T1* | N1** | M0 |
| | T2 | N0 | M0 |
| IIB | T2 | N1 | M0 |
| | T3 | N0 | M0 |
| IIIA | T0 | N2 | M0 |
| | T1* | N2 | M0 |
| | T2 | N2 | M0 |
| | T3 | N1 | M0 |
| | T3 | N2 | M0 |
| IIIB | T4 | N0 | M0 |
| | T4 | N1 | M0 |
| | T4 | N2 | M0 |
| IIIC | Any T | N3 | M0 |
| IV | Any T | Any N | M1 |

*T1 includes T1mi (mi = microinvasion)

**T0 and T1 tumors with nodal micrometastases only are excluded from stage IIA and are classified stage IB.

*Note.* From *AJCC Cancer Staging Manual* (7th ed., p. 349), by S.B. Edge, D.R. Byrd, C.C. Compton, A.G. Fritz, F.L. Greene, and A. Trotti III (Eds.), 2010, New York, NY: Springer, www.springer.com. Copyright 2010 by American Joint Committee on Cancer. Reprinted with permission.

situ carcinoma is designated as Tis and subclassified by type. Microinvasion refers to the extension of cancer cells beyond the basement membrane but with no focus more than 1 mm in greatest dimension. When multiple foci of microinvasion are present, the size of the largest is used for classification (Edge et al., 2010).

## Nodal Status

Lymph node status continues to be the single most important prognostic factor in breast cancer. Histologic examination of lymph nodes is necessary for reliable staging. Clinical staging alone can result in unacceptable false-positive and false-negative status (Lester, 2005; Sheldon, 2005). With negative lymph nodes, the 10-year disease-free survival is approximately 70%–80%. Having 1–3 positive nodes decreases the rate to 35%–40%, and having more than 10 posi-

tive nodes decreases the 10-year disease-free survival rate to 10%–15% (Lester, 2005).

Lymph node dissection can be used to determine both the presence of lymph node metastases and to determine the total number of positive nodes. The objective determines the extent of dissection. Sampling of axillary nodes to determine the presence or absence of nodal metastasis can be accomplished with sentinel lymph node biopsy, which is a minimally invasive technique. This procedure involves the identification and sampling of the first draining node from the breast cancer. Radiotracer, colored dye, or both are used to identify the sentinel node. A complete axillary dissection is recommended for patients with a positive sentinel lymph node and for those with clinically palpable nodes suspicious for metastatic disease. Axillary dissections include the surgical removal of both level I and level II nodes. Complete dissections allow for an accurate count of positive nodes and local control of gross axillary disease. Dissections also provide information about the location of positive nodes (Manasseh & Willey, 2006; Rivers & Hansen, 2007; Santillan et al., 2009).

Lymph node sampling or dissection is not without risks. The extent of axillary dissection affects the risk of lymphedema, sensory disturbances, and other postsurgical effects. Sentinel lymph node biopsy has significantly decreased, but not entirely eliminated, the risk of morbidity from axillary node procedures (Rivers & Hansen, 2007).

## Tumor Size

Tumor size continues to be a reliable prognostic factor. Larger tumor size increases the likelihood of positive axillary nodes and decreases the likelihood of disease-free survival. Tumors less than 1 cm in diameter with node-negative disease have a five-year survival rate of nearly 99% and a

## Table 4-4. Prognostic Factors for Breast Cancer

| Prognostic Factor | Favorable Findings |
|---|---|
| Invasion | In situ disease |
| Lymph node status | Negative |
| Tumor size | Smaller size |
| Histologic grade | Grade 1, well differentiated |
| Lymphvascular invasion | Negative |
| Distant metastasis | Negative |
| Histologic type (invasive carcinomas) | Tubular, cribriform, papillary, mucinous and adenoid cystic, medullary (not atypical medullary) |

*Note.* Based on information from Burstein et al., 2008; Santillan et al., 2009; Shapiro & Barsky, 2009; Wood et al., 2005.

10-year survival rate approaching 90% (Foxson, Lattimer, & Felder, 2011; Lester, 2005). More than 50% of women with tumors larger than 2 cm in diameter will eventually die of the disease (Lester, 2005).

## Histologic Grade

Survival statistics described in terms of histologic grade show that 85% of women with well-differentiated grade 1 tumors, 60% of women with moderately differentiated grade 2, tumors and 15% of women with poorly differentiated grade 3 tumors are alive at 10 years (Lester, 2005). Well-differentiated tumors are a minority. Histologic grade may be useful in identifying potential response to chemotherapy and therefore is useful as both a prognostic and predictive factor (Santillan et al., 2009).

## Hormone Receptor Status

The ER/PR status of tumors is both prognostic and predictive. A majority of invasive breast cancers retain estrogen receptors, allowing estrogen to stimulate tumor cell growth. Patients with ER/PR-positive tumors show better disease-free and overall survival and longer survival after recurrence. Tumors that are ER positive usually exhibit other favorable features. Positive ER status also is predictive of response to hormonal therapy (Burstein et al., 2008; Huston & Osborne, 2005; Santillan et al., 2009).

## HER2 Status

The proto-oncogene ERBB2, also known as HER2/neu, is a transmembrane growth factor receptor and a member of the human epidermal growth factor receptor (HER) family. It is normally present on breast epithelium and is overexpressed in approximately 20%–30% of breast cancers as a result of gene amplification (Sheldon, 2005; Wood et al., 2005). Tumors that overexpress HER2 are associated with higher grade, ER-negative status, higher proliferative indices, and poorer prognosis. As a predictive factor, HER2 overexpression is a predictor of response to trastuzumab. HER2 overexpression also may predict responsiveness to chemotherapy and resistance to endocrine therapy (Burstein et al., 2008).

## Proliferative Rate

Several indices of tumor proliferative rate can be assessed. Flow cytometry can be used to assess ploidy and S-phase fraction. Ploidy refers to the amount of DNA in a tumor. Diploid is normal. Aneuploid is abnormal and can be from both increased or decreased DNA content. The S-phase fraction refers to the number of cells in the S phase of the cell cycle. The mitotic index assesses the number of tumor cells undergoing mitosis and is assessed by reviewing tumors using high-power microscopic fields. Ki-67 and MIB are antibodies that identify antigens expressed by cells in proliferative phases of the cell cycle. Thymidine labeling index measures cells in the S phase of the cell cycle. Higher proliferative rates correlate with poor tumor grades, younger age of patients, ER/PR-negative status, and HER2 overexpression. As a predictive factor, tumors exhibiting high proliferative rates may be more responsive to chemotherapy (Huston & Osborne, 2005; Santillan et al., 2009; Wood et al., 2005).

## Other Factors

Tumor invasion of lymph and vascular systems appears to be a negative prognostic finding but requires specific pathologic criteria for accurate evaluation (Burstein et al., 2008). The presence of tumor cells in the dermal lymphatics is associated with inflammatory carcinoma and is a poor prognostic finding (Lester, 2005). Some histologic types of invasive breast cancer are associated with a better prognosis than others. Favorable diagnoses include tubular, invasive cribriform, and papillary carcinomas, for example. Patient age also appears to be of prognostic value. Younger patients (age 35 and younger) tend to have more high-grade, ER/PR-negative tumors (Burstein et al., 2008).

## Molecular Classification and Profiling

Breast cancer is recognized as a heterogeneous disease. Prognostic and predictive factors have been useful but still lack the ability to provide information about the behavior of breast cancer and to predict clinical outcome and response to treatment. Advances in technology have brought about new methods for classifying breast cancers on a molecular basis. With the use of gene expression microarrays for molecular profiling, breast cancer can be classified in ways that exhibit different clinical outcomes. Five molecular subtypes of breast cancer have been outlined: luminal A, luminal B, HER2, basal, and unclassified (Shapiro & Barsky, 2009). Luminal A and B classifications are described as ER/PR positive and HER2 negative. The HER2 class exhibits HER2 positivity. Basal or basal-like are ER/PR and HER2 negative, positive for cytokeratin 5/6, and positive for epidermal growth factor. Unclassified cancers are negative for all markers (Burstein et al., 2008; Shapiro & Barsky, 2009). The traditional categories of invasive ductal or lobular breast cancer may be molecularly profiled as any one of these five subtypes. The more rare and specific histologic types of breast cancer, such as medullary or metaplastic, primarily belong to one specific molecular classification. The classifications exhibit features that correspond to cell types within the normal breast. Cancers that develop from luminal cells, for example, would be classified as luminal A or B cells. Cancers that develop from basal cells would be classified as basal (Korkola & Gray, 2010).

Gene expression also can be used to profile breast cancer into good-risk or high-risk groups to assist with treatment decision making. Assays available include 21-gene, 70-gene, and 76-gene products and may differ in the requirement for tissue preparation. Assays provide stratification of the tumor as poor versus good prognosis or provide a recurrence score (Burstein et al., 2008; Cianfrocca & Gradishar, 2009; Shapiro & Barsky, 2009). Gene expression profiling tests have limitations, and further investigation and clarification are necessary for optimal use in clinical practice.

## Nursing Implications

Patient education about breast cancer pathophysiology, staging, and prognosis is a very complex and essential nursing process. Education usually begins with a positive biopsy result and includes basic breast cancer information, as well as information on the importance of complete pathologic staging. In the presurgical setting, education about staging is necessary as shared decisions are made regarding surgical treatments, such as the choice between mastectomy and lumpectomy and the lymph node sampling procedure that will be used. Presurgical information also is important to help set the groundwork for a better postsurgical visit, when a multidisciplinary team of surgical, medical, and radiation oncology professionals may present treatment options based on staging and predicted benefit. Nurses caring for patients with breast cancer should have a good understanding of the pathophysiology of breast cancer, classification based on traditional or emerging molecular methods, staging, and prognostic and predictive factors. Decisions in all aspects of the treatment trajectory are made with that information. The best decisions require a multidisciplinary team and patient advocacy.

## Conclusion

The development of breast cancer is a complex process, resulting in both in situ and invasive cancers exhibiting a range of subtypes. Information continues to emerge regarding molecular classification and predictive factors in breast cancer. The TNM staging system has been recently updated and continues to provide an important framework for stage grouping, treatment decisions, and prognosis.

## References

Adriance, M.C., Inman, J.L., Petersen, O.W., & Bissell, M.J. (2005). Myoepithelial cells: Good fences make good neighbors. *Breast Cancer Research, 7,* 190–197. doi:10.1186/bcr1286

Bleiweiss, I.J., & Jaffer, S. (2005). Pathology of invasive breast cancer. In D.F. Roses (Ed.), *Breast cancer* (2nd ed., pp. 98–110). Philadelphia, PA: Elsevier Churchill Livingstone.

Burstein, H.J., Harris, J.R., & Morrow, M. (2008). Malignant tumors of the breast. In V.T. DeVita Jr., S. Hellman, & S.A. Rosenberg (Eds.), *Cancer: Principles and practice of oncology* (8th ed., pp. 1606–1654). Philadelphia, PA: Lippincott Williams & Wilkins.

Caliskan, M., Gatti, G., Sosnovskikh, I., Rotmensz, N., Botteri, E., Musmeci, S., … Luini, A. (2008). Paget's disease of the breast: The experience of the European Institute of Oncology and review of the literature. *Breast Cancer Research and Treatment, 112,* 513–521. doi:10.1007/s10549-007-9880-5

Cianfrocca, M., & Gradishar, W. (2009). New molecular classifications of breast cancer. *CA: A Cancer Journal for Clinicians, 59,* 303–313. doi:10.3322/caac.20029

Conzen, S.C., Grushko, T.A., & Olopade, O.I. (2008). The molecular biology of breast cancer. In V.T. DeVita Jr., S. Hellman, & S.A. Rosenberg (Eds.), *Cancer: Principles and practice of oncology* (8th ed., pp. 1595–1605). Philadelphia, PA: Lippincott Williams & Wilkins.

Edge, S.B., Byrd, D.R., Compton, C.C., Fritz, A.G., Greene, F.L., & Trotti, A., III. (Eds.). (2010). *AJCC cancer staging manual* (7th ed.). New York, NY: Springer.

Ellis, I., Sawyer, E.J., Rampaul, R., & Pineda, C.G. (2006). Phyllodes tumor of the breast. In D. Raghavan, M.L. Brecher, D.H. Johnson, N.J. Meropol, P.L. Moots, & P.G. Rose (Eds.), *Textbook of uncommon cancer* (3rd ed., pp. 209–217). Hoboken, NJ: Wiley.

Estabrook, A., & Giron, G. (2005). Treatment of unusual malignant neoplasias and clinical presentations. In D.F. Roses (Ed.), *Breast cancer* (2nd ed., pp. 699–713). Philadelphia, PA: Elsevier Churchill Livingstone.

Foxson, S.B., Lattimer, J.G., & Felder, B. (2011). Breast cancer. In C.H. Yarbro, D. Wujcik, & B.H. Gobel (Eds.), *Cancer nursing: Principles and practice* (7th ed., pp. 1091–1145). Sudbury, MA: Jones and Bartlett.

Huston, T.L., & Osborne, M.P. (2005). Evaluating and staging the patient with breast cancer. In D.F. Roses (Ed.), *Breast cancer* (2nd ed., pp. 309–318). Philadelphia, PA: Elsevier Churchill Livingstone.

Jaffer, S. (2005). Pathology of special forms of breast cancer. In D.F. Roses (Ed.), *Breast cancer* (2nd ed., pp. 111–133). Philadelphia, PA: Elsevier Churchill Livingstone.

Jemal, A., Siegel, R., Xu, J., & Ward, E. (2010). Cancer statistics, 2010. *CA: A Cancer Journal for Clinicians, 60,* 277–300. doi:10.3322/caac.20073

Kass, R.B., Mancino, A.T., Rosenbloom, A.L., Klimberg, V.S., & Bland, K.I. (2009). Breast physiology: Normal and abnormal development and function. In K.I. Bland & E.M. Copeland III (Eds.), *The breast: Comprehensive management of benign and malignant diseases* (4th ed., pp. 39–58). Philadelphia, PA: Elsevier Saunders.

Korkola, J., & Gray, J.W. (2010). Breast cancer genomes—Form and function. *Current Opinion in Genetics and Development, 20,* 4–14. doi:10.1016/j.gde.2009.11.005

Lester, S.C. (2005). The breast. In V. Kumar, A.K. Abbas, & N. Fausto (Eds.), *Robbins and Cotran pathologic basis of disease* (7th ed., pp. 1119–1154). Philadelphia, PA: Elsevier Saunders.

Manasseh, D.-M.E., & Willey, S.C. (2006). Invasive carcinoma: Mastectomy and staging the axilla. In S.L. Spear (Ed.), *Surgery of the breast: Principles and art* (2nd ed., pp. 122–138). Philadelphia, PA: Lippincott Williams & Wilkins.

Morgan, D.S., & Simpson, J.F. (2006). Non-Hodgkin lymphoma of the breast. In D. Raghavan, M.L. Brecher, D.H. Johnson, N.J. Meropol, P.L. Moots, & P.G. Rose (Eds.), *Textbook of uncommon cancer* (3rd ed., pp. 194–200). Hoboken, NJ: Wiley.

Phillips, J.M., & Price, M.M. (2002). Breast cancer prevention and detection: Past progress and future directions. In K. Jennings-Dozier & S.M. Mahon (Eds.), *Cancer prevention, detection, and control: A nursing perspective* (pp. 389–444). Pittsburgh, PA: Oncology Nursing Society.

Povoski, S., & Barsky, S.H. (2009). In situ carcinomas of the breast: Ductal carcinoma in situ and lobular carcinoma in situ. In K.I. Bland & E.M. Copeland III (Eds.), *The breast: Comprehensive management of benign and malignant diseases* (4th ed., pp. 211–229). Philadelphia, PA: Elsevier Saunders.

Rivers, A., & Hansen, N. (2007). Axillary management after sentinel lymph node biopsy in breast cancer patients. *Surgical Clinics of North America, 87,* 365–377. doi:10.1016/j.suc.2007.01.014

Rosen, P.P. (2009). *Rosen's breast pathology* (3rd ed.). Philadelphia, PA: Lippincott Williams & Wilkins.

Santillan, A.A., Kiluk, J.V., & Cox, C.E. (2009). Assessment and designation of breast cancer stage. In K.I. Bland & E.M. Copeland III (Eds.), *The breast: Comprehensive management of benign and malignant diseases* (4th ed., pp. 429–451). Philadelphia, PA: Elsevier Saunders.

Schnitt, S.J., & Guidi, A.J. (2004). Pathology of invasive breast cancer. In J.R. Harris, M.E. Lippman, M. Morrow, & C.K. Osborne (Eds.), *Diseases of the breast* (3rd ed., pp. 541–579). Philadelphia, PA: Lippincott Williams & Wilkins.

Shapiro, C., & Barsky, S.H. (2009). Infiltrating carcinomas of the breast: Not one disease. In K.I. Bland & E.M. Copeland III (Eds.), *The breast: Comprehensive management of benign and malignant diseases* (4th ed., pp. 231–247). Philadelphia, PA: Elsevier Saunders.

Sheldon, D.G. (2005). Beyond lymph node staging: Molecular predictors of outcome in breast cancer. *Surgical Oncology Clinics of North America, 14,* 69–84. doi:10.1016/j.soc.2004.07.007

Sims, A.H., Clarke, R.B., Howell, A., & Howell, S.J. (2008). The cellular origins of breast cancer subtypes. In J.R. Pasqualini (Ed.), *Breast cancer: Prognosis, treatment, and prevention* (2nd ed., pp. 71–82). New York, NY: Informa Healthcare.

Singh, B. (2006). Pathology of breast disorders. In S.L. Spear (Ed.), *Surgery of the breast: Principles and art* (2nd ed., pp. 66–81). Philadelphia, PA: Lippincott Williams & Wilkins.

Wood, W.C., Muss, H.B., Solin, L.J., & Olopade, O.I. (2005). Malignant tumors of the breast. In V.T. DeVita Jr., S. Hellman, & S.A. Rosenberg (Eds.), *Cancer: Principles and practice of oncology* (7th ed., pp. 1415–1477). Philadelphia, PA: Lippincott Williams & Wilkins.

# CHAPTER 5

# Surgical Management and Reconstruction

Susan G. Yackzan, APRN, MSN, AOCN®, and Judith Hatch, RN, MSN, OCN®, CBCN®, FPMH-NP

## Introduction

With a greater understanding of breast cancer cell growth, lymphatic spread, and metastasis, an evolution in the surgical management of breast cancer has taken place. This evolution is chronicled as a surgical progression from the extensive, radical mastectomy, which was considered standard of care into the mid-20th century, to modified radical mastectomy, total or simple mastectomy, and finally to breast-conserving therapy (BCT) (Jatoi, Kaufmann, & Petit, 2006; Roses, 2005; Sabel, 2009). Progress has been significant, resulting in a situation in which many women and men with breast cancer, especially those with in situ lesions and early-stage disease, have multiple options for surgical management. These options allow for treatment planning that includes the person with breast cancer in the surgical decision-making process.

Surgical management of breast cancer may be a stand-alone treatment modality in some cases, but often it is combined with other treatment modalities. Radiation, chemotherapy, hormonal therapy, and biotherapy are all used in combination with surgery for the treatment of breast cancer. Interdisciplinary care often is provided by nurses, navigators, genetic counselors, clinical trial coordinators, physical therapists, behavioral therapists, and many others who interact with medical oncologists, radiation oncologists, and breast and plastic surgeons in the planning and implementation of treatments. The complexity of breast cancer treatments coupled with the opportunity for patients to participate in treatment decision making provides a unique opportunity and challenge for nursing support, advocacy, and intervention.

## Overview of Breast Surgery for In Situ, Invasive, and Metastatic Disease

Surgery is used throughout the trajectory of benign and malignant breast conditions. Beginning with diagnosis, biopsy procedures provide critical information on the presence of benign, precursor, or malignant lesions. In addition, surgery is essential for staging, identification of prognostic and predictive factors, and treatment of both in situ and invasive breast carcinomas. Surgery also can be used in the metastatic breast cancer setting. Breast surgery, as with any surgery, must be undertaken after careful preoperative evaluation. Preoperative tests such as blood work, chest x-ray, and electrocardiogram may be ordered depending on the age of the patient and other health history. A complete history and physical examination, including bilateral breast examination, review of current medications, and review of family history, are conducted. Comorbid conditions are assessed in light of the effect they may have on surgery, postoperative recovery, and additional treatments under consideration.

## In Situ Disease

Discussion of the surgical management of in situ breast carcinoma includes some consensus practice standards and some controversy. Recommendations and practice differ between the two types of in situ disease, which are lobular carcinoma in situ (LCIS) and ductal carcinoma in situ (DCIS).

LCIS is typically an incidental finding on biopsy and often presents without mammographic abnormality. If LCIS is found on needle biopsy, an open surgical biopsy is indicated to rule out invasive lobular carcinoma or the presence of DCIS (Rosen, 2009). At the time of presentation, LCIS is both multifocal and bilateral in many cases (Burstein, Harris, & Morrow, 2008). Treatment decision making must take into account these presentation patterns. Decision making also includes the controversies in practice theories that view LCIS as either a risk factor for later cancer development or a direct precursor lesion that may progress to invasive lobular carcinoma. With that in mind, treatment options are varied and may include continued surveillance, excision, chemoprevention, or mastectomy (Po-

*The authors would like to acknowledge Dianne D. Chapman, ND, APRN, BC, for her contribution to this chapter that remains unchanged from the first edition of this book.*

voski & Barsky, 2009). If surveillance is chosen, the patient must be educated about the increased risk of subsequent cancer and the importance of adherence to the surveillance regimen. Risk reduction with a chemoprevention agent in combination with surveillance also is an option (National Comprehensive Cancer Network [NCCN], 2010a, 2010b). In cases of pure LCIS, the risk of subsequent invasive cancer is approximately 25% over the next 25–30 years (Schwartz, 2005). If the patient chooses risk-reduction mastectomy, the bilateral nature of LCIS warrants consideration of bilateral mastectomy. A decision to undergo risk-reduction mastectomy should only be made after thorough education and counseling.

As a category, DCIS includes many variants. Some types of DCIS are high grade and very aggressive. Others are low grade and indolent. The overall long-term disease-free survival rates for DCIS are 96%–98% (Allegra et al., 2010). DCIS generally is classified by morphology, grade, and, more recently, molecular markers (O'Sullivan & Morrow, 2007; Virnig, Tuttle, Shamliyan, & Kane, 2010). Classification can be complicated by the presence of more than one cell type within the same intraductal carcinoma lesion. Currently, DCIS is understood to be an intermediate step in the progression of cancer as normal breast cells change and become malignant. Therefore, removal of the lesion is recommended. Surgical procedures for DCIS include excision of the lesion (also known as BCT or lumpectomy), excision of the tumor followed by radiation therapy, and mastectomy (Burstein et al., 2008). All three treatment options are aimed at prevention of both noninvasive and invasive local recurrence (O'Sullivan & Morrow, 2007). Patient preference, extent and type of DCIS, and risk of recurrence are all considerations in the surgical treatment choice.

Most patients with DCIS are candidates for BCT, which involves excision of the DCIS lesion with a margin of healthy tissue. Clear margins are associated with a decreased risk of recurrence (Schwartz, 2005). Recommendations regarding radiation therapy after BCT for DCIS are an area of some controversy, but radiation appears to be beneficial in many situations (NCCN, 2010a). Radiation after excision decreases the risk of recurrence; however, there may be subsets of patients with DCIS for whom the risk of recurrence is so low that no significant benefit would be derived from radiation therapy (Allegra et al., 2010). More research is needed in this area. From a medical perspective, mastectomy is recommended for the management of DCIS when lesions are so large that they cannot be excised with a cosmetically acceptable result or when disease is multifocal. Mastectomy also may be recommended when a patient is unable to undergo radiation therapy after BCT, in those cases when BCT alone would be inadequate, and when attempts at excision with negative margins have been unsuccessful (O'Sullivan & Morrow, 2007). Mastectomy also may be a personal preference. Almost all patients are candidates for mastectomy if they choose that option. Patients also may choose to have a mastectomy with contralateral prophylactic mastectomy

(CPM) with or without reconstruction. In recent years, an increase in the choice of mastectomy and CPM for DCIS has been noted (Tuttle et al., 2009).

Axillary dissection or sentinel lymph node biopsy (SLNB) is not currently recommended for DCIS (NCCN, 2010a). After excision or mastectomy, however, invasive cancer can be found in 15% of patients with DCIS diagnosed by core needle biopsy (Virnig et al., 2010). Those patients found to have invasive carcinoma should have axillary lymph node staging at the time of definitive breast surgery. Because of this possibility, a SLNB is recommended for patients with DICS who choose mastectomy and for those with an excision that might compromise future SLNB (NCCN, 2010a).

## Invasive Disease

Invasive breast cancer often is categorized as early stage or locally advanced. Categorization in this way has both treatment and prognostic implications. Early-stage disease includes stage I and II invasive breast cancers and accounts for the majority of all invasive breast cancer. The primary treatment for early-stage disease is surgery, either BCT or mastectomy depending on the situation and patient preference. Locally advanced disease includes a mix of cancers for which clinical or radiographic evidence shows advanced disease that is confined to the breast and regional lymph nodes (NCCN, 2010a). Locally advanced disease usually includes stage III cancers. In some references, inflammatory cancer is also included in this category (Burstein et al., 2008). Locally advanced disease accounts for about 10% of invasive breast cancers (Palmieri & Perez, 2007). Cancers in this category may be operable or inoperable at presentation. If inoperable at presentation, systemic treatment with chemotherapy, biotherapy, or hormonal therapy may be the initial treatment, and surgery may follow. Some cancers in this category remain inoperable (NCCN, 2010a).

The National Institutes of Health released a consensus statement in the early 1990s on the treatment of early-stage breast cancer (stage I and II). Equivalent survival data for BCT followed by radiation therapy and mastectomy were noted for women with stage I and II breast cancer. In the statement, BCT was recognized as an appropriate treatment for the majority of women with early-stage disease and was even deemed "preferable" because of the preservation of the breast (National Institutes of Health, 1991, p. 394). Mastectomy was the standard surgical treatment prior to that time. Several studies explored the practice adoption of BCT subsequent to the consensus statement publication. Significant and widespread adoption of BCT was expected. However, research on the surgical choice of BCT or mastectomy in women eligible for either procedure has repeatedly shown that mastectomies continue to be performed in substantial numbers, ranging from 30% to more than 50% of cases in reported series (Chagpar et al., 2006; Collins et al., 2009; Farrow, Hunt, & Samet, 1992; Nattinger, Gottlieb, Veum, Yahnke, & Goodwin, 1992).

The first decision to be made regarding surgical treatment of invasive cancer is the confirmation that the patient is a surgical candidate. Asymptomatic patients with early-stage breast cancer do not usually require a metastatic workup before surgical treatment is planned or completed. A metastatic workup may be necessary for those with stage III disease in which metastases are more frequent. Patients with locally advanced and inflammatory breast cancers may be treated with systemic therapy before surgical treatment. After systemic therapy, BCT may be an option for some patients (Burstein et al., 2008).

Invasive breast cancer treatment also includes surgical management of the axilla. Just as with breast surgery, axillary procedures have undergone an evolution. Previously, complete axillary dissection was considered the standard of care for breast cancer and was viewed as a therapeutic intervention in and of itself (Burstein et al., 2008). In more recent years, the therapeutic benefit of axillary dissection has been called into question. The benefit of the procedure for the purposes of staging and prognosis, however, is not in question. The presence or absence of breast cancer in axillary nodes remains the most important prognostic factor in invasive breast cancer (Roses & Giuliano, 2005). Guidelines recommend surgical staging by pathologic assessment of axillary nodes for those with invasive breast cancer (NCCN, 2010a). Lymphatic mapping and sentinel node biopsy has become the preferential method of axillary node assessment. Axillary dissection is indicated for patients with node-positive disease by sentinel node biopsy, patients with palpable lymphadenopathy, and patients with stage III disease (NCCN, 2010a).

## Metastatic Disease

Metastatic disease is primarily treated with systemic therapy including chemotherapy, biotherapy, or endocrine therapy. Surgery may be of benefit in some cases. For patients with an intact primary who are responding to systemic therapy, surgery may be advised, but only if complete resection is possible and other metastases are not immediately threatening (NCCN, 2010a). For those who present with metastatic disease, surgical treatment of the primary tumor may be of some survival benefit. However, the timing of surgery and the best way to select patients who may benefit are not well understood (Burstein et al., 2008).

## Surgical Procedures

Breast cancer surgery is oriented toward the achievement of local control and staging of disease. Local control can be accomplished with either mastectomy or BCT followed by radiation therapy. Axillary lymph node sampling and dissection provide important staging information.

## Mastectomy

The goal of mastectomy is removal of the entire breast. Almost all patients with breast cancer are candidates for mastectomy. Indications for the use of mastectomy over BCT include multicentric disease or diffuse microcalcifications, invasive carcinoma with an extensive DCIS component, positive margins after breast-conserving attempts, cancer recurrence in a previously irradiated breast or a breast with previous BCT, tumor size relative to breast size that would not allow for acceptable cosmetic outcome, and patients for whom radiation therapy is contraindicated or unavailable. Patients also may choose mastectomy over BCT as a matter of personal preference (Manasseh & Willey, 2006). Mastectomy can be performed with or without immediate reconstruction, depending on the tumor characteristics and patient preference. Delayed reconstruction also can be done. If reconstruction is planned, preoperative consultation with a plastic surgeon is essential for planning incision orientation and mastectomy technique. Planning should be conducted jointly for immediate reconstruction cases (Manasseh & Willey, 2006).

Types of mastectomy procedures are outlined in Table 5-1. The extent of dissection and inclusion or exclusion of

| Table 5-1. Types of Mastectomy | |
|---|---|
| Type | Description |
| Total (simple) | Removal of breast tissue from the clavicle to the rectus abdominis sheath, medially to the sternal edge and laterally to the latissimus dorsi muscle<br>No dissection of the axilla<br>Excision including nipple-areolar complex and biopsy scars with margin of healthy tissue |
| Modified radical | Removal of breast tissue as with total mastectomy<br>Removal of level 1 and 2 axillary nodes |
| Skin-sparing | Excision of the nipple-areola complex and minimal amount of skin<br>Possible excision of skin/scar from biopsy<br>Extirpation of remaining breast tissue through open skin area<br>Requires careful handling of skin flaps to prevent necrosis |
| Nipple-sparing | Incision and nipple preservation techniques vary.<br>Retains nipple and areolar complex<br>Removes as much breast tissue as possible<br>Patient consent should include that nipple-areola will be sacrificed if occult tumor is discovered or vascularity is in question. |

*Note.* Based on information from Baron, 2007; Burstein et al., 2008; Carlson, 2006; Garcia-Etienne et al., 2009; Jatoi et al., 2006; Manasseh & Willey, 2006; Rusby et al., 2010; Sabel, 2009.

axillary nodes are important distinctions between the procedures. Total or simple mastectomy is the most common procedure and is illustrated in Figure 5-1. Increased rates of total mastectomy are a result of decreased use of modified radical mastectomy. A combination of increased use of BCT and the decreased need for axillary dissections as sentinel lymph node procedures are increasingly used for lymph node sampling are the reasons for the decreased use of modified radical mastectomy (Sabel, 2009). Modified radical mastectomy combines total mastectomy with removal of axillary level 1 and 2 nodes and is illustrated in Figure 5-2. Skin-sparing mastectomy is a technique that can be used for early-stage cancer when the goal is to preserve as much skin as possible for immediate reconstruction. Skin-sparing mastectomy also may be used for prophylactic mastectomy (Carlson, 2006). Preservation of the skin is more acceptable cosmetically and facilitates an optimally shaped reconstruction in many cases (Rusby, Smith, & Gui, 2010). Nipple-sparing mastectomy was previously termed subcutaneous mastectomy. Nipple-sparing techniques are varied and are planned to maintain blood supply and viability of the retained nipple and areola (Garcia-Etienne, Cody, Disa, Cordeiro, & Sacchini, 2009). Traditional candidates for nipple-sparing mastectomy have been patients undergoing prophylactic mastectomy for risk reduction (Rusby et al., 2010). Patients with DCIS and invasive cancers also may be considered candidates. Criteria vary, but favorable candidates generally have peripheral as opposed to central lesions in the breast, small lesions, and lack of comorbid conditions. Some concern exists that residual breast tissue or tissue retained to increase viability of the nipple may increase

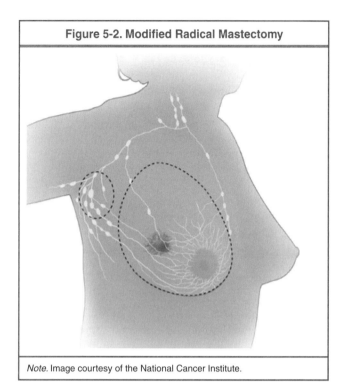

**Figure 5-2. Modified Radical Mastectomy**

*Note.* Image courtesy of the National Cancer Institute.

the recurrence risk (Garcia-Etienne et al., 2009). This is an area of some controversy, and more research is needed. Immediate reconstruction with autologous tissue or an implant may be done after nipple-sparing mastectomy. Patient preference for the procedure is important to subsequent satisfaction with the results (Rusby et al., 2010). Radical (Halsted) mastectomy is no longer performed. Radical mastectomy included removal of the breast and the overlying skin, pectoral major and minor muscles, and axillary contents including level 1, 2, and 3 nodes (Sabel, 2009).

After mastectomy, patients wear a binder to apply compression to the mastectomy site. Patients are encouraged to sit upright and avoid slouching. Range-of-motion exercises for the arm and shoulder usually begin on postoperative day 1, and dressings remain in place for 48–72 hours after surgery. Patients may have one or more drains, depending on the type of surgery. Drains prevent the collection of blood and serum beneath skin flaps and are left in place until drainage is less than 30 ml in a 24-hour period for two consecutive days, usually within 7–14 days. Drains usually are removed at four weeks even with continued output because of infection risk (Sabel, 2009).

Postoperative wound and drain care are of primary concern after mastectomy. Pain management also is a significant concern. Most mastectomy patients experience minimal to moderate pain. More extensive procedures and mastectomy followed by immediate reconstruction may increase postoperative pain (Baron, 2007). After mastectomy, patients are usually discharged within 24 hours, depending on the type of surgery and whether immediate reconstruction was done. Pain

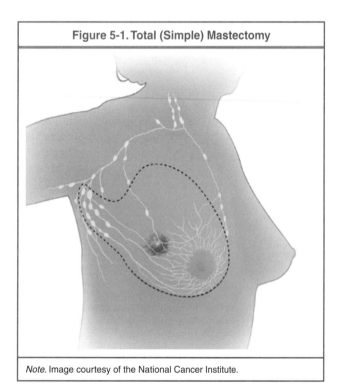

**Figure 5-1. Total (Simple) Mastectomy**

*Note.* Image courtesy of the National Cancer Institute.

management remains important, and patients should have appropriate prescriptions and education to facilitate pain control after discharge. Education about range-of-motion exercises should include instructions for the patient to continue the exercises at home several times a day until full range returns (Baron, 2007). Wound and drain care education must be provided, and patients should know how to contact someone for any questions or problems and if signs of infection occur.

Possible postmastectomy complications include wound infections, seromas, hematomas, incisional pain, or sensory changes (Vitug & Newman, 2007). Serious morbidity from mastectomy is rare. A body mass index (BMI) greater than 30 has been associated with an increased risk of wound complications, as has preoperative hypoalbuminemia and hematocrit greater than 45% (El-Tamer et al., 2007). Postoperative pneumothorax is rare, as is the operative positioning injury of brachial plexopathy. Breast sensations and pain may persist for months to years after surgery. The etiology is unknown but is assumed to be neuropathic (Vitug & Newman, 2007). More extensive surgery can result in more significant complications.

## Breast-Conserving Therapy

BCT is known by many terms, including lumpectomy, wide excision, tylectomy, segmentectomy, segmental excision of the breast, segmental mastectomy, partial mastectomy, tumorectomy, and quadrantectomy (see Figure 5-3). Regardless of the terminology, the goal of BCT is to excise the entire lesion along with a margin of surrounding healthy breast tissue while achieving the best possible aesthetic result. Variables that affect the surgery include tumor size, location, breast size, and tumor characteristics. Recurrence-free survival is associated with tumor-free margins (Roses & Giuliano, 2005). BCT must be followed by radiation therapy to achieve survival rates that are equivalent to mastectomy. For invasive breast carcinomas, axillary staging should be completed at the time of BCT.

Patients who are candidates for BCT include those in whom removal of the tumor with adequate margins can be accomplished with acceptable cosmesis. Patients must have radiation therapy available and be expected to tolerate the regimen. Patients for whom radiation therapy is contraindicated are not candidates for BCT. Examples of patients for whom radiation therapy is contraindicated are patients who are pregnant or who have had prior therapeutic irradiation to the breast. Additional contraindications are multifocal disease and persistently positive margins after excision. A relative contraindication to the procedure is the presence of collagen vascular disease because those patients may not be able to tolerate radiation therapy (Burstein et al., 2008).

The extent of resection is determined by the extent of cancer as assessed clinically or by scans such as mammography, ultrasound, or magnetic resonance imaging. Incisions usual-

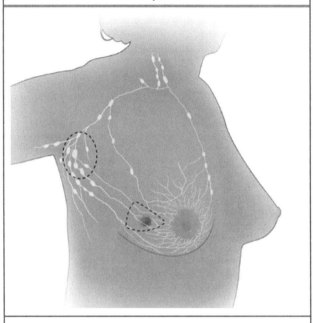

**Figure 5-3. Breast-Conserving Therapy and Axillary Nodes**

*Note.* Illustration by Don Bliss. Used courtesy of the National Cancer Institute.

ly are made directly over the area of tumor and follow normal lines of tension in the skin. Superficial lesions may require some skin excision. For nonpalpable tumors, wire localization can be done preoperatively to guide the resection. Wire localization can be guided by ultrasound or mammography (Sabel, 2009). Surgery that preserves subcutaneous tissue and avoids thick skin flaps helps maintain normal breast contour.

During surgery, margins are examined to look for evidence of gross tumor, and if found, additional tissue is excised. A pathologist also examines the specimen intraoperatively to assess margins. Positive margins are reexcised to achieve a margin of normal tissue around the tumor (Jatoi et al., 2006).

Postoperatively, a detailed pathology analysis of the resected tissue is completed. Margins should be negative or clear of cancer cells. If margins are positive, reexcision should be attempted. A higher radiation boost dose should be considered in cases of microscopically focally positive margins in the absence of an extensive intraductal component (NCCN, 2010a).

BCT usually is completed as an outpatient surgery. Drains are rarely used for BCT but may be necessary for large excisions (Roses & Giuliano, 2005). The dressing usually can be removed the first postoperative day, and patients can resume normal activities within one to two days. Postoperative pain usually is mild to moderate. Because BCT is primarily an outpatient procedure, the patient and home caregivers will need to assess and manage pain on an ongoing basis. A plan for home management, including prescription medications, must be put into place. Patients should know whom to contact for questions and problems. Strenuous physical exercise or activity is discouraged in the immediate postoperative period. Radiation therapy or postoperative chemotherapy can begin after adequate wound healing, usually within one to two weeks.

The most common complications after BCT are seroma, hematoma, and infection. The incidence of these complications is rare. The use of a support brassiere for several days after surgery helps decrease bleeding. The brassiere helps support the weight of the breast, decreasing tension on the suture line, and is especially beneficial for large-breasted patients. Medications and supplements with antiplatelet activity should be avoided for one to two weeks before surgery (Vitug & Newman, 2007). A seroma usually forms in the surgical cavity and reabsorbs eventually (Jatoi et al., 2006). Seromas after BCT can actually preserve the breast contour. If excessive and symptomatic, seromas can be managed by percutaneous aspiration (Sabel, 2009). Infections are rare and typically are managed conservatively (El-Tamer et al., 2007; Sabel, 2009). Altered sensations in the breast usually are not severe but may persist for several years (Baron et al., 2007).

## Sentinel Lymph Node Biopsy and Axillary Node Dissection

Pathologic examination of the lymph nodes is an essential part of breast cancer staging. Results are important for prognosis and for consideration of further treatment recommendations. The axillary nodes are the primary lymphatic drainage for the breast. Up to 40 nodes can be present in the axilla, but this number is widely variable. Axillary nodes are categorized into three levels by their relationship to the pectoralis minor muscle (level 1 nodes are lateral, level 2 nodes are posterior, and level 3 nodes are medial to the pectoralis minor muscle and inferior to the axillary vein). Other nodes that are less commonly involved are Rotter nodes and supraclavicular nodes. Rotter nodes are found between the pectoralis major and minor muscles. Supraclavicular nodes are contiguous with level 3 nodes but lie more medial above the clavicle. These are removed if believed suspicious, especially during intraoperative palpation (Manasseh & Willey, 2006).

As the understanding of axillary spread and less invasive surgery developed, SLNB has been increasingly used. This procedure involves identifying and removing the first draining lymph node or sentinel node. Sentinel lymph node status is a strong predictor of regional lymph node status (Krishnamurthy, 2005). Sentinel lymph node mapping and resection is recommended for patients with stage I and stage II cancer (NCCN, 2010a). Use of the procedure for patients with locally advanced disease or for patients who have undergone preoperative chemotherapy is not as well established (Newman & Newman, 2007). Less arm and shoulder morbidity is associated with SLNB as compared with axillary node dissection (Baron, 2007; NCCN, 2010a). No significant differences have been found in the effectiveness of the procedures in determining the presence or absence of metastases in axillary nodes (NCCN, 2010a).

Identification of the sentinel node or nodes is best done first, before the breast surgery, to prevent disruption of the normal lymphatics. Blue dye, a radioisotope, or a combination is injected at the tumor site, into the subareolar area, or into the skin overlying the tumor (Jatoi et al., 2006). Blue dye can be either isosulfan or methylene blue (Manasseh & Willey, 2006). The radioisotope may be injected 1–24 hours before the procedure, depending on the radioisotope dose, particle size, and volume (Jatoi et al., 2006; Manasseh & Willey, 2006; Newman & Newman, 2007). The radioisotope takes approximately 60–90 minutes to reach the sentinel node (Baron, 2007). A hand-held gamma probe is used to locate the nodes that take up the radioisotope in the axilla. These are known as the "hot" nodes (Manasseh & Willey, 2006). The surgeon injects blue dye while in the operating room to visually identify the lymphatic path and uptake in a node. The dye takes approximately 35 minutes to reach the sentinel node (Jatoi et al., 2006). All nodes that are "hot," blue, or both are removed. On average, 2.1 nodes are removed with the combination technique. After removal, the axilla is inspected for palpable nodes, which are also removed. Sentinel nodes can be examined intraoperatively by frozen section. If they are positive for cancer, the surgeon will proceed with an axillary dissection. Sentinel nodes are further examined by permanent section analysis (Manasseh & Willey, 2006).

An experienced lymph node team is essential for the SLNB procedure. If none is accessible, NCCN guidelines recommend that patients be referred to an experienced SLNB team for the procedure (NCCN, 2010a). Eligibility for the SLNB procedure is generous. Prior breast surgery and multifocal or multicentric disease were thought to be contraindications, but SLNB may be considered appropriate in many cases. Sentinel lymph node identification may be less accurate in patients who are obese and in those whose tumors are larger than 5 cm. The procedure may be contraindicated in patients with significant disruption of lymphatics or those with a history of extensive breast or axillary surgery (Manasseh & Willey, 2006).

Complications from SLNB include allergic reactions to the blue dye used in the procedure, seroma formation, cellulitis, lymphedema, and sensory changes. Rare but significant and life-threatening allergic reactions to isosulfan blue dye have been reported although most allergic reactions are less acute (Newman & Newman, 2007). Morbidity from seroma, cellulitis, and lymphedema is reduced with SLNB as opposed to axillary dissection. Incidence of lymphedema after SLNB is noted in the range of 0%–5%, and although the incidence is less than with axillary dissection, it does exist (Baron, 2007; Burstein et al., 2008; Manasseh & Willey, 2006; McLaughlin et al., 2008). Patients may experience a variety of breast sensations after the procedure that usually improve within three months but may persist for years (Baron, 2007; Baron et al.,

2007). Occasionally, a blue discoloration of the breast from subareolar and dermal injection of blue dye may occur and last for several months (Newman & Newman, 2007).

Axillary lymph node dissection is indicated for suspicious palpable nodes or biopsy-proven positive axillary nodes. Axillary lymph node dissection should include both level 1 and 2 nodes. Level 3 nodes are not removed unless they are suspicious or unless gross disease is present in level 1 and 2 nodes. At least 10 nodes should be removed for adequate staging (NCCN, 2010a). Axillary dissection is beneficial in providing local control for patients with axillary disease and also is important in providing a quantifiable number of axillary nodes, which can be used in decisions regarding additional treatments such as chemotherapy (Chagpar et al., 2007).

A closed-suction drain usually is in place after surgery to decrease the incidence and degree of seroma formation (Roses & Giuliano, 2005). The drains are removed when the drainage is less than 30 ml in 24 hours. The use of a drain is thought to decrease the incidence of seroma formation; however, seroma formation after drain removal is the most common side effect of axillary lymph node dissection. Seromas that are symptomatic and bothersome can usually be treated by percutaneous aspiration (Manasseh & Willey, 2006).

Lymphedema may occur in 10%–30% of patients after axillary lymph node dissection (Baron, 2007; Manasseh & Willey, 2006; McLaughlin et al., 2008; Vitug & Newman, 2007). Incidence rates are highly varied because of the differences in subjective and objective diagnostic criteria and the variations in patient follow-up and duration (Vitug & Newman, 2007). Baseline measurements are essential to objective diagnosis but often are lacking. Lymphedema occurs more often in the upper arm than the forearm, and incidence is greater with more extensive node dissections. Body weight, higher BMI, and history of infection have been associated with an increased incidence of lymphedema in both axillary lymph node dissection and SLNB (McLaughlin et al., 2008).

In addition to seroma formation and lymphedema, complications from axillary dissection include sensory disturbances, shoulder dysfunction, and pain (Rivers & Hansen, 2007). Sensory disturbances are thought to be related to the injury or resection of nerves including the intercostal brachial nerve, which supplies the axilla and upper arm. Other cutaneous nerves also may be injured and cause postoperative sensations. Sensory disturbances can persist for years after axillary lymph node dissection but may not be severe or significantly distressing (Baron et al., 2007). The development of shoulder dysfunction or frozen shoulder may be decreased by judicial and progressive range-of-motion exercise postoperatively. While drains are in place, strenuous and vigorous exercise is not recommended. Patients can be encouraged to begin modest range-of-motion activity on the first postoperative day, such as elevating the affected arm to touch the head. Increasing and progressive range-of-motion exercise may follow (Roses & Giuliano, 2005).

## Reconstruction

Women undergoing mastectomy may wish to consider the option of breast reconstruction. Breast reconstruction is achieved through plastic surgery techniques that attempt to restore a breast mound to near normal shape and size following mastectomy. The various options, the staggered nature of surgical procedures, and the timing of reconstruction after mastectomy are difficult concepts for patients. Lee, Hultman, and Sepucha (2010a) described the decisions of patients with breast cancer regarding reconstruction as "preference sensitive" because they depend primarily on patients' personal preferences and less on medical need when surgeons offer options (p. 563). Five main themes have been reported regarding women's goals and personal concerns with reconstruction: (a) concerns regarding multiple procedures and length of recovery, as well as risk of complications, (b) comfort level with using one's own tissue versus prosthetics, (c) wanting to look natural in clothing, (d) wanting to avoid external prostheses, and (e) considering others' opinions, including physician recommendations (Lee, Hultman, & Sepucha, 2010b).

Women need factual, accurate information to make informed decisions. Information must also be appropriately timed. Meeting with a plastic surgeon before mastectomy may be helpful in making choices based on realistic expectations of achievable outcomes. Premastectomy consults with plastic surgeons also can screen patients who are ineligible for certain procedures. For any woman suspicious for a hereditary cancer syndrome, it may be beneficial to speak with a genetic counselor or advanced practice nurse in genetics before the operation. The risk of genetic predisposition can be assessed so that prophylactic procedures can be discussed. Nurses must advocate for patients by providing an environment that encourages women to vocalize their concerns, expectations, and goals for reconstruction.

### Timing of Reconstruction

Breast reconstruction can be performed at the time of mastectomy or months to years after a mastectomy is performed. Decisions regarding the timing of breast reconstruction must take into account further cancer treatment (radiation), staging (local, regional, or advanced), patient comorbidities, the patient's personal preferences and concerns (finances, avoiding external prostheses), lifestyle risks (tobacco use), and physical characteristics (Lee, Adesiyun, et al., 2010). Treatment of the breast cancer remains the priority, and reconstruction must be planned in a way that will not adversely affect cancer treatment or carry unnecessary risk for the patient (Sabel, 2009). Reconstruction of the nipple-areola complex is usually the last step in reconstruction and is not performed until after other treatments are complete (Rosson et al., 2010).

The benefits of immediate reconstruction include a single hospitalization for both breast surgery and reconstruction and the psychological benefit that can result from a reconstructed, instead of a missing, breast (Baron, 2007). However, the increasing use of immediate reconstruction has brought attention to the complexity of care for patients found to have positive nodes after breast surgery and immediate reconstruction. In those cases, subsequent axillary lymph node dissection and additional treatments such as radiation therapy may be necessary. Radiation therapy after reconstruction may result in two problems. First, the reconstruction may interfere with the delivery of radiation therapy. Second, the radiation therapy may adversely affect the reconstruction (Kronowitz & Robb, 2008). The efforts of a multidisciplinary breast cancer team with coordinated care and exceptional communication in planning surgery are essential to make the best decisions about the timing of reconstruction.

## Types of Reconstruction

Breast reconstruction can be placed in two main categories based on the material used to create the reconstructed breast (see Table 5-2). *Alloplastic* reconstruction uses expanders that are progressively filled with saline and implants that are filled with either silicone or saline. *Autologous* tissue flaps are products of the patient's own tissue and may consist of muscle, skin, and fat. Pedicled autologous flaps are those in which the tissue is partially separated and rotated or moved into position with its vascular supply attached (Sabel, 2009). With a free flap, tissue blood supply is severed, and the flap is repositioned and then anastomosed microsurgically to a blood supply (Hu & Alderman, 2007). Combinations of the two are also used (Baron, 2007).

### Alloplastic Reconstruction: Expanders and Implants

Breast implant reconstruction usually is a multistage process. Utilizing implants for reconstruction is the simplest technical option and initial recovery is less stressful on patients, making this a good choice for older patients and those with comorbidities who might not be able to tolerate long general anesthesia times (Sabel, 2009). In addition, no donor site is needed with this type of reconstruction, which decreases the complexity and potential complications (Wagstaff, Reed, & Caddy, 2010).

### Table 5-2. Types of Breast Reconstruction

| Type | Examples |
|---|---|
| Alloplastic | Silicone gel implant <br> Saline-filled implant |
| Autologous | Transverse rectus abdominis myocutaneous flap <br> Inferior and superior gluteal artery flaps <br> Deep inferior and superficial inferior epigastric flaps |

Implants can be placed through the mastectomy incision and positioned beneath the pectoralis muscle in an immediate, one-step reconstruction procedure, although this is not common (Sabel, 2009). An illustration of a breast implant can be seen in Figure 5-4. In most cases, the muscle and remaining skin must first be stretched to accommodate the implant. This is done gradually with the use of a tissue expander (Baron, 2007). The tissue expander begins as an empty device. It is filled with saline through a resealable port. Additional volumes of normal saline are injected into the tissue expander every one, two, or three weeks over approximately two months in the plastic surgeon's office. The fill amount and duration of injections depend on the desired breast size and tissue expansion. The maximum desired fill is maintained for four to six weeks, and then the tissue expander is exchanged for a permanent implant. Permanent implants can be filled with either saline or silicone gel (Sabel, 2009).

Patients may feel chest fullness or tightness after tissue expansion. Implants will feel full and firm and will not change over time or move like a natural breast when changing positions (Sabel, 2009). The life of the implant varies but typically lasts from 10–15 years before replacement may be required (Hu & Alderman, 2007). A disadvantage of the procedure is the duration of time required for tissue expansion. A second, although usually brief, surgical procedure is required for the exchange of tissue expander and implant. Hematomas and seromas are acute complications. Extrusion of the implant, infection, malposition, and deflation may occur and may require removal of the expander or implant (Rosson et al., 2010; Sabel, 2009). Some degree of contracture develops around all implants. Significant capsular contracture can be a long-term complication causing the breast to become hard and painful (Hu & Alderman, 2007; Sabel, 2009). Visible wrinkling of the implant also can occur over time.

### Autologous Reconstruction

Using the patient's own tissue can result in a softer, ptotic, pliable breast that appears more symmetrical and natural (Serletti, 2008). The tissue is native and therefore is not at risk for a foreign body reaction or capsular contraction (Baron, 2007). Skin, fat, and muscle can all be used for the reconstruction. A goal of current practice is to use as little muscle from the donor site as possible to decrease complications of the procedures and provide better aesthetics (Rosson et al., 2010). These procedures are much more complex than alloplastic reconstructive procedures. They require a longer time in the operating room and a donor site procedure, and the risk of complications is increased (Baron, 2007; Sabel, 2009). Patients with comorbidities, such as vascular disease, that might impair circulation or pulmonary disease that may alter oxygen delivery may not be candidates for these procedures. Active use of nicotine is also a contraindication to many of these

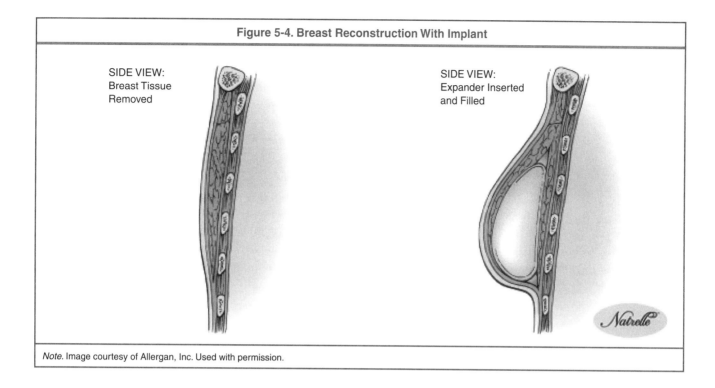

Figure 5-4. Breast Reconstruction With Implant

SIDE VIEW:
Breast Tissue
Removed

SIDE VIEW:
Expander Inserted
and Filled

*Note.* Image courtesy of Allergan, Inc. Used with permission.

procedures (Baron, 2007; Hu & Alderman, 2007). A summary of autologous flap reconstruction procedures is provided in Table 5-3.

The transverse rectus abdominis myocutaneous (TRAM) flap is the most frequently used autologous procedure (Baron, 2007). TRAM flaps may be either pedicle or free flap procedures. In the pedicle TRAM procedure, an area of skin and fat, remaining attached to rectus abdominis muscle, is separated from the abdomen, rotated, and tunneled under the skin to the mastectomy site to form a breast mound (Sabel, 2009). The flap retains its blood supply. In the free TRAM flap procedure, the skin, fat, and rectus abdominis muscle are detached, severing the blood supply to the tissue. The tissue is transferred to the mastectomy site, and blood vessels in the graft are microsurgically anastomosed to thoracic or internal mammary vessels (Hu & Alderman, 2007). Intraoperatively, an arterial vessel in the exposed portion of the flap may be identified and then used for postoperative monitoring by Doppler signal (Sabel, 2009).

Indications for the use of TRAM flaps include patients who have large mastectomy defects or require large amounts of tissue for reconstruction, those who have had prior chest wall irradiation, and those who have a ptotic contralateral breast in whom it would be difficult to achieve symmetry with an implant (Hu & Alderman, 2007). Candidates must have adequate abdominal tissue to use for the flap. The presence of any condition that might compromise blood supply to the flap may exclude a patient from TRAM flaps. Conditions such as diabetes, heart disease, obesity, and smoking are examples (Sabel, 2009). The procedure is contraindicated for patients who have had prior abdominal surgery that may have altered the pedicle or blood supply, including open cholecystectomy, bypass grafts using the internal mammary artery, and abdominoplasty (Hu & Alderman, 2007).

The latissimus dorsi flap (LDF) is another type of myocutaneous (muscle and skin) flap (see Figure 5-5). LDFs may be pedicle or free flaps. For the LDF pedicle flap, skin, fat, and the latissimus dorsi muscle are separated from the patient's back and tunneled under the tissue to the reconstruction site. Free LDFs are completely detached and are transplanted to the mastectomy or breast surgery site. The size of the flap can vary depending on the defect to be reconstructed (Serletti, 2008). LDFs often are combined with a prosthetic implant (Baron, 2007). In those cases, the implant is placed underneath the pectoralis and the latissimus muscle (Serletti, 2008). The donor site for LDFs is left with a scar that may be sizeable and noticeable depending on the extent and location, which is a disadvantage of this procedure.

Indications for the LDF include patients who have had previous implant or TRAM flap failure, those who need reconstruction for a BCT defect, and those who are not eligible for other procedures, such as patients with abdominal obesity or extreme thinness (Baron, 2007; Sabel, 2009). Contraindications to the procedure include prior surgeries that may have interrupted blood supply and severe comorbidities (Hu & Alderman, 2007).

The gluteal flap procedure uses tissue from the buttocks. Gluteal flaps are either superior or inferior depending on the flap blood supply. The superior gluteal artery perforator (S-GAP) flap uses the superior gluteal artery, and flap tissue comes from the upper buttock. The inferior gluteal artery perforator (I-GAP) flap uses the inferior gluteal artery, and flap tissue comes from the lower buttock (Hu & Alderman, 2007). Gluteal flaps consist of skin, fat, and blood vessels with little to no muscle (Sabel, 2009).

S-GAP and I-GAP procedures may be useful for patients who are unable to have a TRAM flap. They are more technically demanding than other procedures and risk injury to or postoperative pain from the sciatic nerve. Surgical time has been reported to be as much as 8–10 hours and includes

**Table 5-3. Autologous Flap Reconstruction**

| Procedure | Technique | Timing | Postoperative Care | Complications |
|---|---|---|---|---|
| Transverse rectus abdominis myocutaneous flap | Rectus abdominis muscle and tissue are either moved as a free flap or rotated and placed into position.<br>Can be a single breast reconstruction using one rectus abdominis muscle or bilateral reconstruction using both.<br>In addition to the muscle, skin and subcutaneous tissue are taken from the lower abdomen, allowing for abdominal contouring (abdominoplasty).<br>Surgery may take 4–6 hours. | Immediate or delayed | Pain management<br>Monitoring of flap for blood flow and signs of thrombosis<br>Drain care<br>Keep patient in semi-Fowler position after surgery to limit tension on the abdomen.<br>Typical inpatient stay of 3–5 days<br>May take 6–8 weeks before patient can return to light activity. | Seroma or hematoma of the breast or abdomen<br>Infection<br>Partial or total flap loss<br>Low back pain<br>Exacerbation of previous back problems<br>Abdominal weakness, bulge, hernia, asymmetry, upper fullness, or upper bulge<br>Umbilical necrosis |
| Latissimus dorsi flap | Latissimus dorsi and tissue overlying the muscle are used. Tissue is raised, rotated, and tunneled into position.<br>If more tissue is necessary, the area of excision can be extended.<br>After muscle has been sutured in position, an implant may be placed beneath the muscle into a pocket. | Traditionally delayed but can be immediate | Pain management<br>Monitoring of flap for blood flow and signs of thrombosis<br>Drain care<br>Normally inpatient stay of 1–2 days<br>Patient can usually return to light activity in 2–4 weeks. | Seroma or hematoma of the breast or upper back donor site<br>Infection<br>Partial or total flap loss<br>Altered shoulder function and strength<br>Implant migration or rupture<br>Capsular contraction of the implant |
| Gluteal perforator flaps (superior or inferior) | Skin, fat, and vessels are removed from the upper or lower buttocks and transferred.<br>Some gluteal muscle may be included in the graft.<br>Requires microvascular surgery.<br>May require vein graft. | Immediate or delayed | Pain management<br>Monitor flap for blood flow and signs of thrombosis<br>Drain care<br>Hospitalization of 4–7 days has been reported (Beshlian & Paige, 2008). | Seroma or hematoma of the breast or buttock<br>Infection<br>Partial or total flap loss<br>Sciatica<br>Flattening of the hip contour |
| Epigastric perforator flap (deep inferior and superficial inferior) | Fat and skin from the abdomen make up the flap tissue.<br>Rectus abdominis muscle is preserved. | Immediate or delayed | Pain management<br>Monitoring of flap for blood flow and signs of thrombosis<br>Drain care | Seroma or hematoma<br>Infection<br>Partial or total flap loss<br>Postoperative abdominal bulge (less common with superficial inferior epigastric perforator flap) |

*Note.* Based on information from Baron, 2007; Beshlian & Paige, 2008; Hu & Alderman, 2007; Rosson et al., 2010; Sabel, 2009; Stermer, 2008.

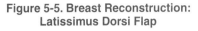

Figure 5-5. Breast Reconstruction:
Latissimus Dorsi Flap

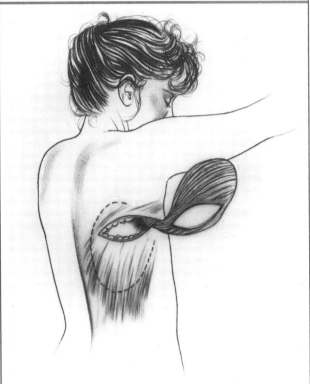

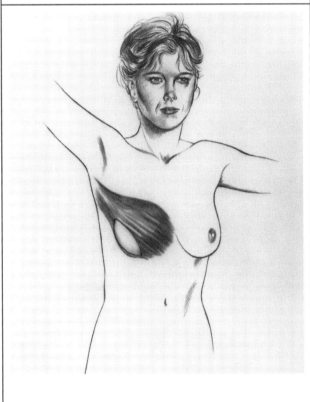

*Note.* Figures courtesy of the National Cancer Institute.

a positioning change from lateral for the flap harvest to supine for insetting of the flap, and microvascular anastomoses (Beshlian & Paige, 2008). The normal buttock contour may be altered with this procedure, but preserving muscle whenever possible helps to diminish that risk (Serletti, 2008). Donor site scars are on the buttocks with these procedures. The S-GAP scar will be on the upper buttock and usually is covered by underwear. The I-GAP scar will be on the lower buttock, usually within the lower buttock crease (Hu & Alderman, 2007). Fat from the buttocks is less pliable than with TRAM flaps, and the reconstruction may be more firm than the natural breast or the result from a TRAM flap procedure (Serletti, 2008).

Deep inferior epigastric perforator (DIEP) and superficial inferior epigastric perforator (SIEP) flaps are modifications of the TRAM flap. Tissue comes from the abdomen for TRAM, DIEP, and SIEP flaps, but the DIEP and SIEP flaps use only skin and fat and preserve the rectus abdominis muscle (Serletti, 2008). The superficial inferior epigastric artery is not always present and may be too small; therefore, the DIEP procedure is more common. Abdominal morbidity is decreased with this procedure because of preservation of the rectus muscle. It also results in less abdominal wall pain and shorter hospitalizations (Rosson et al., 2010; Serletti, 2008).

Other autologous breast reconstruction procedures include lateral thigh flaps and the Taylor-Rubens peri-iliac flap (Sabel, 2009). The Rubens procedure uses tissue from the flank as the donor site and is a good choice for small breast reconstruction. Both procedures may be useful for patients who have had TRAM flaps previously or who desire autologous reconstruction but have inadequate abdominal tissue (Rosson et al., 2009).

Nursing care for patients after autologous reconstruction includes standard postoperative care with the addition of assessment and interventions unique to this population. Postoperative pain may be significant and is the result of surgical procedures that involved both the donor tissue site and the reconstructed breast. Patient positioning for comfort may be a challenge if, for example, tissue was taken from both the right and left buttocks for a bilateral gluteal flap breast reconstruction. An aggressive approach to pain management should be in place, and continued monitoring of pain is necessary. Patients may have multiple drains, wounds, and dressings, and each must be assessed and monitored for signs of infection. Monitoring the graft for tissue perfusion is essential and may include Doppler ultrasound assessment, as well as assessment for color, turgor, and temperature. Interventions to facilitate perfusion of the tissue graft include the use of warm blankets, keeping the patient's room warm, and maintaining hydration and fluid balance. Patients wear a binder postoperatively to provide support for the breast reconstruction, but binders should not cause compression that might impair circulation. Activity may be restricted for several weeks, depending on the procedure and patient recovery. Patients are advised to refrain from heavy lifting. Limited range of motion is allowed postoperatively, depending on the procedure. Patients may be given stretching exercises in the initial postoperative period. Physical therapy may be recommended for strengthening donor sites if muscle was included in the tissue graft (Stermer, 2008).

### Nipple-Areola Complex Reconstruction

The final stage of breast reconstruction is the reconstruction of the nipple-areola complex. This usually is done between six and eight weeks after the breast reconstruction procedure, after the reconstructed breast has stabilized (Hu & Alderman, 2007; Sabel, 2009). Placement of the nipple-areola complex in the correct location and providing comparable appearance and color to the contralateral nipple-areola is essential (Sabel, 2009).

Full-thickness skin grafts can be performed to reconstruct the areola, although tattooing alone will usually result in a good cosmetic outcome. Donor sites for skin grafts include the contralateral areola, medial thigh, mastectomy scar, or TRAM incision (Hu & Alderman, 2007; Sabel, 2009). The graft is sutured into place. A nipple can be created with tab flaps elevated from the breast mound or tissue grafts. The goal is to develop an adequate nipple projection that matches the opposite breast. The area is intradermally tattooed to match pigmentation. Postoperative care includes dressing changes and assessment for signs and symptoms of infection and bleeding, as appropriate to the procedure.

The healthy contralateral breast may require surgical procedures to achieve symmetry. Procedures can be performed at the time of reconstruction or later. Mastopexy (breast lift) may be necessary to achieve an acceptable symmetrical result if a woman has marked ptosis. Breast reduction or augmentation may be recommended. Prophylactic mastectomy with or without reconstruction is also an option for the contralateral breast (Baron, 2007; Hu & Alderman, 2007). Some women use expertly fitted bras and partial prostheses (see Chapter 6).

## The Nurse's Role in the Breast Surgery Setting

Nurses in the breast surgery setting may be caring for patients in operating rooms, ambulatory surgery centers, physician offices, and inpatient units. Nurses may be direct caregivers, navigators, educators, consultants, and counselors and encounter patients before, during, and after surgery. It is important for nurses working with patients with breast cancer to have a good understanding of the rationale behind the procedures used in the surgical management of this disease and to be educated about the indications, advantages, and techniques.

Trends in the surgical management of breast cancer have dramatically changed practice and appear to have swung between the extremes of aggressive and conservative surgical approaches. Best practice questions certainly remain, but current practice allows an opportunity for the patient to make a surgical choice in several situations: BCT or mastectomy? Unilateral or bilateral surgery? Reconstruction or no reconstruction? Alloplastic or autologous reconstruction? Immediate or delayed reconstruction? In situations where a choice exists, healthcare professionals present options and make recommendations, and the patient chooses from the options, making the process one of shared decision making. In this way, consideration can be given to patient preferences and physical, emotional, and rehabilitation needs, as well as tumor characteristics. An optimal treatment plan can be made for and with each patient. The process of making choices can be daunting, especially for patients and families who may be struggling to cope with a new cancer diagnosis. In this setting, significant expertise, advocacy, education, and support from the nurse are essential.

## Conclusion

The surgical management of breast cancer is a significant part of treatment in the noninvasive, early-stage, locally advanced, and metastatic settings. Both breast and lymph node procedures are included in the surgical management of breast cancer. Breast surgery may consist of either BCT or mastectomy. Lymph node procedures include both SLNB and axillary dissection. Breast reconstruction options continue to progress. Both immediate and delayed breast reconstruction procedures are options, and reconstruction can be accomplished with several techniques.

## References

Allegra, C.J., Aberle, D.R., Ganschow, P., Hahn, S.M., Lee, C.N., Millon-Underwood, S., … Zon, R. (2010). National Institutes of Health State-of-the-Science Conference statement: Diagnosis and management of ductal carcinoma in situ, September 22–24, 2009. *Journal of the National Cancer Institute, 102,* 161–169. doi:10.1093/jnci/djp485

Baron, R.H. (2007). Surgical management of breast cancer. *Seminars in Oncology Nursing, 23,* 10–19. doi:10.1016/j.soncn.2006.11.003

Baron, R.H., Fey, J.V., Borgen, P.I., Stempel, M.M., Hardick, K.R., & Van Zee, K.J. (2007). Eighteen sensations after breast cancer surgery: A 5-year comparison of sentinel lymph node biopsy and axillary lymph node dissection. *Annals of Surgical Oncology, 14,* 1653–1661. doi:10.1245/s10434-006-9334-z

Beshlian, K.M., & Paige, K.T. (2008). Inferior gluteal artery perforator flap breast reconstruction. *American Journal of Surgery, 195,* 651–653. doi:10.1016/j.amjsurg.2007.12.041

Burstein, H.J., Harris, J.R., & Morrow, M. (2008). Malignant tumors of the breast. In V.T. DeVita Jr., S. Hellman, & S.A. Rosenberg (Eds.), *Cancer: Principles and practice of oncology* (8th ed., pp. 1606–1654). Philadelphia, PA: Lippincott Williams & Wilkins.

Carlson, G.W. (2006). Invasive carcinoma: Skin-sparing mastectomy. In S.L. Spear (Ed.), *Surgery of the breast: Principles and art* (2nd ed., Vol. 1, pp. 140–147). Philadelphia, PA: Lippincott Williams & Wilkins.

Chagpar, A.B., Scoggins, C.R., Martin, R.C., II, Sahoo, S., Carlson, D.J., Laidley, A.L., ... McMasters, K.M. (2007). Factors determining adequacy of axillary node dissection in breast cancer patients. *Breast Journal, 13,* 233–237. doi:10.1111/j.1524-4741.2007.00415.x

Chagpar, A.B., Studts, J.L., Scoggins, C.R., Martin, R.C., II, Carlson, D.J., Laidley, A.L., ... McMasters, K.M. (2006). Factors associated with surgical options for breast carcinoma. *Cancer, 106,* 1462–1466. doi:10.1002/cncr.21728

Collins, E.D., Moore, C.P., Clay, K.F., Kearing, S.A., O'Connor, A.M., Llewellyn-Thomas, H.A., ... Sepucha, K.R. (2009). Can women with early-stage breast cancer make an informed decision for mastectomy? *Journal of Clinical Oncology, 27,* 519–525. doi:10.1200/JCO.2008.16.6215

El-Tamer, M.B., Ward, B.M., Schifftner, T., Neumayer, L., Khuri, S., & Henderson, W. (2007). Morbidity and mortality following breast cancer surgery in women: National benchmarks for standards of care. *Annals of Surgery, 245,* 665–671. doi:10.1097/01.sla.0000245833.48399.9a

Farrow, D.C., Hunt, W.C., & Samet, J.M. (1992). Geographic variation in the treatment of localized breast cancer. *New England Journal of Medicine, 326,* 1097–1101. doi:10.1056/NEJM199204233261701

Garcia-Etienne, C.A., Cody, H.S., III, Disa, J.J., Cordeiro, P., & Sacchini, V. (2009). Nipple-sparing mastectomy: Initial experience at the Memorial Sloan-Kettering Cancer Center and a comprehensive review of literature. *Breast Journal, 15,* 440–449. doi:10.1111/j.1524-4741.2009.00758.x

Hu, E., & Alderman, A.K. (2007). Breast reconstruction. *Surgical Clinics of North America, 87,* 453–467. doi:10.1016/j.suc.2007.01.004

Jatoi, I., Kaufmann, M., & Petit, J.Y. (2006). *Atlas of breast surgery.* Heidelberg, Germany: Springer.

Krishnamurthy, S. (2005). Pathology of regional lymph nodes. In D.F. Roses (Ed.), *Breast cancer* (2nd ed., pp. 137–144). Philadelphia, PA: Elsevier Churchill Livingstone.

Kronowitz, S.J., & Robb, G.L. (2008). Breast reconstruction. Timing and coordination with adjuvant therapy. In C.E. Butler & N.A. Fine (Eds.), *Principles of cancer reconstructive surgery* (pp. 30–48). New York, NY: Springer.

Lee, B.T., Adesiyun, T.A., Colakoglu, S., Curtis, M.S., Yueh, J.H., Anderson, K.E., ... Recht, A. (2010). Postmastectomy radiation therapy and breast reconstruction: An analysis of complications and patient satisfaction. *Annals of Plastic Surgery, 64,* 679–683. doi:10.1097/SAP.0b013e3181db7585

Lee, C.N., Hultman, C.S., & Sepucha, K. (2010a). Do patients and providers agree about the most important facts and goals for breast reconstruction decisions? *Annals of Plastic Surgery, 64,* 563–566. doi:10.1097/SAP.0b013e3181c01279

Lee, C.N., Hultman, C.S., & Sepucha, K. (2010b). What are patients' goals and concerns about breast reconstruction after mastectomy? *Annals of Plastic Surgery, 64,* 567–569. doi:10.1097/SAP.0b013e3181bffc9b

Manasseh, D.E., & Willey, S.C. (2006). Invasive carcinoma: Mastectomy and staging the axilla. In S.L. Spear (Ed.), *Surgery of the breast: Principles and art* (2nd ed., Vol. 1, pp. 122–139). Philadelphia, PA: Lippincott Williams & Wilkins.

McLaughlin, S.A., Wright, M.J., Morris, K.T., Giron, G.L., Sampson, M.R., Brockway, J.P., ... Van Zee, K.J. (2008). Prevalence of lymphedema in women with breast cancer 5 years after sentinel lymph node biopsy or axillary dissection: Objective measurements. *Journal of Clinical Oncology, 28,* 5213–5219. doi:10.1200/JCO.2008.16.3725

National Comprehensive Cancer Network. (2010a, December). *NCCN Clinical Practice Guidelines in Oncology™: Breast cancer* [v.2.2011]. Retrieved from http://www.nccn.org/professionals/physician_gls/PDF/breast.pdf

National Comprehensive Cancer Network. (2010b, August). *NCCN Clinical Practice Guidelines in Oncology™: Breast cancer risk reduction* [v.2.2010]. Retrieved from http://www.nccn.org/professionals/physician_gls/PDF/breast_risk.pdf

National Institutes of Health. (1991). Early-stage breast cancer. NIH Consensus Conference. *JAMA, 265,* 391–395.

Nattinger, A.B., Gottlieb, M.S., Veum, J., Yahnke, D., & Goodwin, J.S. (1992). Geographic variation in the use of breast-conserving treatment for breast cancer. *New England Journal of Medicine, 326,* 1102–1107. doi:10.1056/NEJM199204233261702

Newman, E.A., & Newman, L.A. (2007). Lymphatic mapping techniques and sentinel lymph node biopsy in breast cancer. *Surgical Clinics of North America, 87,* 353–364. doi:10.1016/j.suc.2007.01.013

O'Sullivan, M.J., & Morrow, M. (2007). Ductal carcinoma in situ—Current management. *Surgical Clinics of North America, 87,* 333–351. doi:10.1016/j.suc.2007.01.006

Palmieri, F.M., & Perez, E.A. (2007). Managing high-risk breast cancer. *Seminars in Oncology Nursing, 23,* 29–36. doi:10.1016/j.soncn.2006.11.005

Povoski, S.P., & Barsky, S.H. (2009). In situ carcinomas of the breast: Ductal carcinoma in situ and lobular carcinoma in situ. In K.I. Bland & E.M. Copeland III (Eds.), *The breast: Comprehensive management of benign and malignant diseases* (4th ed., pp. 211–229). Philadelphia, PA: Elsevier Saunders.

Rivers, A., & Hansen, N. (2007). Axillary management after sentinel lymph node biopsy in breast cancer patients. *Surgical Clinics of North America, 87,* 365–377. doi:10.1016/j.suc.2007.01.014

Rosen, P.P. (2009). *Rosen's breast pathology* (3rd ed.). Philadelphia, PA: Lippincott Williams & Wilkins.

Roses, D.F. (2005). Development of modern breast cancer treatment. In D.F. Roses (Ed.), *Breast cancer* (2nd ed., pp. 333–353). Philadelphia, PA: Elsevier Churchill Livingstone.

Roses, D.F., & Giuliano, A.E. (2005). Surgery for breast cancer. In D.F. Roses (Ed.), *Breast cancer* (2nd ed., pp. 401–452). Philadelphia, PA: Elsevier Churchill Livingstone.

Rosson, G.D., Magarakis, M., Shridharani, S.M., Stapleton, S.M., Jackobs, L.K., Manahan, M.A., & Flores, J.I. (2010). A review of the surgical management of breast cancer: Plastic reconstructive techniques and timing implications. *Annals of Surgical Oncology, 17,* 1890–1900. doi:10.1245/s10434-010-0913-7

Rusby, J.E., Smith, B.L., & Gui, G.P.H. (2010). Nipple-sparing mastectomy. *British Journal of Surgery, 97,* 305–316. doi:10.1002/bjs.6970

Sabel, M.S. (2009). *Surgical foundations: Essentials of breast surgery.* Philadelphia, PA: Elsevier Mosby.

Schwartz, G.F. (2005). Treatment of in situ breast cancer. In D.F. Roses (Ed.), *Breast cancer* (2nd ed., pp. 383–399). Philadelphia, PA: Elsevier Churchill Livingstone.

Serletti, J.M. (2008). Breast reconstruction. Autogenous tissue. In C.E. Butler & N.A. Fine (Eds.), *Principles of cancer reconstructive surgery* (pp. 49–61). New York, NY: Springer.

Stermer, C. (2008). Helping your patient after breast reconstruction. *Plastic Surgical Nursing, 30,* 40–43. doi:10.1097/PSN.0b013e3181dc9498

Tuttle, T.M., Jarosek, S., Habermann, E.B., Arrington, A., Abraham, A., Morris, T.J., & Virnig, B.A. (2009). Increasing rates of contralateral prophylactic mastectomy among patients with ductal carcinoma in situ. *Journal of Clinical Oncology, 27,* 1362–1367. doi:10.1200/JCO.2008.20.1681

Virnig, B.A., Tuttle, T.M., Shamliyan, T., & Kane, R.L. (2010). Ductal carcinoma in situ of the breast: A systematic review of the incidence, treatment, and outcomes. *Journal of the National Cancer Institute, 102,* 170–178. doi:10.1093/jnci/djp482

Vitug, A.F., & Newman, L.A. (2007). Complications in breast surgery. *Surgical Clinics of North America, 87,* 431–451. doi:10.1016/j.suc.2007.01.005

Wagstaff, M.J.D., Reed, M.W.R., & Caddy, C.M. (2010). Breast reconstruction. In M.W.R. Reed & R.A. Audisio (Eds.), *Management of breast cancer in older women* (pp. 213–220). London, England: Springer. doi:10.1007/978-1-84800-265-4

# CHAPTER 6

# Breast Restoration Options Utilizing Prostheses

Michelle A. Casey, CFA, and Suzanne M. Mahon, RN, DNSc, AOCN®, APNG

## Introduction

Restoration of the breast is an important aspect in the care and rehabilitation of all women diagnosed with breast cancer. For most women, local treatment of breast cancer usually involves some surgical treatment of the breast. Many of these women will require at least some degree of breast restoration to improve body image and prevent physical problems. Breast restoration might include surgical procedures to reconstruct a breast (see Chapter 5), as well as the use of prostheses. A major nursing intervention is to assess patients' satisfaction with body image, comfort, and cosmesis, as well as to provide support and refer women to a fitter who may be able to assist with an appropriate bra or prosthesis. Prostheses also are extremely useful in correcting breast disparities that result because of extensive or multiple surgical biopsies or atrophy occurring long-term following lumpectomy and radiation. In some cases, they are useful for improving the outcome of reconstructive surgery. Along with prostheses, many women achieve improved cosmesis with the use of expertly fitted bras and camisoles.

Many mistakenly believe that only women who have a mastectomy will benefit from an expert bra fitting or prostheses. Women who have some breast disparity, either due to lumpectomy and radiation or from reconstruction, should also be regularly referred for evaluation because it is possible and often relatively simple to correct the disparity and improve cosmesis and overall adjustment to body image changes with a proper bra fitting and, in some cases, a small prosthesis. Many women do not even realize this is an option, and they suffer in silence. Nurses can offer referral and encouragement to women in all phases of the breast cancer trajectory to explore options to improve bra fit and breast symmetry.

## Body Image

Breast restoration is central to restoring and improving body image after the surgical management of breast cancer.

Issues related to breast surgery and body image often are discussed in the nursing and medical literature (Ganz, 2008; Helms, O'Hea, & Corso, 2008). Adjustment to changes or disturbances in body image contributes to the quality of life in those diagnosed with cancer (Cidón, 2010; Skrzypulec, Tobor, Drosdzol, & Nowosielski, 2009). Nurses who provide education and information about breast restoration ultimately can help to improve the quality of life for breast cancer survivors and, in many cases, women who have undergone breast biopsy.

Women who undergo lumpectomy and reconstruction may not achieve the cosmesis they anticipated with their surgical choice. Although literature is limited, women undergoing breast-conserving therapy, or lumpectomy and radiation, may not be satisfied with the cosmetic outcome of surgery. In one study, 25% of the subjects (n = 83) who underwent breast-conserving therapy were distressed and dissatisfied with the resulting cosmesis (Markopoulos et al., 2009). Similar results were reported in a study of 110 women undergoing reconstruction (Fernández-Delgado et al., 2008). Nurses should not assume that women who undergo these procedures are satisfied with the outcome.

The concept of body image has several dimensions. Cohen, Kahn, and Steeves (1998) noted that body image includes not only the mental picture of the physical self but also who that person believes she is and how she feels about herself. When a woman looks in the mirror and perceives herself to be attractive, she can be more confident. Breast restoration also helps to reduce or remove the constant reminder that the woman has faced a life-threatening diagnosis. It can allow her to wear attractive clothes comfortably, which ultimately results in improved self-image.

Treatment for breast cancer includes not only treatment for the cancer but treatment of the person as well. Women need instruction, encouragement, and support as they pursue options for breast restoration and need to be reminded that this is important to their long-term well-being and recovery. Often, in the midst of active treatment with chemotherapy and radiation therapy, women neglect this aspect of their care or feel that it is an inappropriate concern. Conversely, pursuing breast restoration should improve self-image and well-being and ultimately will make other aspects of care easier to tolerate. Ganz (2008) emphasized that most women benefit significantly from having a knowledgeable and considerate healthcare provider helping them to better understand the options available for breast restoration, including the use of a prosthesis or reconstructive surgery.

## Prostheses

### Selecting a Fitter

Nursing responsibility begins with supporting women in their decision to explore breast restoration options and referring them to reputable providers. Many more options for breast prostheses are now available. It is no longer satisfactory to "send" women to a place to "get" a prosthesis. Prior to making a referral, it is important to know if a patient's insurance coverage dictates which provider is used. This sometimes influences the referral.

Oncology nurses who discuss the need for breast prostheses with patients must be able to understand what the prosthesis-fitting experience is like for patients. Using this information, nurses can provide anticipatory guidance for patients so that they will know what to expect during the fitting and how they can prepare for it. It is recommended that nurses meet with prosthetic providers in the setting where care is provided. This will allow the nurses to specifically describe how, when, and where the fitting will occur and guide women through the process. In many cases, fitters can provide nurses with a few samples of prostheses and bras to show patients prior to a fitting. This can give them some idea of what to expect and some hope that it is still possible to wear beautiful undergarments.

It takes a tremendous amount of courage for women to have a breast prosthesis fitted, and oncology nurses are well suited to provide support and encouragement for women as they go through the fitting process. Research suggests that the fitting for a prosthesis can be as difficult and emotionally upsetting as the surgical procedure or diagnosis of cancer itself (Roberts, Livingston, White, & Gibbs, 2003).

Nurses need to emphasize that the fitting is a process, probably for life, and not a single, isolated event. Ideally, women will have the fit checked annually. For this reason, it is critical that the woman is comfortable working with the fitter. As a woman's body changes because of treatment or the normal effects of aging, different prostheses or bras might be needed. Nurses who care for women during long-term follow-up can facilitate long-term adjustment to body image by encouraging women to be reevaluated and refitted when changes are needed. Often, these women are not aware of the need for continued evaluation of a prosthesis,

particularly if their surgery was done many years ago when choices were more limited.

Although research is limited, as many as 30% of women are dissatisfied with the external prosthesis for which they have been fitted (Roberts et al., 2003). Dissatisfaction often is linked to the fitting experience, including insufficient time, lack of privacy, fitting by a man, incorrect fit, weight of prosthesis, natural appearance, and attitude of the fitter (Livingston et al., 2005). Dissatisfaction also occurs when the prosthesis is uncomfortable to wear or if clothing and lingerie choices are extremely limited.

### Prosthetic Centers

Oncology nurses often are the first to initiate a referral to a prosthetic center. These nurses must be familiar with the resources in their community and geographic area to make appropriate referrals. Being fitted for any type of breast prosthesis can be a very emotional experience for women, and it is important to ensure that they receive not only a well-fitted prosthesis but also a caring and personal environment for the fitting. Because of the number of measurements and considerations in selecting an appropriate prosthesis, it is often best to discourage mail-order prosthesis options. A fitter typically can provide the woman with a wide variety of options that cannot be explored online or in a catalog.

Nurses must learn who will be providing the fitting for their patients. Certification for fitters is available through each individual breast prosthesis manufacturer. This type of certification typically involves a one-day seminar. In these seminars, content usually includes the principles of taking measurements, the shapes of prostheses, and various bra styles. These seminars are presented by the manufacturers of these items. At the end of the day, participants usually take an open-book test on the content. This training is aimed at familiarizing the fitters with the manufacturer's products and, ultimately, promoting their sale.

Certification by a manufacturer is probably not adequate to ensure the expertise of a fitter. Apprenticeship with an experienced, competent fitter is paramount. Typically, this period of training takes several months. Fitters can come from various educational backgrounds. These might include degrees in education, medical subspecialties, or a social sciences background, or sometimes fitters are long-term survivors of cancer.

Because prosthesis fitters can come from so many different backgrounds, it is important to ensure that women are referred to a fitter who is empathetic, caring, and adequately trained, preferably through an apprenticeship. Excellent interpersonal skills are extremely important to ensure that the fitting process is as easy as possible for patients.

The actual setting where the fitting occurs is another important consideration. Prostheses can be purchased from many different places. Women should be assured that the fitting will occur in a private area. Optimally, the area where the fitting occurs should be feminine and nonclinical in nature.

## Prosthetic Needs and Services Available at the Time of Diagnosis

At the time of diagnosis, some women find it beneficial to learn about the various prosthetic options. As many as 50% of women having a mastectomy may never have been informed that they had the option of learning about prostheses and visiting a fitter prior to surgery. Such a visit may be associated with overall long-term satisfaction with a prosthesis (Glaus & Carlson, 2009). Although this is a busy time for patients, especially prior to surgery, nurses should encourage women to learn about what options are available. Women who are having difficulty deciding between mastectomy and breast-sparing surgery may find it helpful to understand the options for permanent prostheses or reconstruction following mastectomy. For women considering whether to have immediate reconstruction, education about the various prosthetic options, both temporary and long-term, can facilitate decision making. Most reputable fitters are willing to see women during this time frame.

Seeing the fitter prior to surgery helps the woman to establish a relationship with the fitter, as well as to begin to realistically anticipate what will happen in the future. This visit also provides the fitter with an opportunity to provide the patient with a temporary prosthesis to use in the immediate postoperative period. For many women, this can alleviate a significant amount of worry about what to expect right after surgery.

If it is not possible for patients to see the fitter before surgery (which is frequently the case), some prosthetic centers will make a few different types of prostheses and bras available for nurses to show patients in the office or clinic setting prior to surgery. Although this is not a replacement for seeing the fitter, it can give women a much more tangible idea of what to expect and what a prosthesis actually looks and feels like.

Regardless of whether patients see the fitter preoperatively, a discussion regarding prosthesis and bra options can help women to begin to understand and assimilate the process of breast restoration. This anticipatory guidance also will help women to realize that it is normal and appropriate to be concerned about their appearance, despite many other significant treatment issues and decisions that must be dealt with during this time.

## Temporary Prostheses and Postoperative Items

Although it is optimal for women to see the fitter prior to surgery, in reality, this is difficult to achieve. It is, however, important for all women undergoing breast surgery to have access to a temporary prosthesis. A temporary prosthesis is a lightweight, fiber-filled prosthesis that can be worn immedi-

ately following surgery. If worn in a nonsurgical bra, it should be shaped and pinned to the bra to prevent movement. They come in a wide variety of sizes and shapes.

Most temporary prostheses are generically sized. Some, such as those provided through the American Cancer Society (ACS), have an opening through which excess fiber can be removed to achieve a more symmetric appearance in the bra. It is important to assure the woman receiving the prosthesis that almost all women remove some of the filling and that there is nothing wrong with her because she needs to adjust the size. She should be assured that the temporary prosthesis tends to be sized large. It is even more important to assure her that a temporary prosthesis is much different from the one she will eventually use. The permanent prosthesis will stay in place and will therapeutically replace the weight of the breast lost in surgery. A permanent prosthesis will not need continual adjustments.

A temporary prosthesis may be given to patients through ACS's Reach to Recovery program, which also typically includes literature and a visit from a breast cancer survivor (ACS, 2010). Nurses need to become familiar with how the program is administered in their geographic region. This referral usually requires a physician's order. The volunteers receive special training and do not administer medical advice. They will show patients how to use the temporary prosthesis. In some cases, temporary prostheses also may be distributed through a prosthetic center. Nurses working in breast care need to explore what options are readily available in their geographic area and provide assistance to patients in accessing these resources.

Some of the temporary prostheses can range in cost from $6–$80. When available, the Reach to Recovery program provides the temporary prosthesis free of charge. The availability of free or low-cost temporary prostheses makes it unnecessary for women to try to camouflage the physical effects of the surgery in the immediate postoperative period with socks, cotton, washcloths, sanitary pads, shoulder pads, or other novel means.

The temporary prosthesis can be worn in a front-hook leisure bra, a prosthetic camisole, or the woman's own bra. The bra straps can be adjusted to obtain a more symmetric appearance. A leisure bra is a soft, comfortable, front-hook, pocketed bra. In a single mastectomy, it gives support to the unaffected breast and contains the temporary prosthesis. A disadvantage of temporary prostheses is that they tend to move up the chest wall, especially with movement. A leisure bra, camisole, or the woman's own bra can help to anchor the prosthesis.

A prosthetic camisole is a soft, pocketed camisole that can be tucked into pants or skirts and helps to prevent the prosthesis from moving up the chest wall (see Figure 6-1). This camisole also may be useful for women who have drains in place or who find wearing a bra uncomfortable, especially in the immediate postoperative period or during chest wall radiation. Drain pouches are a relatively new development that can ease discomfort in the postoperative period (see Figure 6-2). The drain pouch is made of cotton that attaches with Velcro® (Velcro Industries) strips to the band portion of most bras or camisoles. The drain pouch prevents accidental tugging of the drain and camouflages the drain so it is not a constant reminder.

Some insurance companies will pay a portion of the costs for a leisure bra or prosthetic camisole. Sometimes, however, it is in the woman's best interest to not use all of her benefits for a temporary prosthesis and to save the coverage for a permanent prosthesis. Clarification of benefits is extremely important. Some women will choose to buy the bra or camisole and pay out of pocket. Leisure bras and prosthetic camisoles can be used both in the immediate postoperative period and also long term. Many women wear them while sleeping or relaxing at home.

### Permanent Prostheses

Most women are ready to be fitted for a permanent prosthesis four to six weeks following a mastectomy. This waiting period allows for postoperative swelling and skin sensi-

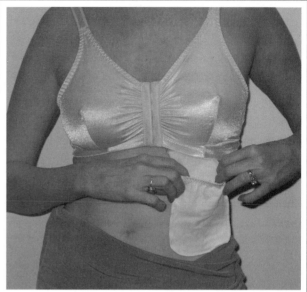

**Figure 6-2. Drain Pouch**

A postoperative drain pouch provides a means for women to secure one or more postoperative drains.

**Figure 6-1. Postoperative Camisole, Drain Pouch, and Temporary Prosthesis**

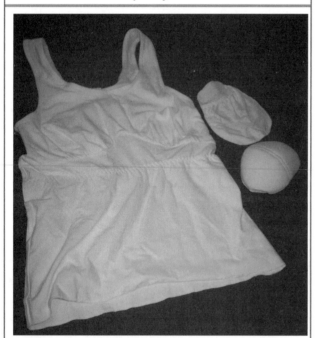

Temporary prostheses are sized based on the woman's bra cup size and, to a lesser extent, the band size. They are available in a variety of shades and sizes. Most require some adjustment and need to be pinned in the bra or placed in a prosthetic camisole. Some women prefer to place the temporary prosthesis in a prosthetic camisole, which might be more comfortable during the immediate postoperative period and sometimes during reconstruction and radiation therapy.

tivity to resolve. Prior to the fitting, it is important to determine insurance coverage and obtain preauthorization (see Figure 6-3). This may take a few days to a week or more depending on the amount of information that is needed and the letters of medical necessity that may be required. The prosthetic center usually can assist women in finding out this information and completing the necessary paperwork. Women also should ascertain that the prosthetic provider is a recognized provider for their insurance company, or the benefits could be significantly reduced or eliminated for prosthetic coverage.

Fitting a permanent prosthesis usually takes at least one to two hours. Some helpful reminders for a woman going to a fitting are included in Figure 6-4. Many prosthetic centers prefer that clients make an appointment to ensure that a fitter will be available. It takes a lot of courage for patients to come for a fitting. It is optimal for the woman to bring a supportive person along for the fitting, such as a sister, spouse, relative, or friend. She also should bring a solid-color, form-fitting shirt or sweater, or some other piece of clothing that she did not think she would be able to wear again, along with any bras she had liked to wear in the past, because often it is possible to continue to use those bras. These bras also provide insight for the fitter on what the woman preferred prior to surgery.

At the fitting, the woman should be taken into a private room. The fitter usually will begin by getting acquainted with the woman. This includes conversing about her surgery, a little about her experiences to date, anticipated treatment, and lifestyle. This conversation will help to relax the woman and,

**Figure 6-3. Questions to Ask About Insurance Coverage**

- Is the fitter an approved provider in the insurance network?
- How much are benefits changed if the woman chooses an out-of-network provider?
- What are the preauthorization requirements?
- Is a prescription adequate, or is a letter of medical necessity required?
- Is there a deductible, and has it been met? What is the out-of-pocket expense amount, and has it been met?
- What percentage of the cost of a form is covered?
- What permanent forms (brands/types) are covered? Are replacement forms covered? Under what circumstances are replacements covered? How often can forms be replaced?
- Is there a charge to see the fitter?
- Are bras covered? Do they need to be a specific type?
- How many bras are covered per year?
- How frequently can bras be replaced?
- Are other garments, such as camisoles, covered?
- Are leisure forms covered (e.g., swimming, exercise, and temporary forms)?

**Figure 6-4. Things to Do and Consider When Going to a Prosthetic Fitting**

- Make an appointment with a fitter.
- Ascertain that the fitter is an approved provider for insurance and that insurance benefits have been verified.
- Bring an objective, supportive person.
- Bring bras that have been previously worn to determine whether they still can be used or adapted with pockets. This affords the fitter some insight into the types of bras the woman has previously preferred to wear.
- Bring a tight-fitting, solid-color top to help to assess for symmetry.
- Bring any items of clothing that the woman desires to wear but is concerned that it may no longer be possible.
- Plan on spending at least an hour at the initial fitting.
- If after a short period of wearing a prosthesis or bra, the fit is not as comfortable as anticipated, contact the fitter to assess if any adjustments need to be made. Realize that the fit of the prosthesis should be assessed on a regular (usually annual) basis.
- Bring an open mind and be willing to try different bras and forms.

more importantly, will provide the fitter with important information about the patient so that she will receive the prosthesis and other items that will best meet her needs and ultimately improve her quality of life. The fitter also can tell the woman about what the fitting process will entail.

Next, the woman will be asked to unbutton or pull up her top so that the fitter can take some general measurements and see what type of bra the woman has chosen in the past. Many women are surprised to learn of the importance of the bra fitting and that a bra is fitted prior to fitting the prosthesis. Fitting the bra first is important because the bra shapes

the unaffected breast and has a big impact on the woman's ultimate comfort.

Typically, the fitter will bring a wide variety of styles of bras into the room. The woman will be asked to remove her top and bra and will try on a variety of bras. These bras often will have pockets to secure the prosthesis. When both the fitter and the woman are satisfied with the bra in terms of appearance and comfort, a selection of prostheses is introduced.

Permanent prostheses come in a variety of shapes and sizes (see Figure 6-5). These include nonattachable prostheses traditionally used in the pocket of a bra. At this point in the fitting, the fitter should talk to the patient about the importance of replacing the weight lost with the surgery. It is extremely important to correctly replace the weight to prevent long-term complications to the back, neck, and shoulder areas. If the weight is not replaced, the body will compensate with shoulder drop on the affected side. Often, in trying to conceal asymmetry, women will curve and drop the affected shoulder. The weight of the permanent prosthesis also keeps the prosthesis in place on the chest wall. Some women, especially older adults, state that the weight is important to restore balance. Insurance companies actually cover the costs associated with a prosthesis because of the need for weight replacement, not for cosmetic or psychological reasons.

Traditional prostheses are made from silicone encased in polyurethane. They are molded into various shapes, densities, weights, and sizes. After a single mastectomy, the first prosthesis is placed in the bra, and the fitter takes a measurement from the center seam to an outer seam and compares it with the unaffected side. This helps to guide the fitter on sizing. The fitter takes a measurement from the collarbone to the nipple area to ensure that projection is equal and there is symmetry. The woman also is observed moving her arms and shoulders. She is questioned about comfort and the general feel. Many different prostheses often need to be tried before a proper fit is achieved. The fitter should always listen to the woman because, ultimately, the woman will select what is best for her. The fitter considers the shape and size of the remaining breast, as well as the amount of tissue on the chest wall and under the arm.

If the woman has had a bilateral mastectomy, it is important to consider any disparities in the chest wall landscape. Women who had a mastectomy many years ago may have less tissue on the chest wall on one side. Sometimes different shaped or sized prostheses need to be used to achieve symmetry. The same consideration may be applicable in women who have had a mastectomy on one side and a lumpectomy on the other. Weight replacement is still important for bilateral mastectomy patients, and time must be taken to adequately assess what feels appropriate for the woman and avoid the misconception of fitting a prosthesis that is too light.

Prostheses are available in many different shapes. Some prostheses are designed for more radical surgeries. These tend to be fuller and have a tail that extends under the arm. Those designed for modified mastectomies taper more grad-

## Figure 6-5. Permanent Prostheses

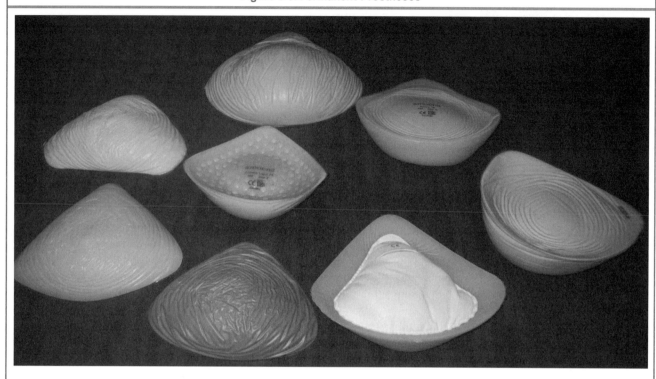

Permanent prostheses come in a wide range of sizes, shapes, colors, and weights.

ually to the chest wall and do not extend as far under the arm (see Figure 6-5).

The prosthesis can be made out of different densities of silicone to simulate the density of the natural breast. If the woman has more ptosis, which occurs naturally with aging, a soft, dual-layer prosthesis might be best. This prosthesis has a firm back and a very soft conformable front, which can simulate a pendulous breast.

The weight of the prosthesis is an extremely important consideration. Some manufacturers whip air into the silicone before it is molded to reduce the weight of the prostheses by 15%–20%. Thus, prostheses come in many different weights, and there is an optimal weight for each woman. Most women will know which feels the best and is balanced. The fitter has to be responsible in this area. It is important not to fit a prosthesis that is too light because therapeutic weight replacement will not be achieved, and the woman will be at risk for developing shoulder drop. The fitter also needs to let the woman help in making this determination. It is best for the fitter not to describe a prosthesis as light or heavy because it may prejudice the decision. Many women will be more comfortable with their decision if they take a prosthesis home and wear it to determine whether it is the right fit. If it truly is uncomfortable, they can exchange it for a different one. Women also need to acclimate their body to the weight from the prosthesis. A typical schedule is for the woman to wear it for two to three hours the first day and then add two hours each day. This helps to reduce minor body aches.

Attachable prostheses are available with rejuvenating silicone on the back of the prosthesis (see Figures 6-6, 6-7, 6-8, and 6-9). This prosthesis should be supported by a bra or camisole. The silicone sticks directly to the chest wall. The woman must be willing to meticulously care for this prosthesis on a daily basis. At night, the prosthesis must be scrubbed with a cleansing solution and a scrub brush to reactivate the silicone. Occasionally this type of prosthesis may not work well for women with heavy perspiration or for intensive swimming.

Today, prostheses are made in a few different shades to better match the skin color of women of different ethnicities. Most manufacturers have prostheses in blush and tawny for African American women. This includes both the attachable and nonattachable types.

Also, some general care instructions exist for all women who wear a permanent prosthesis. The prosthesis should be washed with a mild soap and water and towel-dried daily. Ideally, they are stored in a cradle, which comes with the prosthesis. This cradle supports the shape of the silicone prosthesis and increases its longevity. Most silicone breast prostheses have a two-year warranty against defects, such as gel separation or peeling finish.

For some women, a custom prosthesis is an appropriate choice. This may be the case if they have an uneven or irregular chest wall. In addition, some women will be comfortable only if they have an aesthetic reproduction of their breast. A custom prosthesis may allow the woman to choose the exact skin tone and size. A cast is made of the chest wall, the other breast, and a bra with a prosthesis. A custom prosthesis is bra-specific, so careful bra selection is critical. A cast also is made of the nipple. This form has a nipple, fits the chest wall, and is worn directly against the body, not in a pocket. The woman needs to be at a stable weight. Benefits include that many women like the personalization

**Figure 6-6. Attachable Prosthesis With Rejuvenating Silicone**

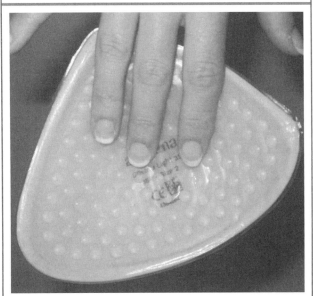

An attachable prosthesis sticks to the skin.

**Figure 6-7. Placement of Attachable Prosthesis**

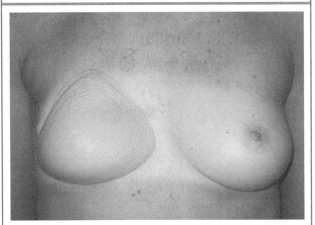

This demonstrates the placement of an attachable prosthesis to the skin. This woman is able to wear this prosthesis with a two-piece swimming suit.

**Figure 6-8. Attachable Prosthesis Supported by a Bra**

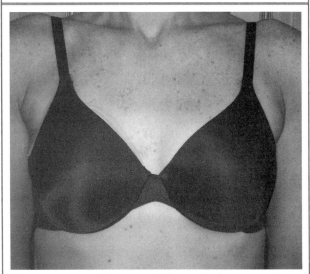

The same woman with an attachable prosthesis supported by a bra. It is important to instruct women who use prostheses that a wide selection of attractive bra styles is available.

**Figure 6-9. Symmetry With Attachable Prosthesis**

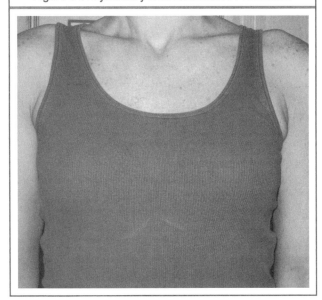

and that it can be worn when swimming. The approximate cost is $3,000, and it sometimes is covered by insurance. Specialized training is needed to fit a custom prosthesis.

## Restoration to Correct Lumpectomy, Reconstruction, and Surgical Disparities

Partial prostheses are available for women who have had lumpectomies, reconstruction, or multiple biopsies or those with congenital disparities. These come in varying shapes, thicknesses, and sizes. Some fitters will custom design prostheses with fiber-filled pads or foam breast cups. Many times, a well-fitted, supportive bra can disguise the disparity and is all that is needed. These principles also are helpful to women undergoing reconstruction using expanders, during which time their prosthesis needs to be changed. After a woman has a lumpectomy and radiation, a disparity often becomes evident after time. This may be due to weight changes or the effects of radiation on the skin. This also can occur in women without breast cancer who have undergone multiple incisional biopsies. Over time a disparity may become evident. Although these women did not anticipate they would need the services of a fitter, their appearance and self-esteem can be greatly enhanced with a well-fitted bra to disguise the disparity. Occasionally a partial prosthesis is needed. They come in a wide variety of shapes and sizes (see Figure 6-10).

For women who choose not to have surgical nipple reconstruction, many ready-made nipples are available, as well as custom-cast nipples. The ready-made nipples come in a variety of circumferences, thicknesses, colors, and nipple projections (see Figure 6-11). The custom-cast nipples are cast from the remaining nipple or are cast prior to surgery, and exact skin tones and projection are selected.

Women who have undergone reconstruction may especially benefit from the services of a fitter. Despite best efforts, breast disparity can sometimes exist. Bras can often correct this. These disparities often are very simple to correct, but women fail to receive these corrective options. Many women expend a lot of energy and experience much frustration as they try to correct these problems with home remedies. Insurance companies are mandated to provide prostheses and bras for any woman who is undergoing breast surgery, but many women are not aware of this. Nurses must educate women about this service to help them to avoid the frustration and discouragement associated with the problem.

The best way to educate women about these options is unclear. Often it is easiest to just ask a woman if her bra is comfortable. Many women do not know that insurance coverage for bras is available. Encouraging women to have the bra fitted properly enables a fitter to suggest other options to correct the disparity. Many women believe that the sole purpose of a

---

**Figure 6-10. Partial Prostheses**

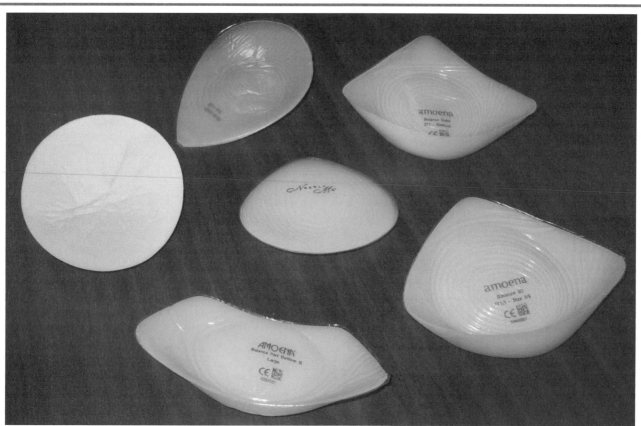

Various shapes and sizes of partial prostheses are available.

## Figure 6-11. Attachable Nipples

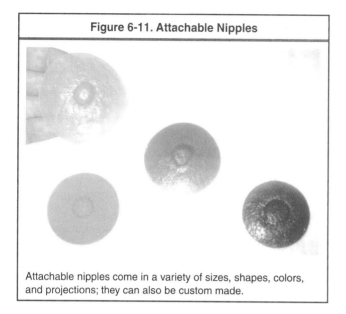

Attachable nipples come in a variety of sizes, shapes, colors, and projections; they can also be custom made.

lumpectomy or reconstruction is to completely eliminate the need for prosthetic services. However, it is impossible, even with the most talented surgeons, to completely eliminate disparities. Weight gain or weight loss also can result in disparity. For many women being treated with lumpectomy and radiation, the disparities magnify with time. Often, refitting the bra will eliminate many problems.

Healthcare providers need to develop strategies and approaches to discuss these issues with women. Asking women whether they have had any trouble with wearing clothes or if they are satisfied with the surgical outcome of the lumpectomy or reconstruction will open the door to providing this education. This needs to be done in a caring, nonjudgmental, nonthreatening, and unhurried manner.

## Insurance Issues

Federal law now mandates that insurance cover the initial breast prosthesis or breast reconstruction. This includes a partial breast prosthesis for women who go through reconstruction and do not desire to have surgery on the unaffected breast. This law also provides for women who have had lumpectomies and need a partial prosthesis to correct disparity. Insurance companies cover different prostheses at varying amounts. Some insurance companies dictate what prostheses will be covered or mandate that a specific provider be used. Medicare covers 80% of each state's allowable amount for the permanent prosthesis every two years, a leisure bra every six months, and a portion of up to six bras per year after the deductible is met. Supplemental policies typically will cover the remaining portion of the allowable amount depending on the policy. Most private insurance covers two bras per year for women who have had breast cancer surgery.

Optimally, women should consult their insurance policy before being fitted to be sure that the facility is an approved provider. Figure 6-3 provides a list of questions to help women to better understand their benefits. Most reputable fitters will precertify or verify benefits before the fitting to provide optimal coverage and choice in forms and other accessories. Often, women will need preauthorization, a prescription, or a letter of medical necessity prior to a fitting. Fitters usually will help women in obtaining the proper paperwork from their oncologist, surgeon, or primary care provider.

Replacement prostheses frequently will be covered when the proper documentation of need is submitted for medical review. Most prostheses have two-year warranties, and few last beyond that time. Weight gain or loss (often as little as 5–10 pounds) also may necessitate a replacement prosthesis. Furthermore, women who were diagnosed many years ago may not be aware of the laws and benefits that may be available to them.

## Accessories

At the time of diagnosis, women frequently think they will have to give up many things because of surgery. This might include activities such as swimming or being able to wear beautiful bras or other lingerie. Pockets can be sewn into bras with adequate support for the prosthesis and for coverage of the breast. This allows women to continue to wear bras they had selected prior to surgery. Additionally, swimsuits are available with a pocket or pockets (see Figure 6-12). These suits typically are more conservatively cut with higher coverage and more material under the arm. Pockets

## Figure 6-12. Swimming Prosthesis in Suit

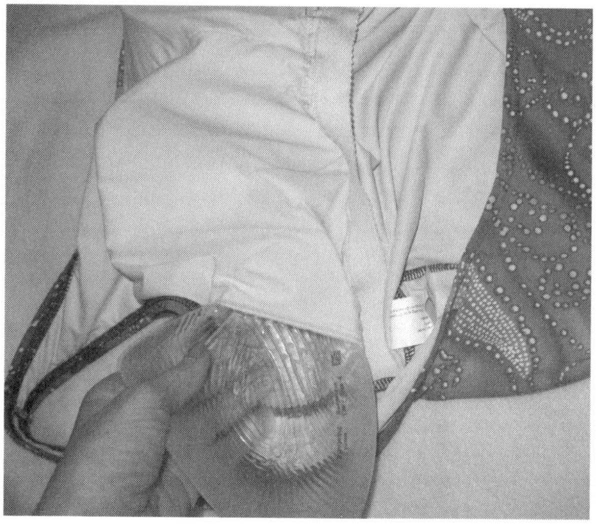

Swimming prosthesis is placed in a pocket in a swimsuit.

also can be sewn into swimsuits that provide adequate coverage of the surgical area. Different types of swimming and exercise forms are available and often are covered by insurance under a separate billing code. These can be made of fiberfill or a firm, durable type of silicone (see Figure 6-13). These forms also are appropriate for women who want to exercise vigorously. Insurance often will pay for these prostheses as well.

---

**Figure 6-13. Swimming and Exercise Prostheses**

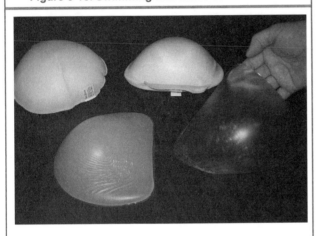

Some swimming and exercise prostheses are fiber-filled; others are made of silicone and may be flesh colored or clear.

---

## Conclusion

Providing women with comprehensive education about breast prostheses and other restoration accessories is a very important but often overlooked responsibility of nurses. Nurses can assist patients with adjusting to body image changes and can facilitate coping by offering encouragement and education about prostheses and what to anticipate during the fitting process. To provide this education and support, nurses must be knowledgeable about the prosthesis resources in the geographic area in which they practice. Optimally, nurses who make the referrals for fittings should know the fitters and have visited the site where the fitting will occur. This helps nurses to provide guidance to patients before the fitting. When the healthcare provider knows the fitter, the result is improved collaboration and more continuity of care.

Women need to realize that the decision to use a prosthesis or have reconstructive surgery is a personal one (Resnick & Belcher, 2002). There is not necessarily a right or wrong answer for any one woman. Women need to feel supported in their decision. Research suggests that women who explore their options carefully prior to surgery, are well educated about all options, and feel they have a major role in all aspects of the decision-making process tend to be more satisfied with whatever choice they make for breast restoration (Glaus & Carlson, 2009). Nurses need to reassure patients and support them in whatever decision they make in order to promote and improve their quality of life.

Unlike in the past, women who will need a full or partial breast prosthesis now have many different options available. Nurses need to be aware of the many options that exist and encourage women that a good fit is possible. Although a prosthesis will never completely replace what was lost with surgery, a well-fitted prosthesis can make an enormous difference in how a woman ultimately adjusts to the cancer diagnosis and the changes in her body image. A well-fitted prosthesis also will help to prevent long-term complications, including shoulder drop. Positive adjustment to these changes in body image ultimately improves the long-term quality of life for women diagnosed with breast cancer.

For women who are weighing the decision of whether to use a prosthesis or undergo reconstruction, it may be helpful to speak with women who have made the choice, are satisfied with their choice, and will not provide medical advice. Having contacts who have had positive experiences with both reconstruction and prostheses may be helpful.

One area in which oncology nurses can have a large impact is in assessment and referral for women who underwent surgery many years ago. Optimally, women should see prosthetic fitters approximately every two years. Changes in weight because of therapy, hormonal manipulation, or aging often necessitate a change in the prosthesis. Many women do not realize that the prosthesis will not last a lifetime and that insurance often will cover replacement costs. Nurses who see women during their follow-up should inquire about the fit of the prosthesis and when patients last saw a fitter for evaluation. Nurses then can encourage women to follow up with the fitter and can make referrals as needed. In addition to ensuring that the woman is wearing a well-fitted prosthesis, this assessment also communicates the nurse's continued care and concern about the survivor's overall well-being.

## References

American Cancer Society. (2010). Reach to Recovery. Retrieved from http://www.cancer.org/docroot/ESN/content/ESN_3_1x_Reach_to_Recovery_5.asp

Cidón, E.U. (2010). Sexual problems after breast cancer: The underreported symptoms. *Gynecologic Oncology, 116,* 147. doi:10.1016/j.ygyno.2009.10.048

Cohen, M.Z., Kahn, D.L., & Steeves, R.H. (1998). Beyond body image: The experience of breast cancer. *Oncology Nursing Forum, 25,* 835–841.

Fernández-Delgado, J., López-Pedraza, M.J., Blasco, J.A., Andradas-Aragones, E., Sánchez-Méndez, J.I., Sordo-Miralles, G., & Reza, M.M. (2008). Satisfaction with and psychological impact of immediate and deferred breast reconstruction. *Annals of Oncology, 19,* 1430–1434. doi:10.1093/annonc/mdn153

Ganz, P.A. (2008). Psychological and social aspects of breast cancer. *Oncology, 22,* 642–646, 650.

Glaus, S.W., & Carlson, G.W. (2009). Long-term role of external breast prostheses after total mastectomy. *Breast Journal, 15,* 385–393. doi:10.1111/j.1524-4741.2009.00742.x

Helms, R.L., O'Hea, E.L., & Corso, M. (2008). Body image issues in women with breast cancer. *Psychology, Health and Medicine, 13,* 313–325. doi:10.1080/13548500701405509

Livingston, P.M., White, V.M., Roberts, S.B., Pritchard, E., Hayman, J., Gibbs, A., & Hill, D.J. (2005). Women's satisfaction with their breast prosthesis: What determines a quality prosthesis? *Evaluation Review, 29,* 65–83. doi:10.1177/0193841X04269640

Markopoulos, C., Tsaroucha, A.K., Kouskos, E., Mantas, D., Antonopoulou, Z., & Karvelis, S. (2009). Impact of breast cancer surgery on the self-esteem and sexual life of female patients. *Journal of International Medical Research, 37,* 182–188.

Resnick, B., & Belcher, A.E. (2002). Breast reconstruction. Options, answers, and support for patients making a difficult personal decision. *American Journal of Nursing, 102*(4), 26–33.

Roberts, S., Livingston, P., White, V., & Gibbs, A. (2003). External breast prosthesis use: Experiences and views of women with breast cancer, breast care nurses, and prosthesis fitters. *Cancer Nursing, 26,* 179–186.

Skrzypulec, V., Tobor, E., Drosdzol, A., & Nowosielski, K. (2009). Biopsychosocial functioning of women after mastectomy. *Journal of Clinical Nursing, 18,* 613–619. doi:10.1111/j.1365-2702.2008.02476.x

# CHAPTER 7

# Radiation Therapy

Connie J. Ferraro, RN, BSN, OCN®, and Phillip J. Catanzaro, MD, PhD

## Introduction

Recently, numerous advances have occurred in radiation therapy (RT), especially in fractionation schedules and concurrent chemotherapy and radiation regimens, that have had a major impact on breast cancer treatment. Nurses are key to providing quality care, education, and support to women receiving RT for breast cancer.

RT uses x-rays to cure, control, or palliate cancer (Buchholz & Hunt, 2010). Radiation has the ability to produce free radicals in tumor tissue, and in an oxygenated milieu, will result in tumor or cell death. This is important because a well-oxygenated tumor demonstrates a much greater response to radiation than a poorly oxygenated tumor (Buchholz & Hunt, 2010). The goal of RT is to achieve maximum tumor cell kill while minimizing injury to the normal tissues in the regional area (Haffty, Buchholz, & Perez, 2008).

## History

RT has been used for the treatment of breast cancer for more than a century (Buchholz & Hunt, 2010). In the early 1900s, RT was first used to treat chest wall recurrences in patients with breast cancer after mastectomy, as well as for primary treatment in patients with advanced breast cancer (White & Wilson, 2002). In 1948, Francoise Baclesse, from the Curie Foundation in Paris, reported improved long-term disease-free survival rates of advanced-stage patients treated with RT (brachytherapy) alone (Baclesse, 1949).

These successful applications of RT played a major role in promoting the concept of breast-conserving therapy (BCT) as an alternate to mastectomy (Baclesse, 1949). European studies in the 1960s showed that RT to treat T1, T2, and less advanced T3 tumors yielded comparable results as mastectomy (Pierquin et al., 1991). Several other prospective randomized trials, especially within the United States, have since confirmed that lumpectomy plus RT to the breast yields equiv-alent local control as mastectomy. As a result, BCT plus RT has been established as an alternative to mastectomy (Buchholz & Hunt, 2010).

## Selection of Patients for Breast-Conserving Therapy

Selection of patients for BCT requires an interdisciplinary team approach including the active participation of the patient. This includes discussing the risks and benefits of both options (mastectomy or BCT plus RT) for the local control of an early-stage breast cancer (Foxson, Lattimer, & Felder, 2011). The goal of BCT plus RT is to maintain local control and a low rate of recurrence while retaining a sensate breast and good cosmesis (Foxson et al., 2011; White & Wilson, 2002).

In evaluating patients for BCT plus RT, absolute and relative contraindications exist (Bernice, 2005). Absolute contraindications to BCT include first and second trimester of pregnancy, two or more gross malignancies in separate quadrants of the breast, persistent positive margins, active collagen vascular disease, especially scleroderma, and prior chest RT. Dormant collagen vascular diseases are usually a relative contraindication (Bernice, 2005).

Relative contraindications for BCT plus RT include young age. It is difficult to define young age. Most would argue that patients in their 30s have a higher incidence of recurrence following BCT plus RT. An additional relative contraindication that must be considered relates to the patient's breast size in comparison to tumor size. For example, a very large tumor in a small breast may result in disfigurement of the breast with lumpectomy alone, and that particular individual may benefit from mastectomy followed by reconstruction. On the other hand, very large breasts may pose a technical challenge for delivering RT and can be associated with an increase in skin-related toxicity. However, this should not be considered an absolute contraindication for BCT (Buchholz & Hunt, 2010; Foxson et al., 2011; Gray, McCormick, Cox, & Yahalom,

1991; White & Wilson, 2002). Finally, those with an extensive family history of genetic breast cancer and *BRCA1* and *BRCA2* carriers have similar results as unaffected individuals with BCT plus RT, and it is not a contraindication (Buchholz & Hunt, 2010).

The local recurrence rate following BCT alone is approximately 13% at 10 years (Foxson et al., 2011), a percentage that varies directly with the size of the margin. Indeed, RT is not a substitute for clear margins. BCT plus RT is considered the standard of care for ductal carcinoma in situ (DCIS) (Leonard & Swain, 2004). Three prospective studies indicated that the addition of RT to BCT in patients with DCIS resulted in an approximate 50% reduction in breast cancer recurrence (Leonard & Swain, 2004). In summary, BCT plus RT remains the standard of care for both noninvasive as well as invasive breast cancers (Buchholz & Hunt, 2010).

## Postmastectomy Radiation

Postmastectomy RT is the use of RT to the chest wall as well as the lymphatic drainage chains in the axillary, supraclavicular, and internal mammary nodal areas (Bernice, 2005; White & Wilson, 2002). Numerous studies have indicated that postmastectomy RT reduces local recurrence rates; the effect on overall survival benefit is controversial (White & Wilson, 2002). Indications for postmastectomy RT are as follows (National Comprehensive Cancer Network [NCCN], 2011).

- Patients with four or more positive lymph nodes or extracapsular nodal extension
- Patients with tumors greater than 5 cm
- Patients with positive or close margins of resection (less than 1 mm)
- Patients with nipple or skin involvement of the tumor

In patients who choose to undergo immediate reconstruction, the risk of complications, especially cosmetic, has been shown to increase with the addition of postmastectomy RT. Poor cosmesis is a special risk for individuals who opt for implant placement rather than tissue expanders. Cosmetic results are somewhat improved with the use of tissue expanders or vascularized flap technique in combination followed by RT (Pomahac, Recht, May, Hergrueter, & Slavin, 2006).

## Dose Considerations

RT is painless and is delivered in only a few minutes each day. It is important to stress to the patient that she will not become radioactive during her treatment. The entire time in the treatment room is about 10 minutes, most of which involves proper orientation of the patient to receive RT.

RT is used to treat all stages of breast cancer and uses high-energy x-rays (photons) and electrons. Particle radiation, which includes alpha particles and neutrons, is available for the treatment of breast cancer but is not commonly used at this time. All forms of RT have the ability to destroy cancer cells by interfering with cellular division (White & Wilson, 2002). Tumor cells are especially sensitive to free radicals during cellular division (Buchholz & Hunt, 2010).

The penetration of RT varies with beam energy. Generally, photons are deeply penetrating and have both an entrance point and an exit point, exposing all tissue in its path. Electrons will penetrate to a certain depth, depending on their energy. This property of electrons allows combinations of photons and electrons to treat the breast while at the same time avoiding the normal structures of the lung and heart (Buchholz & Hunt, 2010).

RT affects only the areas treated (Bruner, Haas, & Gosselin-Acomb, 2005). Dose is expressed in radiation absorbed dose (rad) or gray (Gy) and centigray (cGy) (1 cGy = 1 rad and 1 Gy = 100 rad or 100 cGy) (Bruner et al., 2005). The term used to describe a daily dose of RT is commonly called a fraction. Generally, the dose required for control of microscopic disease is 50–60 Gy (White & Wilson, 2002).

Photon and electron RT, described previously, are commonly referred to as external beam radiation therapy (EBRT), which is the most commonly administered method of delivery. It uses a linear accelerator (White & Wilson, 2002).

EBRT is delivered to the entire breast following BCT and to the chest wall following mastectomy. In either case, 45–50 Gy of photon irradiation is delivered to the chest wall/breast in 1.8–2 Gy fractions (treatments are designated as fractions) (Bruner et al., 2005).

Following BCT, an additional electron treatment (called a *boost*) of 10–16 Gy is delivered to the tumor bed. Following a mastectomy, generally a 10 Gy electron boost delivered to the scar (Bedwinek, 1993; Buchholz & Hunt, 2010). The rationale for the boost treatment is that most recurrences in the breast occur within 2 cm of the primary tumor in BCT or around the scar following mastectomy (Gordils-Perez, Rawlins-Duell, & Kelvin, 2003). Surgical clips placed at the time of resection, which demarcate the lumpectomy cavity, are crucial for correct placement of the electron beam component of therapy (Buchholz & Hunt, 2010).

Depending on tumor size and locoregional extent, treatment of the chest wall may be accompanied by the supraclavicular lymph nodes or the internal mammary lymph node chain. These areas depend on the location of the tumor and the number of axillary nodes that are positive. Previously, RT was directed to the dissected axilla following mastectomy. That practice did not improve local control or survival; it resulted in complications, including lymphedema of the arm, that might be severe. The practice of treating the axilla is no longer done with the rare exception of tumor remaining in the axilla after lymph node dissection (Buchholz & Hunt, 2010).

RT to the breast usually begins four to six weeks after conservative surgery, to allow for adequate healing time of the surgical wound (Gordils-Perez et al., 2003). However, initiation of RT might be safely delayed in patients who require chemotherapy, which commonly precedes RT. Delays in initiation of RT beyond 12–16 weeks (in the absence of chemotherapy) have been associated with an increase in breast relapse rates (Buchholz et al., 1993). Some even recommend a postchemotherapy, pre-RT mammogram in patients who have chemotherapy causing a delay of RT for a period of time greater than 16 weeks (White & Wilson, 2002).

## Treatment Planning

Prior to initiating RT for breast cancer, several steps must occur.
- Initial nurse/clinician consultation and examination
- Patient education regarding the treatment regimen
- Treatment planning, also called simulation
- Dosimetry and physics calculations and verification
- Treatment port setup verification
- Initiation of treatment

The initial phase of the treatment process is to obtain adequate identification of the patient. For this reason, a photograph of her face is initially obtained, and a bar code is produced. This bar code is recognized by the computer in the linear accelerator to deliver only the planned treatment to the proper patient. During the process of simulation (i.e., recreation of treatment conditions), a special treatment planning computed tomography (CT) scan will be obtained with the patient in treatment position (see Figure 7-1). Following

this, the radiation oncologist and the dosimetrist (an individual trained to produce computerized treatment plans for RT) will decide on the appropriate treatment volume. Once the plan is complete, the physician and medical physics team will review the entire plan so that it adequately targets the area at risk while at the same time limiting x-ray exposure to healthy surrounding structures, such as the lungs and the heart. It is customary that the patient's skin is marked with tiny tattoos so that each treatment can be aimed at precisely the same region.

On the initial treatment day, each step is reviewed. A series of x-rays (portal films or ports) are taken to verify that they represent the intended treatment area. The physician verifies these ports before administration of the first treatment (White & Wilson, 2002).

Most patients are treated in a supine position (with rare exceptions) with the arm raised above the shoulder and resting on an immobilizing device to ensure proper positioning for each treatment (Buchholz & Hunt, 2010) (see Figure 7-2). It is common for the patient's treatment course to

### Figure 7-2. Computed Tomography Simulator

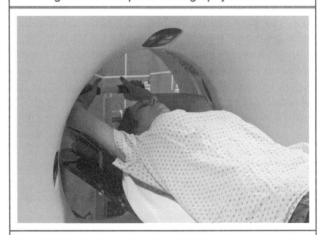

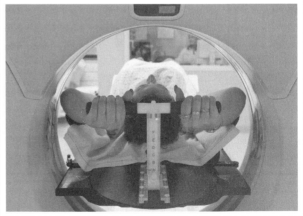

*Note.* Photos courtesy of the Cleveland Clinic Center for Medical Art and Photography. Used with permission.

### Figure 7-1. Computed Tomography Scan for Treatment Planning

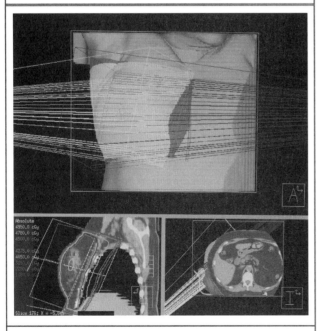

*Note.* Image courtesy of the Cleveland Clinic Center for Medical Art and Photography. Used with permission.

undergo routine quality assurance checks, with port films being repeated on a five- to seven-day cycle. As previously stated, treatment consists of approximately five to six weeks of treatment to the entire breast, followed by a boost to the surgical site for approximately one to one and a half weeks (White & Wilson, 2002).

## Various Techniques Used in Radiation Therapy and Partial Breast Irradiation

Until recently, EBRT was the most common form of RT delivery; however, it requires approximately six or more weeks of treatment. This might be impossible or very difficult when the patient lives a long distance from the treatment center. In the past, many of these patients were advised to undergo mastectomy (White & Wilson, 2002).

With this motivation, studies have now afforded women the opportunity to undergo an accelerated course of partial-breast irradiation (PBI). PBI was suggested as a substitute for whole breast RT following BCT. It is clear that the RT following BCT is necessary, but many women who undergo BCT are unable, for logistical reasons as well as because of the cost, to undergo a complete course of EBRT. Accordingly, PBI using intracavitary brachytherapy has been suggested as a substitute for whole breast RT. At the present time, although this is a promising modality of treatment, it is still considered experimental, and the results are being evaluated (Gordils-Perez et al., 2003). In addition to the brachytherapy approach, an approach with EBRT using a three-dimensional (3-D) conformal planning system has been suggested. The interstitial brachytherapy protocol is carried out by the Radiation Therapy Oncology Group (RTOG) 95-17, and the 3-D conformal treatment is per RTOG 0319 (Vicini, Pass, & Wong, 2003). Some have used an intracavitary approach with the MammoSite® (Cytyc Corp.) applicator (see Figure 7-3).

The MammoSite RT System is a dual-lumen, closed-ended catheter with an inflatable balloon at one end. At the opposite end of the catheter is both a red and blue port. The blue port is the fluid port used for filling and deflating the balloon. The red port is the obturator and radiation source port. MammoSite catheters are currently available in two balloon sizes. Balloon shapes can be either spherical or elliptical. Catheters are chosen so that the balloon size and shape approximates the size and shape of the lumpectomy cavity.

The MammoSite catheter may be placed at the time of lumpectomy or as a later procedure under ultrasound guidance. The balloon is placed into the lumpectomy cavity and filled with a mixture of saline and contrast. The catheter protrudes from the breast, is covered by a dressing, and can be worn within a bra or other garment for comfort. Contrast inside the balloon allows for the use of a CT scan to confirm placement. Balloon contact or conformance with the entire

### Figure 7-3. MammoSite® Catheter for Placement in the Breast

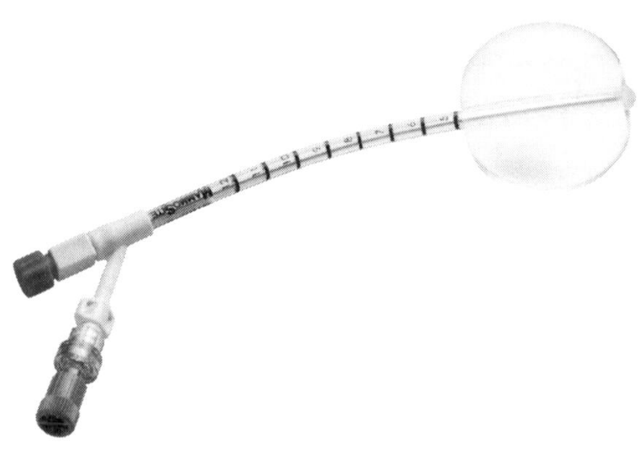

Note. Figure courtesy of Hologic. Used with permission.

interior surface of the lumpectomy cavity is necessary. Additionally, a distance of at least 5 mm from the applicator to the skin edge is necessary to minimize radiation dermatitis (Sanders, Scroggins, Ampil, & Li, 2007). Patients are treated with high-dose iridium-192 radiation on an outpatient basis and typically receive a total dose of 34 Gy. The radiation dose is given as twice-daily fractions of 3–4 Gy for a total of 10 treatments over five to seven days (Sanders et al., 2007).

As with any indwelling device, a risk of infection is associated with the MammoSite catheter. Antibiotic prophylaxis may be considered at the time of catheter placement. Dressing changes should be done daily, as well as whenever the dressing becomes soiled or saturated. Routine daily dressing changes may be done during daily RT treatment visits. Use of an antibacterial cleansing agent and antibiotic ointment may be recommended. The site should be assessed at each visit for signs of infection, and patients should be educated to report any fever or other sign of infection. Patients and caregivers should receive training about catheter care and dressing change supplies in the event that dressing changes need to be done at home. Patients are instructed to keep the catheter clean and dry and should not shower or submerge the catheter in water (Sanders et al., 2007).

Early experience with MammoSite has been favorable, but further study and longer follow-up are needed. Trials comparing accelerated PBI and EBRT are ongoing and consider the issues of dwell position as well as short- and long-term toxicities (Hogle, Quinn, & Heron, 2003; Sanders et al., 2007).

Side effects include occasional pain and a sensation of heaviness or engorgement in the breast. Reduction of edema and healing might require one year's time. In severe cases, patients may need to use analgesics such as acetaminophen or prescription-strength ibuprofen. Return visits start usually at two and six weeks after treatment.

The eligibility criteria for using either 3-D conformal or MammoSite treatment include all invasive histologies except lobular carcinoma. Lesions must be less than 3 cm in greatest dimension, and the patient must have three or fewer positive lymph nodes. Margins must be negative according to the National Surgical Adjuvant Breast and Bowel Project definition (margins free of tumor cells). There must be no extensive intraductal component, and brachytherapy catheter placement is usually done within six weeks of surgery (Vicini et al., 2003).

The physics and dosimetry of both of the setup procedures can be found in the RTOG protocols discussed previously. It should be noted that the external beam treatment is 3-D conformal and not intensity-modulated radiotherapy. This delivers 38.5 Gy in a fraction per day separated by six hours and is given on five consecutive days (Vicini et al., 2003).

Accelerated PBI delivers RT to the lumpectomy site only in patients with early-stage breast cancer (stage I or II) (Gordils-Perez et al., 2003). The total elapsed treatment time is significantly decreased to a five-day (one week) treatment course. Accelerated PBI usually is delivered with 3-D conformal therapy or the MammoSite brachytherapy (Jeruss et al., 2006).

## Palliative Radiation for Metastatic Disease

Unfortunately, some patients are unable to obtain a disease-free state after initial therapy or present with metastatic disease. The primary goal of RT in the metastatic setting is to palliate symptoms such as pain and to improve functional status (White & Wilson, 2002).

The three most common sites of breast cancer metastases are the chest wall, bone, and brain (Buchholz & Hunt, 2010). RT is directed at the particular site of metastases, and a dose of 30–37.5 Gy (two to three weeks of daily treatment) is typically administered. When treating the bone, local treatment is aimed at relieving pain and preventing fractures of weight-bearing bones. If a lytic lesion has involved more than 50% of the cortex of a weight-bearing bone, standard protocol involves a combination of surgery and radiotherapy, with surgery preceding radiotherapy (White & Wilson, 2002). Education of the patient about weight-bearing restrictions is vital.

Occasionally, a bony metastasis in the spine can produce a spinal cord compression, a true oncologic emergency that requires treatment with surgery and/or RT along with cortical steroids. Approximately 10% of patients with metastatic cancer will have a spinal cord compression. The thoracic spine is affected most often because it is the longest section of the vertebral column, and perhaps it is related to the pattern of drainage from the primary tumor site of the breast (White & Wilson, 2002). Generally, the total RT dose of therapy is 30 Gy given over a two-week period of time.

When dealing with brain metastases, whole brain treatment uses EBRT to a dose of 37.5 Gy. If appropriate, it may be followed by a single stereotactic radiosurgery treatment (Gamma Knife® [Elekta AB] treatment) (Haffty et al., 2008). Steroids and anticonvulsants may be necessary to control symptoms. The most common side effects of whole brain RT include fatigue and temporary alopecia. The patient and her family should be prepared for this.

## Nursing Care of Patients Receiving Radiotherapy

Nursing care of patients receiving RT should focus on all of the needs and problems that are associated with a cancer diagnosis, be patient specific, and address specific radiation issues. Issues specific to RT nursing care and education (Foxson et al., 2011) include

- Diagnosis and acceptance of treatment
- Clearing misconceptions patients may have regarding RT
- Potential side effects of therapy
- Anticipated length of the treatment period
- Preparation (physical and psychological) for treatment
- Transportation needs
- Symptomatic relief of side effects of treatment
- Nutritional support
- Social and financial assistance
- Clarification of variations in the treatment plan
- Acceptance and continuation of treatment despite immediate discomforts
- Continued follow-up after completion of treatment.

During a course of RT to the breast, certain side effects are expected. It is important to tell patients that the appearance of side effects and their severity are individual and cannot be predicted by patient age or extent of disease. Side effects usually appear within 10–14 days of treatment initiation and might not disappear until after completion of treatment (Haffty et al., 2008; Witt, 2005). Nurses fill a uniquely important role in dealing with the acute effects of RT. Accordingly, nurses need to make themselves aware of these potential side effects and their management (see Table 7-1).

Acute side effects (occurring within a week to months) of therapy include fatigue, slight change in breast size, radiation dermatitis, and tenderness in the treated breast. Chronic (occurring after months to years) side effects include extensive fibrosis compromising cosmesis, lymphedema, radiation pneumonitis, brachial plexopathy, rib fractures, and, rarely, secondary cancer (Bruner et al., 2005).

Women need to be informed that it is possible to become pregnant after RT, but they are advised to wait until two years after RT before becoming pregnant. In the event that lactation occurs in the treated breast (this is rare), the patient should be instructed to nurse only at the untreated breast. The rationale for this is to reduce the risk of mastitis in the treated breast, which is difficult to treat (Buchholz & Hunt, 2010).

**Table 7-1. Radiation Therapy Side Effects and Management**

| Side Effect | Presentation | Treatment |
|---|---|---|
| Brachial plexopathy | Numbness or difficulty moving the affected arm; most often has surgical cause | Pain management; refer to occupational and/or physical therapy. |
| Change in breast size | Slight swelling of the breast in the acute phase, followed by slight decrease in breast size in the chronic phase | Reassure the patient that this is a normal postoperative/post-treatment presentation; obtain a surgical consult if necessary. Many women benefit from a bra fitting and partial prosthesis (see Chapter 6). |
| Fatigue | Lack of energy, increased sleep time; usually appears in the third week of treatment and lasts 2–3 weeks after treatment | Allow for periods of rest throughout the day; instruct the patient to plan and prioritize activities. Light exercise, proper diet, and social activities may help to combat fatigue. |
| Lymphedema | Swelling of the affected upper extremity. Most common in women with 11 or more nodes resected. (Not as much of a radiation-induced side effect anymore because axillary nodes are rarely treated.) | Instruct the patient to keep her arm elevated above the level of the heart, avoid hypervolemia, wear a compression arm stocking, and refer to the lymphedema clinic should the need arise. |
| Radiation dermatitis | Radiation Therapy Oncology Group stages 1. Dull erythema, dry desquamation, decreased sweating 2. Tender or bright erythema; patchy, moist desquamation; moderate edema 3. Confluent moist desquamation, pitting edema, skin peeling in skin folds 4. Ulceration, hemorrhage, necrosis | General skin care guidelines • Maintain skin integrity by washing with a gentle soap and patting to dry. • Keep the treated skin dry until itching occurs. • Once itching occurs, moisturize with lotion (recent studies indicate that there is no preference on lotion type). Continue to moisturize for three weeks after completion of treatment. • Take diphenhydramine for mild pruritus. • Consider hydrocolloid dressings for large areas of moist desquamation. • Wear loose-fitting garments. • Avoid underwire bras. • Do NOT apply tape to treatment area. • Protect the skin from exposure to direct sunlight. • Avoid the use of cooling and heating pads or electric blankets. |
| Radiation pneumonitis | Cough, fever, and/or shortness of breath accompanied by radiographic changes consistent with a noninfectious infiltrate in the underlying volume of lung that was irradiated. Risk is definitely proportionate to the volume of lung that was in the treatment field. | Place the patient on steroids as soon as possible. Promote good pulmonary hygiene, adequate hydration, and humidification. |
| Rib fracture | Rib pain and radiographic findings of fracture on treated side. Rare occurrence without trauma to site. | Pain management |
| Tenderness in the treated breast | Pain often is described as being sharp and superficial to the skin; especially around the scar site. | Instruct the patient to use over-the-counter pain relievers as needed. Applying mild pressure to the site may also be effective. |

*Note.* Based on information from Bernice, 2005; Bruner et al., 2005; Buchholz & Hunt, 2010; Haffty et al., 2008; Krumm et al., 2002.

## Conclusion

Education of patients with breast cancer involves good communication between patients and healthcare providers. It is imperative that nurses present patients with accurate information. With the advent of the Internet as a patient resource as well as the ever-growing number of pa-

tient advocacy groups, patients have never had more opportunities to take control of their disease and to be informed, empowered survivors. Nurses need to make it a priority as healthcare providers to further their own education and maintain their stance as a primary resource for patients. Nurses should use the patient resource available from NCCN, the *NCCN Guidelines for Patients™:*

*Breast Cancer* (see www.nccn.com/patient-guidelines .html).

The future of medicine certainly will see advances in the field of RT. Nursing care, based on research and empirical data, needs to focus on preventing and treating the side effects of treatment, including those of biologic, physical, psychological, and sociologic origins.

## References

Baclesse, F. (1949). Roentgen therapy as the sole method of treatment of cancer of the breast. *American Journal of Roentgenology and Radiation Therapy, 62,* 311–319.

Bedwinek, J. (1993). Breast conserving surgery and irradiation: The importance of demarcating the excision cavity with surgical clips. *International Journal of Radiation Oncology, Biology, Physics, 26,* 675–679. doi:10.1016/0360-3016(93)90287-6

Bernice, M. (2005). Nursing care of the client with breast cancer. In J.K. Itano & K.N. Taoka (Eds.), *Core curriculum for oncology nursing* (4th ed., pp. 492–511). St. Louis, MO: Elsevier Saunders.

Bruner, D.W., Haas, M.L., & Gosselin-Acomb, T.K. (Eds.). (2005). *Manual for radiation oncology nursing practice and education* (3rd ed.). Pittsburgh, PA: Oncology Nursing Society.

Buchholz, T.A., Austin-Seymour, M.M., Moe, R.E., Ellis, G.K., Livingston, R.B., Pelton, J.G., & Griffin, T.W. (1993). Effect of delay in radiation in the combined modality treatment of breast cancer. *International Journal of Radiation Oncology, Biology, Physics, 26,* 23–35. doi:10.1016/0360-3016(93)90169-V

Buchholz, T.A., & Hunt, K.K. (2010). Breast-conserving therapy: Conventional whole breast irradiation. In J.R. Harris, M.E. Lippman, M. Morrow, & C.K. Osborne (Eds.), *Diseases of the breast* (4th ed., pp. 507–521). Philadelphia, PA: Lippincott Williams & Wilkins.

Foxson, S.B., Lattimer, J.G., & Felder, B. (2011). Breast cancer. In C.H. Yarbro, D. Wujcik, & B.H. Gobel (Eds.), *Cancer nursing: Principles and practice* (7th ed., pp. 1091–1145). Sudbury, MA: Jones and Bartlett.

Gordils-Perez, J., Rawlins-Duell, R., & Kelvin, J.F. (2003). Advances in radiation treatment of patients with breast cancer. *Clinical Journal of Oncology Nursing, 7,* 629–636. doi:10.1188/03. CJON.629-636

Gray, J., McCormick, B., Cox, L., & Yahalom, J. (1991). Primary breast irradiation in large-breasted or heavy women: analysis of cosmetic outcome. *International Journal of Radiation Oncology, Biology, Physics, 21,* 347–354. doi:10.1016/0360-3016(91)90781-X

Haffty, B.G., Buchholz, T.A., & Perez, C.A. (2008). Early stage breast cancer. In E.C. Halperin, C.A. Perez, & L.W. Brady (Eds.), *Principles and practice of radiation oncology* (5th ed., pp. 1175–1281). Philadelphia, PA: Lippincott Williams & Wilkins.

Hogle, W.P., Quinn, A.E., & Heron, D.E. (2003). Advances in brachytherapy: New approaches to target breast cancer. *Clinical Journal of Oncology Nursing, 7,* 324–328. doi:10.1188/03 .CJON.324-328

Jeruss, J.S., Vicini, F.A., Beitsch, P.D., Haffty, B.G., Quiet, C.A., Zannis, V.J., ... Kuerer, H.M. (2006). Initial outcomes for patients treated on the American Society of Breast Surgeons MammoSite clinical trial for ductal carcinoma in-situ of the breast. *Annals of Surgical Oncology, 13,* 967–976. doi:10.1245/ASO.2006.08.031

Krumm, S.L., Bucholtz, J., Ziegfeld, C., Burks, K., Wainstock, J.M., DeClue, C.B., ... Shockney, L.D. (2002). Nursing care. In W.L. Donegan & J.S. Spratt (Eds.), *Cancer of the breast* (5th ed., pp. 763–792). St. Louis, MO: Elsevier Saunders.

Leonard, G.D., & Swain, S.M. (2004). Ductal carcinoma in situ, complexities and challenges. *Journal of the National Cancer Institute, 96,* 906–920. doi:10.1093/jnci/djh164

National Comprehensive Cancer Network. (2011, May). *NCCN Clinical Practice Guidelines in Oncology™: Breast cancer* [v.2.2011]. Retrieved from http://www.nccn.org/professionals/ physicians_gls/pdf/breast.pdf

Pierquin, B., Huart, J., Raynal, M., Otmezguine, Y., Calitchi, E., Mazeron, J.J., ... Julien, M. (1991). Conservative treatment for breast cancer: Long-term results (15 years). *Radiotherapy and Oncology, 20,* 16–23.

Pomahac, B., Recht, A., May, J.W., Hergrueter, C.A., & Slavin, S.A. (2006). New trends in breast cancer management: Is the era of immediate breast reconstruction changing? *Annals of Surgery, 244,* 282–288. doi:10.1097/01.sla.0000217626.88430.c3

Sanders, M.E., Scroggins, T., Ampil, F., & Li, B.D. (2007). Accelerated partial breast irradiation in early-stage breast cancer. *Journal of Clinical Oncology, 25,* 996–1002. doi:10.1200/ JCO.2006.09.7436

Vicini, F.A., Pass, H., & Wong, J. (2003). A phase I/II trial to evaluate three dimensional conformal radiation therapy (3D-CRT) confined to the region of the lumpectomy cavity for stage I and II breast carcinoma (9/30/03). Unpublished raw data, William Beaumont Hospital, Royal Oak, MI. Retrieved from http://www.rtog.org/ members/protocols/0319/0319.pdf

White, J.R., & Wilson, J.F. (2002). Radiation therapy for breast cancer. In W.L. Donegan & J.S. Spratt (Eds.), *Cancer of the breast* (5th ed., pp. 639–655). St. Louis, MO: Elsevier Saunders.

Witt, M.E. (2005). Nursing implications of radiation therapy. In J.K. Itano & K.N. Taoka (Eds.), *Core curriculum for oncology nursing* (4th ed., pp. 748–762). St. Louis, MO: Elsevier Saunders.

# CHAPTER 8

# Systemic Therapy

Seth Eisenberg, RN, ADN, OCN®

## Introduction

With the possible exception of ductal carcinoma in situ, breast cancer is considered a progressive disease with aggressive metastatic qualities. Although local management strategies (surgery and radiotherapy) have an important role in therapy and are detailed elsewhere in this book, systemic therapy is required to cure or slow disease progression (Conzen, Grushko, & Olopade, 2008).

The current dogma of modern systemic therapy began to emerge in the late 1970s when combinations of antineoplastic agents were first shown to have generally superior efficacy over sequential single agents (Smalley, Murphy, Huguley, & Bartolucci, 1976). Since that time, tremendous knowledge has been gained regarding specific subtypes of breast cancer, the role of biomarkers, signaling pathways, and drug resistance.

The extreme heterogeneity of breast cancer has necessitated a wide variety of treatment options when compared with other neoplasms. This varied molecular nature has prompted it to be viewed as a collection of biologically discrete diseases rather than a singular homogeneous cancer. Treatment strategies typically are based on a number of characteristics. These include receptor status (estrogen receptor [ER], progesterone receptor [PR], and HER2); tumor size and presence of metastatic disease; and patient-specific characteristics (age, menopausal status, comorbidities, and prior therapy) (Crane-Okada & Loney, 2007; Di Cosimo & Baselga, 2010; Petrakis & Paraskakis, 2010). While all of these are important in determining appropriate therapy, ER/PR and HER2 play a major role. Figure 8-1 illustrates the diversity of systemic treatment options.

Although the development of systemic treatment has evolved toward the use of more targeted therapies, clinicians continue to rely on some of the same cytotoxic agents that have been in use for the past four decades. Chemotherapy plays an integral role in the treatment of metastatic breast cancer (MBC), advanced local disease, high-risk node-negative disease, and triple-negative breast cancer (TNBC) (Crane-Okada & Loney, 2007; Frye, Mahon, & Palmieri, 2009; Mahon & Palmieri, 2009). Endocrine therapy can be used with or without chemotherapy in the adjuvant setting, where the primary goal of treatment is to prevent disease recurrence and to slow disease progression in patients with MBC (Conzen et al., 2008).

Systemic therapy can consist of single agents or combinations of medications (Beslija et al., 2009). Sequential single-agent therapies—where one medication is used until it becomes ineffective—are also an option. Combination therapy generally is chosen based on synergistic complementary mechanisms of action, preferably with different side effects. Therapy selection also may be based on the potential for cross-resistance (Tkaczuk, 2009). Because the goals of systemic therapy range from curative to palliative, these goals may affect the selection of agents based on toxicity profiles and associated quality-of-life concerns.

Genetic profiling also has revealed specific subgroups defined by gene expression: luminal A, luminal B, HER2, and basal-like (Cheang et al., 2009; Sotiriou & Pusztai, 2009). Luminal A are low-proliferative, ER-positive tumors; luminal B are high-proliferative, ER-positive tumors; ER/PR/HER2-negative tumors are considered triple-negative or sometimes referred to as basal-like; and HER2-amplified tumors are responsive to HER2 therapy (Pusztai, 2009). Recent evidence points to outcomes based on gene expression profiling. In particular, patients with luminal B–type tumors have worse overall survival and are associated with increased expression of HER2 genes, although less than a third are HER2 positive (Cheang et al., 2009). Each of these subgroups shapes the types of therapy used in clinical settings. Ongoing international research into biomolecular pathways has allowed for the development of newer and increasingly more effective forms of systemic therapy.

*The author would like to acknowledge Susan G. Yackzan, APRN, MSN, AOCN®, for her contribution to this chapter that remains unchanged from the first edition of this book.*

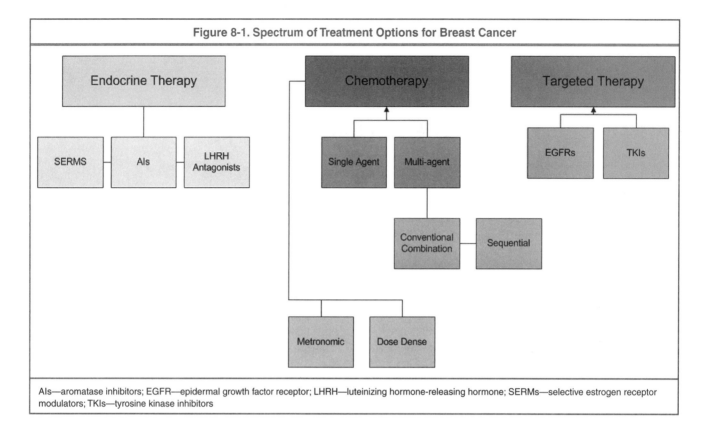

Figure 8-1. Spectrum of Treatment Options for Breast Cancer

AIs—aromatase inhibitors; EGFR—epidermal growth factor receptor; LHRH—luteinizing hormone-releasing hormone; SERMs—selective estrogen receptor modulators; TKIs—tyrosine kinase inhibitors

The timing of treatment plays an important role, as therapy may be given in neoadjuvant, adjuvant, or palliative care settings (Mathew, Asgeirsson, Jackson, Cheung, & Robertson, 2009; Shenoy et al., 2009). Preoperative systemic therapy may be able to decrease tumor size, facilitating subsequent resection (Mathew et al., 2009). Adjuvant therapy can eradicate micrometastases and prevent recurrence (Conzen et al., 2008).

The development of drug resistance is a significant concern with all systemic therapies. A number of mechanisms are thought to be responsible, and it is likely that several interrelated factors are involved. Overexpression of HER2 has been associated with hormone receptor resistance. Signaling between members of the HER family, which includes HER1 (epidermal growth factor receptor [EGFR]), HER2, and HER4, is implicated along with the PI3K/AKT/mTOR pathway, which controls cellular activities including proliferation, growth, and metabolism (Di Cosimo & Baselga, 2010; Serra et al., 2008). Research is currently under way to exploit signaling pathways. Additional information can be found in the Drug Resistance section.

One consequence of the complex heterogeneity of breast cancer is the inherent difficulty in comparing the overall survival (OS) or disease-free survival (DFS) results between different therapies and associated studies. Some patients, such as those with TNBC, will have a worse prognosis based on the absence of these tumor markers regardless of the therapy used for treatment and therefore cannot be compared to ER/PR-positive women. Conflicting results from seemingly identical trials also can be attributed to these differences in molec-

ular subtypes, which may not have been detected or accounted for during study accrual (Pusztai, 2009). Finally, most clinical trials have excluded patients older than age 70, despite the fact that these patients generally have less aggressive disease when compared to younger women (Petrakis & Paraskakis, 2010). Therefore, it should be noted that systemic therapies cannot be evaluated out of context. This overarching caveat should be kept in mind when evaluating the results of different clinical trials comparing systemic therapies.

## Endocrine Therapy

ERs on the surface of breast cancer cells are stimulated by the presence of estrogen, which in turn stimulates tumor growth (Crane-Okada & Loney, 2007; Mouridsen, Rose, Brodie, & Smith, 2003). Ovarian production of estrogen and progesterone normally decline after menopause, at which time the ovaries, along with the adrenal cortex, secrete androgens, which are converted to estrogen. It has been well established that estrogen production can be blocked surgically through oophorectomy, adrenalectomy, or hypophysectomy (Legha, Davis, & Muggia, 1978). However, these latter two surgical approaches have since fallen out of favor because of overall lack of efficacy and severe side effects. Pharmaceutical alternatives commonly are used and will be discussed as follows.

Even without gonadal production, estrogen continues to be made in the breast tissue, muscle, skin, and fat and particularly in breast tumors themselves (Mouridsen et al., 2003). Other sources of estrogen production include estrone sulfate, which is produced by aromatase, and fatty esters of estrogens, which are formed by combining low-density lipoproteins and estradiol and are thought to function as hormonal reserves (Mouridsen et al., 2003; Santen, Brodie, Simpson, Siiteri, & Brodie, 2009).

It is estimated that 60% of premenopausal and 80% of postmenopausal women with breast cancer are ER/PR positive (Goel, Sharma, Hamilton, & Beith, 2009; Montemurro & Aglietta, 2009). Breast cancer in older postmenopausal women also tends to be hormone receptor sensitive (Petrakis & Paraskakis, 2010), and the tumors themselves have an increased affinity to estrogen (Santen et al., 2009). ER and PR positivity are not static; expression can change as a result of therapy or the disease itself (Arpino et al., 2005). Endocrine therapy is currently recommended for most ER/PR-positive patients regardless of age, tumor stage, and menopause status, although the choice of specific agents will vary (National Comprehensive Cancer Network [NCCN], 2011).

Many of the endocrine therapies are oral agents. Although this fosters independence—patients do not have to be treated in a hospital or outpatient setting—it does have considerable potential to affect compliance. Regardless of the drug, noncompliance tends to be greater with oral agents than with IV chemotherapy or radiotherapy (Ma et al., 2008). Poor compliance may be due to intolerable drug side effects but also may occur for other reasons, including coincident maladies not related to the medication and high prescription costs (Ward, 2010). Ma et al. (2008) studied adherence to breast cancer treatment for patients receiving radiotherapy, chemotherapy, and oral tamoxifen therapy and found noncompliance rates of 4%, 7%, and 37%, respectively. Similarly, in a double-blind study comparing tamoxifen to placebo for a period of five years, the researchers found that 31% of the patients in the tamoxifen arm had discontinued their medication prior to the end of the study. Even more striking, 21% of the patients in the placebo arm had stopped their therapy as well (Bramwell et al., 2010). Although compliance was not an end point of the study design, it highlights the importance of patient education and follow-up, particularly because it is well documented that endocrine therapy can have long-term benefits when taken as prescribed (Ward, 2010).

Although not all ER/PR-positive patients will respond to endocrine therapy, several strategies can be used to impede estrogen-dependent tumor growth (Johnston, 2010; Mouridsen et al., 2003). Blocking of the estrogen receptors can be accomplished through the use of selective estrogen receptor modulators (SERMs) (Fabian, 2007). Aromatase inhibitors (AIs) can suppress estrogen production without interfering with downstream steroid production (Mouridsen et al., 2003). Estrogen production also can be affected by luteinizing hormone-releasing hormone (LHRH) agonists, which act to chemically ablate ovarian function (Goel et al., 2009). Estrogen receptors can be downregulated by the use of the es-

trogen receptor antagonist fulvestrant, which competitively binds to the ER (Fabian, 2007; Valachis, Mauri, et al., 2010).

## General Side Effects

One common side effect associated with endocrine therapy is hot flashes, which are possibly linked to a relationship between estrogen deprivation and serotonin receptors (Mortimer, 2010). Hot flashes have been treated with some success using selective serotonin reuptake inhibitors (SSRIs) such as fluoxetine or paroxetine (Mortimer, 2010). Venlafaxine has also shown some benefit. The antiepileptic drug gabapentin can decrease symptoms as well (Loprinzi et al., 2009). Further research in this area of symptom management is warranted.

Decreased estrogen levels also are associated with diffuse arthralgias, notably with the AIs. Because estrogen receptors do not exist in the joints but are present in the brain, it has been postulated that antiestrogen therapy may reduce the threshold to inflammatory joint pain (Mortimer, 2010). This side effect is particularly distressing in a population of women who may already be suffering from joint pain from a variety of etiologies. AI-induced joint pain is typically worse in the morning, but no rationale has been proposed. No specific treatment has been suggested, but a positive correlation between increased vitamin D levels and decreased pain has been suggested (Mortimer, 2010).

Sexual issues related to endocrine therapy include decreased libido, arousal, and orgasm; vaginal dryness; and dyspareunia (Mortimer, 2010). It is important for nurses to be comfortable discussing sexuality-related side effects without regard for patient age or sexual preferences. General principles include first establishing a trusting relationship in a comfortable environment, involving the partner in discussions, and offering information on lubricants and positions that may enhance sexual fulfillment (Barton-Burke & Wilkes, 2006; Katz, 2007).

As opposed to the SERMs, all of the AIs can increase the incidence of fractures or skeletal-related events (Santen et al., 2009). Detailed information regarding the prevention and treatment of skeletal-related events can be found in the Supportive Therapy: Bisphosphonates section.

## Tamoxifen

First synthesized in 1966 and approved by the U.S. Food and Drug Administration (FDA) in 1977, the oral drug tamoxifen (Nolvadex®, AstraZeneca) belongs to a group of antiestrogens referred to as SERMs, which block estrogen by competitively binding to the receptors (Crane-Okada & Loney, 2007; Legha et al., 1978). It also is believed to disrupt cellular proliferation by the inhibition of transforming growth factor-beta (Wilkes & Barton-Burke, 2010).

For the past two decades, tamoxifen has been the gold standard treatment for hormone-sensitive breast cancer in postmenopausal women (Giobbie-Hurder, Price, & Gelber, 2009). Used alone or in combination with systemic chemotherapy, tamoxifen has been shown to reduce the risk of death (Giob-bie-Hurder et al., 2009). However, the maximum length of tamoxifen therapy is limited to five years because of drug resistance and resultant disease progression.

Tamoxifen can be used to decrease the risk of ipsilateral breast cancer recurrence following breast-conserving therapy for ductal carcinoma in situ, sequentially (prior to chemotherapy) in adjuvant settings for both pre- and postmenopausal women, and as initial therapy for recurrent or metastatic disease (NCCN, 2011).

Estrogen receptors can be found in other physiologic locations aside from breast tissue. One undesirable effect of tamoxifen is its ability to both stimulate and inhibit estrogen receptors (Santen et al., 2009). This stimulation can lead to the development of endometrial cancer, which is also believed to be a result of DNA damage and hormone-specific effects (Laxmi et al., 2010; Mouridsen et al., 2003). The estrogen agonist effect of tamoxifen is believed to be partially responsible for disease recurrence when the drug is administered for more than five years (Fabian, 2007). These undesired characteristics, along with inevitable drug resistance, have fostered the development of antiestrogen alternatives and the third-generation AIs. These newer medications do not have stimulatory properties, and the AIs are thought to be more effective than tamoxifen in patients who are ER positive but PR negative (Fabian, 2007).

Additional side effects of tamoxifen include osteoporosis, thrombotic events, cataracts, and leg cramps (Crane-Okada & Loney 2007; Visvanathan, Lippman, Hurley, & Temin, 2009). Patients who do not tolerate tamoxifen may have better success by switching to one of the AIs. A listing of side effects can be found in Table 8-1.

As a prodrug that utilizes the CYP2D6 pathway and the hepatic cytochrome P450 enzyme system for metabolism, tamoxifen has a number of noteworthy possible drug interactions. These include cyclophosphamide, letrozole, glucocorticoids, and some oral antibiotics (Wilkes & Barton-Burke, 2010). In a study of 2,430 women being treated with tamoxifen and a variety of SSRIs, Kelly et al. (2010) demonstrated a statistically significant increase in breast cancer–related death rates for patients who used both tamoxifen and the SSRI paroxetine, a CYP2D6 inhibitor. For this reason, nurses should be vigilant in performing a thorough assessment of concurrent medications. Fluoxetine is also a CYP2D6 inhibitor; however, the study lacked sufficient power to prove an unfavorable outcome with concurrent use. Further research with these two medications is needed. Drug interactions also have been demonstrated with St. John's wort (Wilkes & Barton-Burke, 2010).

Because tamoxifen increases the risk of deep vein thrombosis, nurses should instruct patients to avoid activities that can lead to venous pooling. Patients also should be taught to assess their skin for development of a rash and to report symptoms to their medical provider (Wilkes & Barton-Burke, 2010).

Tamoxifen resistance is a significant concern. Evidence suggests that an increase in EGFRs, EGFR2 (also known as

**Table 8-1. Common Side Effects of Oral Endocrine Therapy**

| Medication | Side Effect |
|---|---|
| Anastrozole | Asthenia<br>Elevated gamma-glutamyltransferase and cholesterol<br>Fatigue<br>Fetotoxicity<br>Headache<br>Hot flashes<br>Pharyngitis<br>Skeletal-related events |
| Exemestane | Alopecia<br>Arthralgias<br>Fatigue<br>Fetotoxicity<br>Headaches<br>Hot flashes<br>Hypertension<br>Increased sweating<br>Skeletal-related events<br>Weight gain |
| Letrozole | Arthralgias<br>Dizziness<br>Elevated liver transaminases and cholesterol<br>Fatigue<br>Fetotoxicity<br>Hot flashes<br>Night sweats<br>Skeletal-related events<br>Weight gain |
| Tamoxifen | Dermatologic reactions (e.g., rash)<br>Hot flashes<br>Increased incidence of endometrial cancer<br>Menstrual irregularity<br>Nausea, vomiting, anorexia<br>Sexual dysfunction<br>Thromboembolic events (e.g., deep vein thrombosis)<br>Transient bone or tumor pain with initial dosing<br>Weight loss |

*Note.* Based on information from AstraZeneca Pharmaceuticals, 2009a; Novartis Pharmaceuticals Corp., 2010; Pharmacia & Upjohn, 2011; Wilkes & Barton-Burke, 2010.

HER2/neu), insulin-like growth factor-1 receptors, or tyrosine kinase receptor activation can potentiate tamoxifen resistance (Cristofanilli et al., 2010; Dalenc et al., 2010). Laboratory studies using the tyrosine kinase inhibitor lapatinib have shown the potential to restore lost ER signaling (Johnston, 2010). Research continues to look at signaling pathways and their role in resistance.

The future of tamoxifen therapy as the gold standard is currently under scrutiny because of favorable results from the use of third-generation AIs (Janni & Hepp, 2010; Valachis, Mauri, et al., 2010). Currently, the NCCN guidelines support using either tamoxifen or an AI as initial therapy in hormone receptor–positive, postmenopausal women (NCCN, 2011).

## Raloxifene

Another antiestrogen, raloxifene (Evista®, Eli Lilly and Co.), was initially approved for managing osteoporosis. Subsequently, the large, double-blind, multicenter Study of Tamoxifen and Raloxifene (STAR) trial was designed to compare the efficacy and side effects of raloxifene to tamoxifen for the prevention of invasive breast cancer in women at risk (Visvanathan et al., 2009; Vogel, 2009). Eligible participants were postmenopausal women older than 34 with a predicted breast cancer risk of at least 1.66%. The initial study showed both drugs to be equally effective in chemoprevention. Six years later, a follow-up of 19,490 participants showed raloxifene to be approximately 76% as effective as tamoxifen but with fewer side effects, specifically thromboembolic events, cataracts, and the development of endometrial cancer (Vogel et al., 2010). The future role of raloxifene is currently being debated, and it remains to be seen precisely what role it will play in breast cancer treatment.

## Fulvestrant

Fulvestrant (Faslodex®, AstraZeneca Pharmaceuticals) is an antiestrogen that does not share the agonist properties of tamoxifen. In laboratory models, fulvestrant has been shown to differ from tamoxifen by having a higher ability to antagonize estrogen-regulated genes, and it has the added benefit of halting cellular growth during the $G_0$ phase (AstraZeneca Pharmaceuticals, 2004; Frasor et al., 2004). Blocking of the MAKP pathway also occurs (Howell, 2006) in addition to degradation of both estrogen and progesterone (Valachis, Mauri, et al., 2010). Efficacy in ER/PR-positive women has been demonstrated in a number of trials including comparisons to tamoxifen (Howell, 2006; Howell et al., 2004). The Evaluation of Faslodex versus Exemestane Clinical Trial (EFECT) study was a double-blind, placebo-controlled, randomized trial that compared the efficacy and tolerability of fulvestrant to the AI exemestane (Aromasin®, Pfizer Inc.) (Chia et al., 2008). In the study, 693 postmenopausal women with advanced breast cancer were enrolled at 138 international centers. Patients received either an intramuscular injection of fulvestrant or placebo or oral exemestane or placebo. The study's primary end point was time to progression (TTP). This study also examined side effect–related quality of life and found that both medications were well tolerated.

Aside from injection-site pain, hot flashes, nausea, and fatigue were the most common adverse events. Fulvestrant has thus far not been associated with an increase in endometrial cancer. Because of its unique mechanism of action, it also is not believed to have cross-resistance to other antiestrogens (Valachis, Mauri, et al., 2010).

Although both drugs in the EFECT study demonstrated efficacy for this population, the median TTP was less than four months, and 70% of the women had disease progression by six months. The authors concluded that a number of confounding factors may have contributed to the lower-than-anticipated response rates, and additional studies using fulvestrant are under way. It is FDA approved for the treatment of postmenopausal ER-positive women with disease progression after treatment with antiestrogen therapy (AstraZeneca Pharmaceuticals, 2004).

## Aromatase Inhibitors

The enzyme aromatase is a significant biologic component responsible for the production of estrogen (Santen et al., 2009). Research in the 1970s demonstrated that aromatase was found not only in breast tissue but in adipose tissue as well and that nongonadal tissues were a significant source of estrogen production (Santen et al., 2009). Other studies demonstrated that malignant breast tumors themselves produced endogenous aromatase, providing the rationale for further developing AIs (Nabholtz, 2008).

The first-generation AI aminoglutethimide (AG) opened the door to a new class of medications and a drug that researchers hoped would be superior to tamoxifen, which was also under development during this time. However, AG was not sufficiently specific in its mechanism of action and consequently had significant toxicities (Nabholtz, 2008). In the late 1980s, the second-generation AI formestane was shown to be more potent and more specific than AG but failed to show benefit over tamoxifen.

By the early 1990s, the current third-generation oral AIs were developed. Three AIs are FDA approved: exemestane (Aromasin), letrozole (Femara®, Novartis Pharmaceuticals Corp.), and anastrozole (Arimidex®, AstraZeneca Pharmaceuticals). Whereas SERMs prevent binding of estrogen to the receptor, AIs act to stop estrogen production by preventing the conversion of testosterone and androstenedione to estrogen through inhibition of the P450 cytochrome aromatase (Fabian, 2007; Nabholtz, 2008).

Two specific types of AIs exist: androgen analogs or type I AIs, and nonsteroidal (type II) AIs. The only type I currently available is exemestane, which works by interfering with enzymatic binding. Letrozole and anastrozole belong to the type II category and are competitive inhibitors (Nabholtz, 2008). Because of a negative feedback loop resulting in increased levels of both luteinizing hormone and follicle-stimulating hormones, which causes ovarian stimulation, AIs are only effective in postmenopausal women or premenopausal women with loss of ovarian function (Nabholtz, Bonneterre, Buzdar, Robertson, & Thürlimann, 2003; Santen et al., 2009).

Several international studies have demonstrated efficacy of the AIs. The Breast International Group (BIG) 1-98 trial was conceived as a double-blind phase III study comparing tamoxifen to letrozole. Patients were to receive tamoxifen or letrozole for five years, or two years of tamoxifen followed by three years of letrozole, or two years of letrozole followed by three years of tamoxifen. More than 8,000 patients were enrolled in the combined arms. During an interim analysis at 51 months, patients receiving letrozole had better DFS when compared to the tamoxifen arm. Based on this information, the study was then modified by the unblinding of patients who had been randomized to the tamoxifen-alone arm. A significant DFS advantage was again seen with letrozole at 76 months (Giobbie-Hurder et al., 2009; van de Velde, Verma, van Nes, Masterman, & Pritchard, 2010). It should be noted that there was no statistically significant difference in OS between these two groups and no improvement in DFS in patients randomized to receive letrozole following two years of tamoxifen. Similarly, the Arimidex, Tamoxifen, Alone or in Combination (ATAC) Trial, which compared tamoxifen to anastrozole, also demonstrated an overall superiority for the latter (ATAC Trialists' Group, 2008). A total of 9,366 women were randomized to receive anastrozole or tamoxifen as monotherapy or anastrozole plus tamoxifen. The third arm was stopped because of lack of improved efficacy after initial analysis. However, of the remaining patients in the anastrozole versus tamoxifen arms, improvement in DFS was observed.

Depending on individual patient selection, AIs can be used as an upfront therapy (i.e., before tamoxifen), switching therapy (where patients are initially treated with one agent and then changed to an AI), and extended therapy after completion of five years of tamoxifen (van de Velde et al., 2010). Switching therapies in particular have shown tremendous promise by improving both DFS and OS (Janni & Hepp, 2010; van de Velde et al., 2010).

Little evidence exists to support using one AI over another, and it is difficult to compare trial results because of lack of study homogeneity. Further research is needed to grasp a better understanding of individual agents and how they should best be used (NCCN, 2011).

### Anastrozole

Results from studies focusing on postmenopausal women indicate that AIs are superior to tamoxifen (Janni & Hepp, 2010). The North American and Tamoxifen or Arimidex Randomized Group Efficacy and Tolerability (TARGET) trials were randomized, double-blind, multicenter trials that compared the efficacy of tamoxifen to anastrozole for first-line treatment of advanced breast cancer in 1,021 women (Nabholtz et al., 2003). Anastrozole was superior to tamoxifen when looking at TTP (11.1 months versus 5.6 months, $p = 0.005$). The TARGET trial demonstrated that anastrozole was equal to tamoxifen, although only 45% of the participants were ER/PR positive. However, both groups reported significantly lower side effects, particularly thrombosis and vaginal bleeding. The ATAC trial included more than 5,000 post-

menopausal women and was designed to compare anastrozole alone and in combination with tamoxifen as adjuvant treatment for a period of five years. Results showed an increase in DFS but no OS benefits (ATAC Trialists' Group, 2008). Subsequent analysis also showed DFS efficacy extending beyond five years and again a reduction in side effects such as endometrial cancer and thromboembolic events. However, an increase in skeletal-related events was reported (ATAC Trialists' Group, 2008).

Side effects of anastrozole include hot flashes, fatigue, vaginal dryness, nausea, vomiting, and headache (Wilkes & Barton-Burke, 2010). Additional side effects are included in Table 8-1.

### Letrozole

The MA.17 trial included 1,579 women who were randomized to receive either letrozole or placebo after completing five years of tamoxifen therapy (Goss et al., 2008). Follow-up was done at 30 and 54 months, although the study was unblinded at first analysis when data showed a significant difference in DFS for patients who had been randomized to receive letrozole. As would be expected with AIs, more fractures were noted with the letrozole group than with the placebo. However, the risk of developing metastatic disease was reduced by 61% (Goss et al., 2008). Side effects of letrozole include somnolence and dizziness, hot flashes, and nausea (Wilkes & Barton-Burke, 2010).

### Exemestane

Less research has been published on the efficacy of exemestane, an oral inactivator of aromatase (Deeks & Scott, 2009). The Intergroup Exemestane Study was a randomized switching protocol whereby patients receiving tamoxifen would either continue therapy for five years or switch to exemestane at two years and continue for three additional years (Coombes et al., 2007). A total of 4,724 patients were enrolled at multiple sites between 1998 and 2003. An interim analysis performed at a median of 55 months showed a small decrease in breast cancer–related deaths in the exemestane arm. Similar to the other AIs, side effects of exemestane include decreased bone mineral density (BMD), hot flashes, fatigue, and insomnia (Deeks & Scott, 2009; Wilkes & Barton-Burke, 2010).

## Luteinizing Hormone-Releasing Hormone Agonists

Also known as gonadotropin-releasing hormone, LHRH plays a role in estrogen production (Hackshaw et al., 2009). In premenopausal women, LHRH agonists can effectively suppress ovarian production of estrogen and may be considered a viable alternative to oophorectomy (Goel et al., 2009). By inhibiting pituitary gonadotropin, LHRH agonists produce a chemically reversible menopause (Goel et al., 2009; Wilkes & Barton-Burke, 2010).

### Goserelin

A number of trials have compared the efficacy and quality of life of these agents with that of tamoxifen alone, tamoxifen with chemotherapy, chemotherapy alone, and AIs. The International Breast Cancer Study Group Trial VIII examined the efficacy of goserelin (Zoladex®, AstraZeneca Pharmaceuticals) in premenopausal node-negative women (International Breast Cancer Study Group, 2003). A total of 1,065 women were randomized to goserelin alone, chemotherapy alone, or chemotherapy followed by goserelin. OS for all three arms of the study were equivalent, although DFS for ER-negative patients was better for women who received chemotherapy (84% versus 73%). The Zoladex in Premenopausal Patients (or ZIPP) study also looked at the use of goserelin in premenopausal women with early breast cancer. This multicenter study included 2,706 women who were randomly assigned to receive two years of goserelin, tamoxifen, both drugs, or neither (Hackshaw et al., 2009). Analysis at 15 years confirmed earlier conclusions that the greatest benefit was noted in patients who received goserelin alone compared to the control group; adding goserelin to tamoxifen produced a statistically insignificant improvement. Goserelin was more effective in patients who were ER positive.

The most common side effect of goserelin noted in these trials was hot flashes. Other side effects include headache, sweating, acne, depression, vaginitis, and edema (AstraZeneca Pharmaceuticals, 2009b). Unlike typical injectable medications, goserelin is a pellet that is deposited deep into the subcutaneous abdominal tissue. The preassembled syringe uses a special large-bore needle. Discomfort can be decreased by first injecting the area with a local anesthetic such as 1% buffered lidocaine (Wilkes & Barton-Burke, 2010). Nurses should be well versed on the administration of this drug and should explain the procedure thoroughly to the patient prior to injection.

### Leuprorelin Acetate

The LHRH agonist leuprorelin acetate (Lupron Depot®, Abbott Laboratories) was first used as an effective treatment for men with prostate cancer and is being studied in premenopausal women with breast cancer. For the Takeda Adjuvant Breast Cancer Study with Leuprorelin Acetate (or TABLE) study, Schmid et al. (2007) randomized 599 patients to receive leuprorelin acetate or chemotherapy. At a follow-up of 5.8 years, DFS was equal. They reported a trend for lower breast cancer–related mortality for the leuprorelin acetate arm (28.9% versus 39.5%).

Leuprorelin acetate is administered by intramuscular injection into the gluteus. Hot flashes and increased sweating were commonly reported side effects during the trials. Postmarketing side effects also include headache, dizziness, breast tenderness, and peripheral edema (Wilkes & Barton-Burke, 2010).

The current NCCN guidelines recommend the use of LHRH agonists as one method of ovarian ablation, but the optimal frequency and duration have yet to be firmly established (NCCN, 2011). AIs are recommended in postmenopausal women who have been treated with tamoxifen and for women who have not received antiestrogen treatment (or for whom it has been more than one year since treatment). Many questions remain unanswered regarding the optimal use of endocrine therapy, particularly the AIs (Ward, 2010), and more studies with LHRH agonists are needed.

## Chemotherapy

### Background

Despite its inherent lack of specificity, chemotherapy continues to play a central role in the systemic treatment of breast cancer. As a group, all antineoplastic agents work by interfering with cellular division, although the mechanism of action varies between classes of drugs.

Chemotherapy agents can be classified based on how they assert their effect during the cell cycle. Cell cycle–specific drugs are active during the S, M, or G phase and include paclitaxel, methotrexate, and fluorouracil. Other antineoplastics are cell cycle nonspecific and include cyclophosphamide, cisplatin, and doxorubicin.

One inherent weakness in the effectiveness of chemotherapy is tied to the Gompertzian model of tumor growth. As the size of the tumor increases, the growth fraction (number of dividing cells) slows, with a smaller percentage of dividing cancerous cells. Because chemotherapeutic agents act during cellular replication, their effectiveness diminishes as cellular reproduction slows (Barton-Burke & Wilkes, 2006). Accordingly, chemotherapy is most effective in smaller tumors with a higher growth fraction. In addition, effectiveness of all chemotherapy is dependent on the cell kill hypothesis, which states that with each dose of chemotherapy, only a percentage of malignant cells will be killed, thus necessitating subsequent doses (or cycles) of treatment (Barton-Burke & Wilkes, 2006). Because of the inherently toxic nature of chemotherapy, rest periods, which allow the recovery of normal cells (e.g., hematopoietic cells), are built into cycles. Evidence suggests that breast cancer cells proliferate more rapidly than is generally associated with Gompertzian kinetics (Venturini et al., 2005), providing the impetus for alternative dosing strategies.

When to begin treatment, and when to stop, is a conundrum. For early-stage breast cancer, adjuvant therapy should be initiated quickly, as delays can result in an increased risk of disease recurrence and subsequent relapse (McArthur & Hudis, 2007a). In general, with anthracycline-based regimens, six cycles have shown superior efficacy to four cycles (McArthur & Hudis, 2007b). The optimal number of cycles remains unclear. Bonadonna et al. (2005) reported on long-term survival for patients who had received combination therapy with cyclophosphamide, methotrexate, and fluorouracil

(CMF). With a median follow-up of 25 years, analysis confirmed that patients who had received 12 cycles did not fare any better than those who had received 6.

However, for patients with MBC experiencing disease progression or intolerable side effects, treatment should be changed or stopped completely (Palmieri, Frye, & Mahon, 2009). Decisions to pursue further treatment should involve a thorough discussion with the patient and family. Nurses can provide emotional support to patients and families during these difficult times.

## Regimens

The use of chemotherapy for breast cancer has evolved over the decades and continues to be evaluated through an unprecedented number of international trials. Single-agent therapy used during the 1960s evolved during the 1970s when it was discovered that combination chemotherapy used for the treatment of other solid tumors could be more effective than single agents. Canellos et al. (1974) reported on the success of combining CMF and prednisone for the treatment of advanced breast cancer. This novel regimen was able to reduce large tumors prior to surgery. Accordingly, a number of chemotherapy combinations or regimens have evolved. The fluorouracil, doxorubicin, and cyclophosphamide (FAC) regimen, which is one of the oldest combinations, produced responses in patients with MBC, which had previously been rare. This regimen was later compared to other combinations including cyclophosphamide, doxorubicin, and fluorouracil (CAF) and doxorubicin, and cyclophosphamide (AC) (Fisher et al., 1990). By the 1990s, the novel agent paclitaxel had demonstrated improved efficacy over many of the older regimens and was later combined with AC. New combinations continue to be studied as researchers look for more effective and less toxic regimens.

How chemotherapy is used depends on the extent of disease, ER/PR status, and the timing of treatment (neoadjuvant or adjuvant). In general, chemotherapy often is beneficial regardless of tumor size, patient age, and number of positive nodes (Conzen et al., 2008). Groundbreaking work by Allegra and colleagues in the 1970s demonstrated that tumors in patients who were ER negative were more responsive than those who were ER positive (Allegra, Lippman, Thompson, & Simon, 1978). Indeed, chemotherapy is the treatment of choice for patients whose tumors do not express estrogen, progesterone, or HER2 receptors, known as TNBC (Isakoff, 2010). TNBC occurs in approximately 25%–30% of all breast cancers and tends to be highly aggressive (Burness, Grushko, & Olopade, 2010; Gucalp & Traina, 2010). Chemotherapy remains the treatment of choice for patients with bulky, visceral disease and those experiencing symptoms caused by the primary tumor or metastases (Beslija et al., 2009).

Treatment includes the use of taxanes and anthracycline agents (Perez, Moreno-Aspitia, Thompson, & Andor-

fer, 2010). The relatively new agent ixabepilone (Ixempra®, Bristol-Myers Squibb Co.) has shown promise in this setting, particularly with women who were deemed taxane-resistant (Perez, Patel, & Moreno-Aspitia, 2010). Also, preclinical and early clinical evidence suggests that the platinum compounds may be particularly effective with TNBC, and trials are currently under way (Isakoff, 2010; Perez, Moreno-Aspitia, et al., 2010). In addition, the use of EGFR inhibitors is showing promise for TNBC, although benefits will most likely occur when it used in conjunction with chemotherapy (Burness et al., 2010). This class of drugs will be discussed in detail.

Although in some settings the use of taxanes in combination with an anthracycline has mostly supplanted CMF and FAC, no one combination of agents, dosages, or regimen frequency can be applied to all patients (Conzen et al., 2008; Palmieri et al., 2009). It often is difficult to predict which disease variables will influence overall survival. Hence, numerous chemotherapy regimens have been used on a wide variety of patients and with varying degrees of success. Single-agent therapy remains a viable option for patients with less aggressive or locally advanced disease (Andreetta, Minisini, Miscoria, & Puglisi, 2010).

Much experience has been gained with the use of chemotherapy in the adjuvant setting. The NCCN guidelines continue to recommend a combination of an anthracycline (e.g., doxorubicin) and a taxane-based regimen as first-line therapy (NCCN, 2011). Unfortunately, up to 90% of patients with MBC who have been treated with these agents will develop drug resistance with resultant disease progression (Palmieri et al., 2009).

For many patients, combination therapy is extensively used, as it provides increases in TTP and progression-free survival (PFS) (Andreetta et al., 2010). However, combination therapy for women with MBC has not been proven superior to sequential single agents in terms of OS (Andreetta et al., 2010), and it is well established that multidrug therapy also increases the number and degree of toxicities (NCCN, 2011). There is not a wealth of data on the sequential use of second-line agents after primary treatment has failed (Tkaczuk, 2009). Therefore, no gold standard has emerged for the treatment of MBC.

Much less is known about the optimal role of chemotherapy for older adult patients with breast cancer, and little agreement exists as to the best possible course of treatment (Petrakis & Paraskakis, 2010). Organ damage, particularly cardiotoxicity, remains a significant concern if doxorubicin is part of the regimen (Bernardi et al., 2008). Mucositis tends to be more severe in older patients. Nausea and vomiting, discussed in detail later, also can be worse, which is particularly troublesome in patients whose oral fluid intake may already be insufficient. Pharmacokinetic changes due to age or polypharmacy can produce unexpected toxicities (Crivellari et al., 2007). Single-agent therapy may be better tolerated than combination therapy, although healthy patients may tolerate therapies identical to those offered to younger patients

(Petrakis & Paraskakis, 2010). Treatment with low-dose regimens also has been explored, but no large-scale studies have thus far demonstrated overall benefits (Crivellari et al., 2007).

## Dose-Dense Therapy

Different approaches to the timing of chemotherapy are being used in the clinical setting. A number of studies have examined the role of dose-dense therapy, which can be defined as giving higher dosages of chemotherapy per cycle or giving the same dosage more frequently (Citron, 2004). This type of treatment is feasible by incorporating colony-stimulating factors into chemotherapy regimens (Sugarman et al., 2009). Historical evidence for potential efficacy was derived from observations that women who had received at least 85% of their planned dose of CMF had better OS than those who did not, supporting the theory of attempting to deliver the maximum tolerated dose (Bonadonna et al., 2005; Bonadonna, Valagussa, Moliterni, Zambetti, & Brambilla, 1995; Citron, 2004). Additional evidence is supported by the observed trend for greater survival when CMF cycles were reduced from 28 days to 21 days (Mayers, Panzarella, & Tannock, 2001). The Cancer and Leukemia Group B (CALGB) 9741 trial compared the administration of doxorubicin, cyclophosphamide, and paclitaxel (AC+T) given every two or every three weeks (Citron et al., 2003). The study also examined the combination given sequentially and included the granulocyte colony-stimulating factor filgrastim. DFS was the primary end point of the study. Of the 1,973 patients who were treated, DFS and OS were longer in the dose-dense arms regardless of tumor size, ER status, and number of positive nodes. The authors also reported a relatively low incidence of chemotherapy-associated toxicities.

This approach has also been applied to the treatment of older women. Zauderer, Patil, and Hurria (2009) reported on a retrospective study of 162 patients with a mean age of 66 (range 60–76) who received AC+T every two weeks for four cycles. A total of 22% of the patients were unable to complete the planned four cycles because of allergic reactions, neutropenic fever, and patient preference. Sixty-seven patients (41%) experienced at least one grade 3 or 4 hematologic toxicity. Although age alone was not correlated with toxicity risk, more blood transfusions were required for patients 70 years of age or older. The need for transfusions coincides with an association between patients with low baseline hemoglobin levels and grade 3 or 4 hematologic toxicities. This study was not designed to look at survival benefit but concluded that dose-dense therapy was feasible in older patients.

Sugarman and colleagues reported on a pilot of dose-dense sequential cyclophosphamide followed by paclitaxel on a 14-day cycle (Sugarman et al., 2009). The primary end points were absence of neutropenic fever and neutropenia on planned treatment days. Only 60% of the patients were able to complete therapy.

The Prospective Observational European Neutropenia Study (or POENS) investigation revealed that patient variables, specifically older age and lower weight, were significant risk factors for developing neutropenia and that the prophylactic use of colony-stimulating factors decreased the incidence of neutropenia and therefore prevented interruption of treatment or dose reduction (Schwenkglenks et al., 2010).

This highlights a potential liability of dose-dense therapy unless it is supported by the inclusion of growth factors (Aapro, Crawford, & Kamioner, 2010). Filgrastim and pegfilgrastim can be beneficial for dose-dense administration of various regimens. Both the American Society of Clinical Oncology and NCCN guidelines recommend colony-stimulating factors for patients who are receiving chemotherapy regimens with at least a 20% risk of developing febrile neutropenia (Aapro et al., 2010; Kearney & Friese, 2008; NCCN, 2010). See Figure 8-2 for examples of commonly used chemotherapy regimens shown to cause neutropenia.

In clinical practice, the use of colony-stimulating factors is inconsistent (Renwick, Pettengell, & Green, 2009). Clinicians may use filgrastim, which requires daily subcutaneous dosing, or pegfilgrastim, which involves only one injection. Both drugs are generally initiated 24 hours after the end of chemotherapy and have equal efficacy (Quirion, 2009). Colony-stimulating factors are associated with additional cost and side effects, both of which can affect patient compliance and antineoplastic treatment options. Bone pain commonly occurs and may be relieved by the use of nonsteroidal anti-inflammatory agents (if not contraindicated) (Wilkes & Barton-Burke, 2010). Injections can be painful if given too quickly.

## Metronomic Therapy

Metronomic chemotherapy uses frequent (weekly) lower dosages of chemotherapy (Greenberg & Rugo, 2010; Kerbel & Kamen, 2004). Although it is based on some of the same rationale as dose-dense therapy, metronomic dosing offers less toxicity and targets the endothelial cells of tumor angiogenesis, as opposed to targeting rapidly proliferating cells in gen-

---

**Figure 8-2. Chemotherapy Regimens Associated With 20% or Greater Risk of Febrile Neutropenia**

- Doxorubicin, cyclophosphamide → docetaxel
- *Doxorubicin, cyclophosphamide → paclitaxel
- Docetaxel, doxorubicin, cyclophosphamide
- *Docetaxel, doxorubicin, cyclophosphamide
- *Epirubicin, cyclophosphamide
- Doxorubicin, docetaxel
- Doxorubicin, paclitaxel
- Paclitaxel → doxorubicin, cyclophosphamide

* Dose-dense regimens

*Note.* Based on information from Kearney & Friese, 2008; National Comprehensive Cancer Network, 2010.

eral (Kerbel & Kamen, 2004). A groundbreaking animal study by Browder et al. (2000) demonstrated that while the maximum tolerated dose of cyclophosphamide was able to exert cytotoxic and antiangiogenic effects in mice, the neovasculature was repaired during the traditional rest period between cycles. When doses were administered closer together, apoptosis of the tumor's endothelial cells would occur, subsequently resulting in tumor death. These results led to the assertion that if chemotherapy for general cancer treatment was delivered more frequently, vascular repair would be less likely. Browder's experiments also demonstrated efficacy against mouse tumors with cyclophosphamide resistance. In the clinical setting, metronomic therapy is similar to maintenance therapy for acute lymphoblastic leukemia (Kerbel & Kamen, 2004).

Several antineoplastic agents, including methotrexate and paclitaxel, have demonstrated antiangiogenic properties in vitro. Studies have been conducted with various agents to examine the effectiveness and tolerability of metronomic dosing. In a small study of 64 patients with MBC, oral cyclophosphamide was administered daily along with twice-daily oral methotrexate on days 1 and 2. Two patients achieved a complete response, and 12 achieved a partial response. Twenty-six percent of the patients continued to respond at 52 weeks. Overall, the treatment was well tolerated with minimal alopecia and neutropenia (Colleoni et al., 2002). Another small trial using metronomic cyclophosphamide, capecitabine, and the vascular endothelial growth factor (VEGF) monoclonal antibody (MoAb) bevacizumab for women with MBC produced 1 complete response and 21 partial responses (Dellapasqua et al., 2008). Eight patients had stable disease for greater than six months. The researchers noted better responses in patients who were ER positive, which is thought to be due to a less aggressive tumor variant. Few patients had side effects greater than grade 3 (according to the Common Terminology Criteria for Adverse Events version 3).

Mauri et al. (2010) performed a meta-analysis of 11 studies administering taxanes on a weekly schedule versus every three weeks. Six of the studies used paclitaxel, four used docetaxel, and one used nanoparticle albumin-bound paclitaxel (nab-paclitaxel). Allowing for the heterogeneity of the studies, the authors concluded that weekly paclitaxel was superior in terms of OS compared to the every-three-week regimen. The same was not true for patients who had received docetaxel, although only three small studies were examined. Weekly taxane infusions also were associated with fewer side effects, such as peripheral neuropathy (PN) and neutropenic fever.

In a study of 4,950 women who were randomized to receive either paclitaxel or docetaxel weekly or every three weeks, researchers concluded that both PFS and OS for the weekly paclitaxel was superior to the three-week schedule (Sparano et al., 2008). However, contrary to the previously described studies, 27% of the patients in the weekly arm had grade 2–4 peripheral neuropathy, which was greater than the other three cohorts.

Although metronomic therapy is included as an option in the NCCN guidelines for breast cancer, its precise role in breast cancer treatment has yet to be established. Larger controlled studies evaluating the effectiveness and toxicity of conventional current and novel agents are warranted.

## General Considerations

A discussion of chemotherapy would not be complete without addressing the general issues associated with the administration of these agents. Side effects can range from mild to debilitating, depending upon the drug, dosage, treatment schedule, and individual patient variables.

### Nausea and Vomiting

Nausea and vomiting are common side effects of chemotherapy, and some of the most commonly used drugs for the treatment of breast cancer (e.g., cyclophosphamide and doxorubicin) are considered moderately or highly emetogenic (Wilkes & Barton-Burke, 2010). Despite tremendous progress with the incorporation of newer classes of antiemetics into treatment regimens, nausea remains the singularly most distressing side effect for patients receiving chemotherapy (Shih, Wan, & Chan, 2009).

Risk factors for experiencing nausea have been identified and include patients who have received prior chemotherapy, exhibit anxiety, are younger in age, or have a history of motion sickness (Shih et al., 2009; Wilkes & Barton-Burke, 2010). Interestingly, a history of alcohol use connotes a decreased risk, although the mechanism is not well understood.

Both NCCN and the American Society of Clinical Oncology have produced guidelines regarding the appropriate selection of antiemetics depending on the potential emetogenicity of the particular agent or agents. General recommendations include use of the substance P/neurokinin 1 (NK-1) receptor antagonist aprepitant or its IV counterpart fosaprepitant, the glucocorticoid dexamethasone, a selective serotonin 5-HT$_3$ receptor antagonist such as ondansetron or granisetron, and the benzodiazepine lorazepam.

Nurses play an important role in preventing and treating nausea and providing accurate patient education. Patients should understand the rationale for filling antiemetic prescriptions and adhering to dosing schedules—even in the absence of nausea. The use of an anxiolytic, such as lorazepam, can be effective in preventing anticipatory nausea (Barton-Burke & Wilkes, 2006). Additional interventions are found in Figure 8-3. Nurses must be aware of the side effects of antiemetics. Aprepitant can cause constipation, diarrhea, or hiccoughs (Wilkes & Barton-Burke, 2010). Because aprepitant can interact with many other medications via the CYP3A and CYP2C9 and P450 hepatic isoenzyme pathways (Wilkes & Barton-Burke, 2010), nurses should obtain a detailed medication history and consult with a clinical pharmacist as needed. All of the selective serotonin 5-HT$_3$ receptor antagonists

**Figure 8-3. Interventions for Preventing or Reducing Chemotherapy-Induced Nausea and Vomiting**

- Administer antiemetics prior to chemotherapy.
- Attempt to control nausea with the first treatment.
- Have patients avoid noxious odors.
- Discourage eating heavy or fatty foods.
- Experiment with small meals prior to or after treatment.
- Suck on hard candy during treatment.
- Provide distractions during treatment.
- Provide emotional support.

*Note.* Based on information from Barton-Burke & Wilkes, 2006.

can cause headache and constipation, and dolasetron can prolong electrocardiogram intervals (Wilkes & Barton-Burke, 2010). Of all the selective serotonin 5-HT$_3$ receptor antagonists, only palonosetron is FDA approved for the prevention of both acute and delayed nausea and vomiting.

### Alopecia

A diagnosis of breast cancer carries tremendous implications for a patient's self-image. Adding to the consequences of body-altering surgery, chemotherapy often results in alopecia. Hair loss can have a profound effect on sexual identity and interpersonal relationships and, along with nausea, is considered one of the top three most burdensome side effects of chemotherapy (Hesketh et al., 2004). Alopecia can lead to anxiety and depression, which can further influence decisions to continue therapy. Hair loss also affects family members, particularly children who may struggle with accepting a mother's appearance, or may adversely affect normal socialization with peers, including attending school functions or carpooling (Hesketh et al., 2004).

Rapidly dividing hair follicles are sensitive to drugs that cannot distinguish between abnormal and normal cells. The damage, though temporary, is the result of matrix cell reproduction (Trüeb, 2009). Agents associated with alopecia include cyclophosphamide, paclitaxel, and the anthracyclines. Doxorubicin in particular can result in alopecia in more than 80% of patients (Barton-Burke & Wilkes, 2006). Varying degrees of hair loss can affect all parts of the body, including eye lashes and brows. Hair may begin to fall out within two to three weeks of initiating therapy; regrowth often occurs within two to three months after completion of therapy (Barton-Burke & Wilkes, 2006).

Prevention of alopecia has been attempted by the application of cold to the scalp. Results, however, have been mixed. One small study designed to assess the psychological components of ice cap versus no ice cap reported a 52% success rate (van den Hurk, Mols, Vingerhoets, & Breed, 2009).

It has long been believed that scalp cooling might lead to an increased risk of scalp metastasis. However, a recent retrospective study by Lemieux and colleagues did not support this theory. Of 640 patients with breast cancer, scalp metasta-

sis developed in 1.1% of those who had used cooling at a median follow-up of 5.8 years (Lemieux, Amireault, Provencher, & Maunsell, 2009). Of the seven patients who developed scalp metastases, none had received taxane therapy, and all had evidence of metastatic disease in other sites in addition to the scalp. Four of the seven had stage III breast cancer. The authors concluded that scalp cooling was not associated with significant risk of scalp metastases. Grevelman and Breed (2005) reviewed 53 studies published between 1973 and 2003 and examined the efficacy of scalp cooling. Success rates varied considerably and were influenced by cooling time: 76% effective for scalp cooling longer than 1.5 hours post-treatment versus 71% if less than 1.5 hours. The presence of liver function abnormalities also was correlated with decreased success. Extreme lack of homogeneity and weak study designs make aggregated conclusions difficult. Benefit also varied depending on drug or drugs used, whether single-agent or combination therapy, and prior therapy. The optimal degree of hypothermia was not identified, nor has this variable been accurately studied. While recognizing the potential for scalp metastasis, the authors concluded that scalp cooling should still be considered. However, because of the lack of well-designed randomized trials, this intervention remains controversial. Topical agents such as minoxidil have been tried without success, and a number of agents designed to block keratinocyte apoptosis are being explored (Hesketh et al., 2004).

Nurses should emphasize that alopecia is a temporary condition and that regrowth will occur. Patients and family members should be encouraged to verbalize their feelings. One approach to reduce the visual trauma is to suggest that patients cut their hair prior to or at the start of treatment. The head should be washed with a mild shampoo (such as baby shampoo), and sunscreen with a sun protection factor higher than 15 should be used to protect the head when uncovered. Patients can shift the focus to emphasize other aspects of their physical appearance, such as clothing and makeup, and use scarves, hats, and wigs (Barton-Burke & Wilkes, 2006).

### Secondary Malignancies

Both doxorubicin and cyclophosphamide are associated with an increased risk of myelodysplastic syndrome or acute leukemia (Martin et al., 2009; McArthur & Hudis, 2007a). Although it is unclear what role genetic predisposition plays in the development of secondary malignancies, cyclophosphamide is classified as a known carcinogen (Eisenberg, 2009). Although the risk is relatively small, patients must be aware of it prior to beginning therapy.

### Risks to Nursing Personnel Handling Chemotherapeutic Agents

Finally, any discussion of chemotherapy should reinforce the importance of using adequate safety precautions for nurses administering hazardous drugs. Exposure to chemotherapy continues to be a major concern for nurses handling hazardous drugs (Eisenberg, 2009). It has been demonstrated to cause a number of reproductive issues, in addition to harming the off-spring of exposed individuals (Martin, 2005). National guidelines for the safe handling of hazardous drugs have been published by the Oncology Nursing Society, the National Institute for Occupational Safety and Health, and the American Society of Health-System Pharmacists, and readers are encouraged to utilize these recourses (Polovich, Whitford, & Olsen, 2009).

## Specific Chemotherapeutic Agents

Although a comprehensive review of all chemotherapeutic agents used for breast cancer is beyond the scope of this chapter, pertinent information for commonly used agents is presented. As illustrated in Table 8-2, the number of chemotherapy agents used singly or in combination is impressive and will continue to grow as newer agents and combinations are evaluated.

### Cyclophosphamide

First synthesized in 1958 as an analog to nitrogen mustard (Anders & Kemp, 1961), the alkylating agent cyclophosphamide causes cross-linkage of DNA (Barton-Burke & Wilkes, 2006). It has been extensively used for a multitude of solid and hematologic malignancies and continues to be an integral part of many breast cancer treatment regimens. Cyclophosphamide is available in both oral and IV formulations. The oral form should be taken with food. White blood cell (WBC) nadir occurs within 7–14 days, although the duration may be longer when it is used in combination with other chemotherapy agents. Hemorrhagic cystitis and cardiomyopathy can occur, although these typically are seen only in high-dose regimens, such as those used in stem cell transplantation.

### Doxorubicin

Doxorubicin, approved by the FDA in 1974, is a member of the anthracyclines, which also includes epirubicin, idarubicin, and daunorubicin. Doxorubicin intercalates DNA base pairs, inhibits DNA and RNA synthesis, and has an affinity for binding to lipid-containing cellular membranes (Wilkes & Barton-Burke, 2010). As early as 1974, doxorubicin demonstrated activity in breast cancer (Blum & Carter, 1974) and, like cyclophosphamide, has shown activity in a number of other neoplasms. WBC nadir occurs 10–14 days after administration.

Anthracyclines have well-documented cardiac toxicities associated with cumulative doses greater than 450–550 mg/m² (Wilkes & Barton-Burke, 2010). This life-threatening side effect becomes even more onerous for women who are HER2 positive and receive trastuzumab (Herceptin®, Genentech, Inc.), which is also associated with cardiac dysfunction (Beslija et al., 2009).

Doxorubicin is a powerful vesicant and causes severe tissue necrosis if extravasated. The degree of cellular destruction is

**Table 8-2. Common Chemotherapy Agents Used in Breast Cancer**

| Single Agents | |
| --- | --- |
| **Drug Classification** | **Drug Name** |
| Anthracyclines | Doxorubicin<br>Epirubicin<br>Liposomal doxorubicin |
| Taxanes | Paclitaxel<br>Docetaxel<br>Nab-paclitaxel |
| Antimetabolites | Capecitabine<br>Gemcitabine |
| Microtubule inhibitors | Vinorelbine |
| Alkylating agents | Cyclophosphamide |

| Combination Chemotherapy | |
| --- | --- |
| **Regimen** | **Regimen Name** |
| Cyclophosphamide, doxorubicin, and fluorouracil | CAF/FAC |
| Fluorouracil, epirubicin, and cyclophosphamide | FEC |
| Doxorubicin and cyclophosphamide | AC |
| Epirubicin and cyclophosphamide | EC |
| Doxorubicin and docetaxel | AT |
| Doxorubicin and paclitaxel | AT |
| Cyclophosphamide, methotrexate, and fluorouracil | CMF |
| Docetaxel and capecitabine | – |
| Gemcitabine and paclitaxel | GT |
| Ixabepilone and capecitabine | – |

*Note.* From *NCCN Clinical Practice Guidelines in Oncology™: Breast Cancer* [v.2.2010], by National Comprehensive Cancer Network, 2010. Retrieved from http://www.nccn.org/professionals/physician_gls/PDF/breast.pdf. Adapted with permission.

intensified because the drug is not metabolized in tissues and can persist for weeks to months (Langer, Sehested, & Jensen, 2000). Nursing administration of all vesicants must follow strict protocols for prevention of extravasation. This includes proper vein selection, venipuncture technique, or implanted port access; positive blood return; patient assessment; and follow-up instructions (Schulmeister, 2007, 2009). One antidote currently is FDA approved for anthracycline extravasation. Dexrazoxane for injection (Totect®, TopoTarget) demonstrated a proven efficacy of 98% in two clinical trials (Mouridsen et al., 2007) and is available in a three-day kit. Doxorubicin is red in color and may cause the urine to change color as well. Patients need to be instructed that this is a normal part of excretion and is not related to bleeding. Nausea and vomiting are common with all anthracyclines, and hand-foot syndrome (HFS) can occur with the liposomal formulation.

### Fluorouracil

Fluorouracil is a pyrimidine antimetabolite that inhibits DNA synthesis by impeding the formation of thymidine synthetase. Administration of methotrexate subsequent to fluorouracil enhances effectiveness; however, side effects are potentially increased. Leucovorin also increases the effectiveness of fluorouracil. WBC nadir occurs 10–14 days following administration. Patients should be instructed not to take folic acid during therapy. Although nausea is not as severe as with other chemotherapies, antimetabolites tend to cause gastrointestinal mucosal toxicity resulting in mucositis and diarrhea. Changes in nail integrity can result in cracking, and visual side effects such as photophobia and conjunctivitis also can occur (Wilkes & Barton-Burke, 2010).

### Methotrexate

A folic acid antagonist, methotrexate works by blocking dihydrofolate reductase. Because methotrexate is albumin bound, the use of other albumin-bound medications, such as phenytoin and tetracycline, should be avoided. In addition, omeprazole can result in elevated methotrexate levels. As with fluorouracil, folic acid should not be taken because of decreased methotrexate activity (Wilkes & Barton-Burke, 2010). WBC nadir occurs four to seven days after administration. Mucositis, diarrhea, and photosensitivity can occur.

### Paclitaxel and Docetaxel

As relative newcomers, the taxanes, paclitaxel and docetaxel, have become instrumental in systemic breast cancer therapy. Taxanes are commonly used for the treatment of invasive breast cancer (Gradishar et al., 2009; NCCN, 2011). They work by causing polymerization of the microtubules, thus interfering with normal mitosis (Chevallier et al., 1995; Slichenmyer & Von Hoff, 1991). A number of trials have documented the efficacy of both drugs (Seidman, Reichman, et al., 1995; Seidman, Tiersten, et al., 1995; Valero et al., 1995). The National Surgical Adjuvant Breast and Bowel Project (NSABP) B-28 trial examined DFS and OS by administering four cycles of paclitaxel after four cycles of AC in patients with locally advanced breast cancer (Mamounas et al., 2005). A total of 2,587 patients were randomized to receive either AC or AC followed by T (paclitaxel). Ninety-eight percent of the patients completed the AC arm; only 75.9% completed the AC→T arm. Predominant toxicities related to the taxane arm were grade 3 neurosensory toxicity (18%) and arthralgia or myalgia (12%). Of interest, eight patients developed acute leukemia or myelodysplastic syndrome. At a median follow-up of 64 months, the paclitaxel arm demonstrated a 17% improvement in DFS and a 7% improvement

in OS. Improved outcomes with taxanes also were seen in the CALGB 9344 study, which examined escalating doses of doxorubicin against standard AC plus T (Henderson et al., 2003).

Recently, Moulder et al. (2010) explored the administration of a 3-hour paclitaxel infusion versus a 96-hour infusion to test the hypothesis that longer infusion times, with subsequent prolonged drug-tumor contact, would provide better outcome. The researchers randomized 107 patients to both arms. Patients in the 96-hour arm suffered more hematologic toxicities, mucositis, myalgias, and PN. No significant differences in response rates were seen.

Because taxanes are not readily soluble in water, special vehicles are required. Paclitaxel is mixed with polyoxyethylated castor oil (Cremophor® EL, BASF Corp.); docetaxel requires polysorbate 80 (Tween® 80, ICI Americas, Inc.). Both of these vehicles are responsible for potentially life-threatening allergic hypersensitivity reactions characterized by bronchospasm, dyspnea, wheezing, abdominal or chest pain, itching, hypotension, and tachycardia. Therefore, premedication with corticosteroids such as dexamethasone, diphenhydramine, and an $H_2$ antagonist such as ranitidine is required (Wilkes & Barton-Burke, 2010). Owing to these severe reactions, paclitaxel has traditionally been infused over three hours; however, with sufficient premedication, some regimens allow for 60- or 90-minute infusions, as seen in dose-dense therapy. Docetaxel should be infused over one hour.

Nurses must have emergency equipment available prior to initiating therapy. Baseline vital signs and frequent assessments are needed during the infusion. It is recommended that patients who have had a severe anaphylactic reaction not be rechallenged (Wilkes & Barton-Burke, 2010).

Both drugs require di(2-ethylhexyl) phthalate (DEHP)-free bags and tubings (or glass bottles and polyethylene-lined tubings) because the vehicles can leach the plasticizer DEHP. A 0.22 micron or smaller filter must be attached to the administration set (BASF Corp., 2008; ICI Americas, Inc., 2006).

Taxanes can interact with numerous other medications via the CYP28C and CYP3A4 pathways (see Table 8-3). Paclitaxel

### Table 8-3. Taxane-Drug Interactions

| Interaction | Drug/Substance |
|---|---|
| Can decrease paclitaxel levels | Carbamazepine<br>Phenytoin |
| Can increase paclitaxel levels | Fluconazole<br>Ciprofloxacin<br>Doxycycline<br>Erythromycin<br>Grapefruit juice<br>Verapamil |

*Note.* Based on information from Wilkes & Barton-Burke, 2010.

can decrease the renal clearance of doxorubicin and therefore should be given afterward (Wilkes & Barton-Burke, 2010).

Although the toxicities of the taxanes are similar, docetaxel is noted for causing erythema, desquamation, onycholysis, and HFS. (See the Capecitabine section for further discussion of HFS.) Onycholysis involves changes to the nails and includes discoloration and splitting. The latter may be accompanied by subungual bleeding and potential loss of the nail (Scotté et al., 2005). It can affect the hands and feet. Based on the same theories supporting use of ice caps for the prevention of alopecia, Scotté and colleagues conducted a phase II study of 45 patients using frozen gloves to prevent skin toxicities of the hands (Scotté et al., 2005). All patients received docetaxel for a variety of tumors. The frozen gloves successfully prevented onycholysis compared to an incidence of 29% for patients whose hands were unprotected. In another study, the same author enrolled 50 patients receiving docetaxel to test the efficacy of a frozen sock to reduce or prevent nail toxicities (Scotté et al., 2008). The frozen sock successfully prevented toenail toxicity; the incidence of toxicity was 21% for unprotected feet. The author noted that the frozen sock did not prevent erythema or desquamation; therefore, devices should be explored that apply cold only to the toes.

Docetaxel also can cause fluid retention characterized by pedal edema, which may progress to generalized edema and associated weight gain. These effects can often be mitigated by using 8 mg of dexamethasone twice daily for three days prior to therapy (Wilkes & Barton-Burke, 2010). Progressive edema with respiratory compromise can occur. Thorough nursing assessments should be performed. Patients should be instructed to notify the patient care team if symptoms develop and need to understand the importance of taking oral dexamethasone as ordered.

PN is a common, potentially debilitating side effect, with an incidence of up to 60% (Wilkes & Barton-Burke, 2010), although symptom reporting varies widely, in part because of its subjective nature and the lack of universally accepted assessment tools (Paice, 2009). Researchers have yet to determine the precise mechanism for PN. It has been hypothesized that because microtubules are also found in neuronal axons, the same disruption responsible for cancer cell death also results in damage to nerve fibers (Donovan, 2009). In addition, there is a dying-back of the nerve, which begins distally (Loven et al., 2009). The risk of developing taxane-induced PN is increased for patients who receive other neurotoxic agents or have diabetic neuropathy, vitamin $B_{12}$ deficiencies, or a history of alcohol abuse (Donovan, 2009; Stein, 2010). Symptoms include decreased sensation, particularly to painful stimuli or temperature, tingling and numbness, pain, weakness, and loss of or diminished reflexes (Donovan, 2009).

Very little research exists on the effective prevention of PN. Animal models using the amino acid acetyl-L-carnitine have shown promise, but no large, well-controlled studies have been conducted (De Grandis, 2007; Jin, Flatters, Xiao, Mul-

hern, & Bennett, 2008). Small trials using vitamin E and the amino acid glutamine have shown mixed results (Loven et al., 2009; Paice, 2009). Symptomatic treatment of PN has included opioids, corticosteroids, tricyclic antidepressants, and anticonvulsants—all with varying results (Donovan, 2009; Paice, 2009). Nonpharmacologic interventions such as acupuncture also may be of some benefit.

It is important that nurses provide education regarding taxane-associated PN before initiating therapy and that they assess patients regularly. Development of PN should be reported to the medical provider, as a dose reduction for paclitaxel or cessation of docetaxel therapy will be required (Bristol-Myers Squibb Co., 2000; sanofi-aventis, 2010).

## Newer Agents

### Nab-Paclitaxel

The nanoparticle albumin-bound form of paclitaxel, nab-paclitaxel (Abraxane®, Abraxis BioScience, LLC), was developed to circumvent allergic reactions associated with the solvent polyoxyethylated castor oil (Cremophor EL). Preclinical studies demonstrated better efficacy than paclitaxel (Gradishar et al., 2005, 2009). Albumin is beneficial because it easily carries hydrophobic molecules and can be transported across tumor membranes by way of caveolin-1. Elevated levels of this protein have been associated with breast tumors (Roy, LaPlant, Gross, Bane, & Palmieri, 2009).

Three hundred patients were randomly assigned to receive one of three different nab-paclitaxel doses (twice weekly or once every three weeks) or docetaxel every three weeks. PFS was longer for one of the nab-paclitaxel groups. Grade 4 neutropenia was greater in patients who received docetaxel (75% versus 9% for the highest weekly nab-paclitaxel dose). In addition, febrile neutropenia and fatigue also were more severe. PN was equal among all four arms, but resolution was quicker in the nab-paclitaxel arm.

### Gemcitabine

Gemcitabine, an antimetabolite initially approved for the treatment of pancreatic cancer, is also indicated for breast, ovarian, and lung cancers. Roy and colleagues investigated nab-paclitaxel in combination with gemcitabine (Roy et al., 2009). The study enrolled 50 women with MBC from 22 different centers. They reported a 50% response rate with a median duration of 6.9 months. The regimen was well tolerated, and incidence of PN was low.

### Capecitabine

Clinical trials have demonstrated the potential efficacy of using the oral agent capecitabine, a fluoropyrimidine prodrug of fluorouracil. Capecitabine has a unique mechanism of action in that it is terminally converted to fluorouracil by the enzyme thymidine phosphorylase, which is present in neoplastic cells at a concentration of up to 10 times greater than in normal tissues (Aprile, Mazzer, Moroso, & Puglisi, 2009). The drug also is believed to be synergistic with other antineoplastic agents and with leucovorin (Aprile et al., 2009) and may have an affinity for ER-positive tumors (Wardley et al., 2010).

In 2002, O'Shaughnessy et al. published the results of a pivotal phase III study comparing docetaxel and capecitabine to docetaxel alone in 503 women with MBC. The study showed a statistically significant OS advantage for the capecitabine arm (hazard ratio [HR] = 0.775 (p < 0.0126; 95% CI, 0.634–0.947). At one year, the survival rate was 57% compared to 47% (O'Shaughnessy et al., 2002). Although the combination was reported to be generally well tolerated, the incidence of HFS was greater in the combination arm.

In the neoadjuvant phase III GeparQuattro study, researchers investigated concurrent capecitabine plus docetaxel versus sequential docetaxel followed by capecitabine. The third arm, which received docetaxel alone, functioned as a control group (von Minckwitz et al., 2010). All of the 1,186 patients had previously completed four cycles of cyclophosphamide and the anthracycline epirubicin prior to being randomized. Patients receiving the concurrent therapy required a 25% dose reduction of docetaxel. Even with the reduction, the incidence of febrile neutropenia and HFS was highest in this arm. By design, the sequential arm required a longer duration of therapy (36 weeks versus 24 weeks), which affected patient compliance and ultimately may have affected efficacy. In their conclusion, the authors reported no difference in presurgical benefit between the three arms and did not recommend adding capecitabine to this regimen in the neoadjuvant setting.

Tanaka et al. (2010) explored the combination of oral cyclophosphamide with capecitabine for patients with MBC. Although the study sample was small (N = 45), the combination was well tolerated and produced PFS and OS rates comparable to more toxic regimens, with the added benefit of being an entirely oral regimen.

Comparatively few studies have been done using capecitabine as single-agent therapy, and the results have been less clear. In one multicenter study of older patients with stage I, II, and III breast cancer, it was shown to be inferior to standard treatment with either CMF or AC (Muss et al., 2009). Although Venturini et al. (2007) concluded that monotherapy was efficacious in 631 patients with advanced breast cancer, weakness in the study design limits interpretation of the data.

HFS, also referred to as palmar-plantar erythrodysesthesia, is a known side effect of capecitabine. Affecting the palms of the hands and sometimes the soles of the feet, the syndrome begins with altered tactile sensation and progresses to painful erythema and edema (Gressett, Stanford, & Hardwicke, 2006). The exact mechanism is not known, but drug metabolites in the dermis have been postulated (Bellmunt, Navarro, Hidalgo, & Solé, 1988). Upon examination, tissues display dilated blood vessels with WBC infiltration indicative of an inflammatory process. Studies with fluorouracil have shown that women are at higher risk for developing HFS, although

this has not been demonstrated with capecitabine (Gressett et al., 2006). HFS currently has no known treatment; cessation of the causative agent generally is indicated. However, some possible benefit has been observed using pyridoxine for prophylaxis in one small study (Mortimer et al., 2003).

Additional side effects of capecitabine include neutropenia, nausea and vomiting, and fatigue. Because capecitabine can potentiate the effects of warfarin, the anticoagulant may need to be adjusted accordingly. Capecitabine should be taken within a half hour of eating (Wilkes & Barton-Burke, 2010).

Research on the optimal use of capecitabine for breast cancer continues. Capecitabine is FDA approved for the treatment of MBC after anthracycline failure in combination with docetaxel and as monotherapy for patients resistant to both paclitaxel and anthracycline-containing regimens (Roche Pharmaceuticals, 2005).

### Ixabepilone

Ixabepilone is part of a new family of antineoplastics known as epothilone B analogs, whose mechanism of action is similar to the taxanes (Stein, 2010). Ixabepilone prevents cell division during the $G_2/M$ phase by binding to the beta tubulin structures. One strategic advantage of the epothilones is a decreased susceptibility to drug resistance, particularly with other taxanes.

Ixabepilone has shown favorable results as monotherapy and in combination with other antineoplastic agents. In their phase II study, Perez and colleagues demonstrated the efficacy of ixabepilone in patients with MBC who had become resistant to taxanes, anthracyclines, and capecitabine (Perez et al., 2007). Additional studies have supported these results when given alone (Thomas, Tabernero, et al., 2007) or in combination with other antineoplastic agents (Perez, Patel, et al., 2010; Thomas, Gomez, et al., 2007). Ixabepilone has also shown encouraging results in patients with TNBC whose tumors may express higher levels of βIII-tubulin and are associated with taxane resistance (Perez, Patel, et al., 2010).

As with the taxanes, ixabepilone is poorly soluble and requires the solvent polyoxyethylated castor oil and can cause potentially life-threatening hypersensitivity reactions (Frye et al., 2009). Similar premedications used with paclitaxel are recommended, although corticosteroids are only required for patients who have had a prior reaction to medications containing polyoxyethylated castor oil (Stein, 2010).

Similar to the taxanes, ixabepilone can cause neutropenia and PN. The incidence of PN is up to 65%, and it generally is seen within the first three cycles of treatment. Ixabepilone should be infused within six hours after being mixed, using DEHP-free tubings and a 0.2–1.2 micron filter. Unlike other antineoplastics, it must be diluted in lactated Ringer's (Wilkes & Barton-Burke, 2010) or in 0.9% sodium chloride buffered with sodium bicarbonate (Kossoff, 2010). Ixabepilone can interact with other medications (e.g., ketoconazole, voriconazole) through the CYP3A4 pathway, resulting in increased ixabepilone levels. Because of a greater risk of toxicity, the manufacturer does not recommend using ixabepilone in combination with capecitabine for patients with abnormal hepatic function (aspartate transaminase or alanine aminotransferase greater than 2.5 times the upper limit of normal, or bilirubin greater than 1 times the upper limit) (Bristol-Myers Squibb Co., 2010).

## Signaling Pathways: Targeted Therapies

The HER family has four tyrosine kinase receptors: HER1 (EGFR or ErbB1), HER2 (ErbB2 or HER2/neu), HER3 (ErbB3), and HER4 (ErbB4). Cellular survival is closely dependent on these receptors and their associated pathways. Abnormal regulation of signaling pathways plays an important role in angiogenesis and the subsequent proliferation of tumor cells. Extracellular membrane proteins responsible for signaling include the HER family and insulin-like growth factor 1 receptor (Wong, 2009). Intracellular transduction proteins include Ras, Raf, and mitogen-activated protein kinase (MAPK). Within MAPK, three subtypes exist: p38, ERK, and JNK (Haagenson & Wu, 2010).

Breast cancer cells frequently have increased levels of MAPK, which is also associated with more aggressive disease (Bianchi et al., 2009). A second intracellular pathway includes the proteins phosphoinositide 3-kinase (PI3K), AKT (signaling molecule AKT), and mammalian target of rapamycin (mTOR). It is important to note that these pathways do not function in isolation. Research suggests that activation of Ras or PI3K can influence each other (Gossage & Eisen, 2010).

HER receptors contain both an extracellular and an intracellular domain with respective ligand binding. Although several ligands have been identified for HER1, HER3, and HER4, specific ligands for HER2 have not been identified, which has thus far limited the development of ligand-specific agents (Rosen, Ashurst, & Chap, 2010).

Tumorigenesis can be potentially halted by interfering with complex protein-mediated pathways. As such, anticancer agents targeting these pathways are radically different from conventional chemotherapy, particularly in terms of their specific side effect profiles. Currently, these targeted therapies can be divided into two major groups: MoAbs, which target the extracellular domain, and tyrosine kinase inhibitors (TKIs), which target the intracellular domain (Burness et al., 2010). Because it is believed that no single pathway is responsible for solid tumor growth, it is likely that targeted therapies will need to be able to block multiple pathways or be used in combination with other agents (Gossage & Eisen, 2010). Combining targeted agents can provide synergism as they focus on different pathways or different points along the same pathway. This is a particularly salient concept as signaling pathways display complex feedback loops; disabling only one pathway can cause other pathways to compensate, rendering the treatment ineffective. Preclinical research is continuing to explore the use of various combinations of agents to block multiple pathways and effectively shut down feedback loops while maintaining tolerable toxicity profiles (Di Cosimo & Baselga, 2010).

## Human Epidermal Growth Factor Receptors

Approximately 20%–25% of women with breast cancer have HER2 overexpression (Brufsky, 2010). HER2 overexpression can result in angiogenesis and tumor metastasis. These patients generally have a poorer prognosis due to aggressive disease with increased tumor angiogenesis, poor differentiation, and a high proliferative index (Lurje & Lenz, 2009; Patani & Mokbel, 2010). Preclinical studies also implicate HER2 overexpression in the development of ER resistance (Di Cosimo & Baselga, 2010). The ErbB signaling pathway can be blocked through the use of MoAbs, such as trastuzumab, or the TKIs, such as lapatinib and gefitinib.

### Trastuzumab

Trastuzumab, a recombinant, humanized anti-HER2 MoAb, was developed in 1990 and approved in 1998 for the treatment of women with HER2-positive breast cancer (Brufsky, 2010). It works by attaching to the extracellular domain of HER2-positive cells and causing receptor inhibition, interruption of downstream signaling, apoptosis, and decreased angiogenesis (Patani & Mokbel, 2010). Trastuzumab also inhibits the PI3K pathway.

Early phase II and phase III clinical trials demonstrated the tolerability and effectiveness of trastuzumab. Slamon et al. (2001) randomized 469 patients with MBC to receive chemotherapy (either cyclophosphamide and an anthracycline, or paclitaxel), or the same chemotherapy plus trastuzumab. The median TTP was 4.6 months for the chemotherapy-only arms and 7.4 months with the addition of trastuzumab (p < 0.001). The OS was 50% versus 32% (p < 0.001).

Subsequently, trastuzumab has been studied in combination with several chemotherapeutic agents, including docetaxel, paclitaxel, capecitabine, and carboplatin. Studies have also been performed with ER-positive patients receiving endocrine therapy with letrozole and anastrozole. The interest in combining trastuzumab with endocrine therapy stems from laboratory models suggesting that crosstalk between HER2 and ER pathways can induce endocrine therapy resistance (Kaufman et al., 2009). In the TAnDEM study, Kaufman and colleagues randomized 207 patients with MBC to receive trastuzumab and anastrozole or anastrozole alone. Patients in the trastuzumab arm had improved PFS (5.8 months versus 2.9 months). Superior TTP also was observed (4.6 months versus 2.4 months).

The side effects of trastuzumab are mild, particularly in comparison to chemotherapy. However, cardiac abnormalities (left ventricular systolic dysfunction and congestive heart failure [CHF]) are a particular concern. Although the exact mechanism of injury is unknown, it is thought to be due to disturbances in EGFR signaling within cardiac tissue (Ewer & Ewer, 2008). This is a different mechanism than the cardiac damage seen with anthracyclines and does not appear to be cumulative (Moss, Starbuck, Mayer, Harwood, & Glotzer, 2009). The incidence of dysfunction varies and is dependent on specific variables, including concurrent and past chemotherapy and patient selection. In a five-year analysis of the NSABP B-31 trial, 4% of the patients receiving cyclophosphamide and doxorubicin followed by paclitaxel and trastuzumab developed cardiac dysfunction, and 19% required cessation of trastuzumab because of cardiac dysfunction (Tan-Chiu et al., 2005). However, none of the 31 patients who had developed CHF died from cardiac-related causes, and 26 patients were eventually symptom free once therapy had ceased. Other studies in which anthracyclines were not included have shown a relatively low rate of occurrence. Robert et al. (2006) reported cardiotoxicity in 2 of 92 evaluable patients who received trastuzumab with carboplatin and paclitaxel. Accordingly, the NCCN guidelines recommend combining taxanes, vinorelbine, and capecitabine as first-line therapy for patients with HER2-positive disease (NCCN, 2011).

Recently, Untch et al. (2010) reported on using the anthracycline epirubicin in place of doxorubicin, with cyclophosphamide and trastuzumab. The Herceptin, Cyclophosphamide, and Epirubicin (HERCULES) study was a randomized phase II trial designed to assess the cardiac toxicity of two dose levels of epirubicin, thought to have potentially less cardiac toxicity than doxorubicin. At two years, the researchers determined that the incidence of cardiotoxicity was equal to non-doxorubicin-containing regimens for the lower-dose epirubicin arm (1.7%); the incidence increased to 5% for the higher-dose arm (Untch et al., 2010).

Risk factors for developing cardiac toxicity include patients older than age 50, those with preexisting cardiac disease or who are taking antihypertensive medications, and those who have had extensive prior treatment with anthracyclines (Patani & Mokbel, 2010). Based on these risks, some authors advocate taking a cautious approach to incorporating trastuzumab into treatment regimens based solely on HER2 positivity (Ewer & Ewer, 2008; Moss et al., 2009; Ring, 2010).

Astute nursing assessment is paramount and should include pulmonary symptoms (complaints of shortness of breath, presence of rales) and checking for weight gain and edema (Mahon & Palmieri, 2009). A baseline assessment of cardiac function, including electrocardiogram and echocardiography or multigated acquisition, is valuable in ruling out patients with cardiac disease (Moss et al., 2009). Some patients may benefit from beta-blockers or angiotensin-converting enzyme inhibitors for cardioprotection.

The first dose of trastuzumab is usually administered over 90 minutes. As a humanized MoAb, infusions generally are well tolerated. However, patients should be observed for the development of fever and chills. In the absence of reactions, subsequent doses can be given over 30–60 minutes (Wilkes & Barton-Burke, 2010). Trastuzumab is incompatible with dextrose-containing solutions.

## Pertuzumab

Despite trastuzumab's effectiveness, resistance to the drug typically occurs during the course of treatment. The investigational drug pertuzumab, a recombinant humanized MoAb, binds to a different HER2 epitope than trastuzumab and therefore is believed to have a complementary mechanism of action. In a small phase II study of HER2-positive women who had progressed while receiving trastuzumab, researchers reported an objective response rate of 24%, with 7.6% achieving a complete response (Baselga et al., 2010). Side effects included manageable diarrhea and skin toxicities. No cardiac abnormalities were observed. In a small pilot (N = 11) designed to assess the cardiac toxicity of trastuzumab combined with pertuzumab, Portera et al. (2008) reported cardiac toxicity in 54% of the participants, although most patients were asymptomatic. Further research is needed to determine the overall efficacy and toxicity profile of pertuzumab both alone and in combination with trastuzumab.

## Trastuzumab-DM1

The concept of conjugating a MoAb with a cytotoxic agent is not new; the anti-CD33 MoAb gemtuzumab ozogamicin is conjugated with the antitumor antibiotic calicheamicin and was approved by the FDA for the treatment of acute myeloid leukemia in 2000. However, trastuzumab-DM1 (T-DM1) is the first such agent for the treatment of breast cancer. T-DM1 is composed of trastuzumab attached to maytansine, an investigational antimicrotubule chemotherapy agent (Murphy & Fornier, 2010). Two small studies have demonstrated a moderate response rate, and further studies are ongoing.

## Bevacizumab

In December 2010, the FDA voted to remove breast cancer as an indication for bevacizumab. The initial E2100 phase III trial allowed for accelerated approval by the FDA pending replication of the findings in additional studies. However, recent analysis of the subsequent AVADO and RIBBON1 trials failed to demonstrate that the drug prolongs overall survival in patients with breast cancer or provides a sufficient benefit in slowing disease progression to outweigh the significant risk to patients (FDA, 2010). However, because the medication remains available for other oncology indications and may be included in off-label breast cancer treatment regimens, it has been included in this text.

The VEGF inhibitor bevacizumab initially demonstrated efficacy in the treatment of breast cancer when used in combination with chemotherapy. In their pivotal E2100 phase III trial, Miller et al. (2007) randomized 722 patients to receive paclitaxel alone or in combination with bevacizumab. The addition of bevacizumab produced longer DFS (11.8 months versus 5.9 months; HR = 0.60; p < 0.001). The investigators reported little change in the frequency and severity of side effects, although the incidence of grade 3 or 4 infection, neuropathy, and fatigue were somewhat higher with the addition of bevacizumab. In a recent meta-analysis of bevacizumab in patients with MBC, Valachis and colleagues analyzed five studies totaling 3,163 patients (Valachis, Polyzos, et al., 2010). PFS for patients who had received the MoAb with chemotherapy was significantly higher than those receiving chemotherapy alone (HR = 0.070; 95% CI = 0.060–0.082; p = 0.00000093). The results also suggested that drugs such as bevacizumab are more efficacious when used for initial, up-front treatment.

Different theories exist on how bevacizumab works in conjunction with chemotherapy. *Vessel normalization* suggests that tumor vasculature may be transiently improved by VEGF medications, thereby providing better tumor penetration from chemotherapy. Another theory is based on the concept that many of the chemotherapeutic agents used for breast cancer (e.g., paclitaxel) can cause mobilization of endothelial progenitor cells, which ultimately support tumor growth. Medications such as bevacizumab can prevent this effect (Kerbel, 2009). It has been suggested that eliminating potential rebound regrowth of tumor vasculature during periods of rest between chemotherapy cycles (as is done with metronomic therapy) would be an effective strategy, and evidence of this hypothesis has been supported clinically (Dellapasqua et al., 2008).

One concern specific to bevacizumab is its potential use in the neoadjuvant setting, where it could cause impaired wound healing following surgery (Greenberg & Rugo, 2010). The drug should be stopped prior to surgery and held for at least four weeks postoperatively, although no universal agreement exists because of the limited information in this setting (Bose et al., 2010; Wilkes & Barton-Burke, 2010). Ongoing trials are evaluating the role of bevacizumab with many chemotherapy regimens in adjuvant and neoadjuvant settings.

Although infusion reactions are rare, the first dose of bevacizumab should be infused over 90 minutes. Infusions can be decreased to 60 minutes followed by 30 minutes if well tolerated at each step (Wilkes & Barton-Burke, 2010). Hypertension, resulting from blockage of nitric oxide production with subsequent blood vessel dilation, is the most common side effect and occurs in 15%–60% of patients (Greenberg & Rugo, 2010; Wilkes & Barton-Burke, 2010). It usually is not acute and develops after subsequent doses. However, an accurate baseline blood pressure is required, and vital signs should be checked before each infusion. A black box warning exists for gastrointestinal hemorrhage, although the incidence has been reported to be 0.5% for patients with breast cancer (compared to 2.4% in those treated for colorectal cancer). Proteinuria can occur, and physicians may require baseline and/or serial urinalysis to be performed. Patients receiving concurrent therapy with paclitaxel have an increased risk of CHF (Wilkes & Barton-Burke, 2010).

## Tyrosine Kinase Inhibitors

### Lapatinib

Several oral TKIs are currently FDA approved for the treatment of various cancers. Lapatinib is approved for patients with HER2-positive MBC after failure with a taxane and anthracycline. As a member of the small molecule agent family, lapatinib is a unique dual kinase inhibitor of HER1 and HER2 (Jones & Buzdar, 2009). Its mechanism of action includes competing for adenosine triphosphate binding sites and interfering with ERK1/2 and PI3K pathways. Early results from studies indicate that lapatinib does not possess cross-resistance with trastuzumab (Konecny et al., 2006).

Efficacy in combination with capecitabine has been demonstrated in a phase III randomized study that compared capecitabine alone to capecitabine and lapatinib in patients who had disease progression after receiving trastuzumab with an anthracycline and taxane. The combination arm had 49 disease-progression events compared to 72 for the capecitabine-only arm (HR = 0.49; 95% CI; p < 0.001) (Geyer et al., 2006).

Blackwell et al. (2010) studied the potential efficacy of combining lapatinib with trastuzumab in HER2-positive patients who had disease progression after receiving trastuzumab. A combined total of 296 patients were randomized to receive trastuzumab and lapatinib, or lapatinib alone. Median PFS was 12 weeks for the combination arm versus 8 weeks for the lapatinib arm (HR = 0.71; 95% CI, 0.52–0.98; p < 0.027) (Blackwell et al., 2010). The researchers concluded that the combination corroborated preclinical evidence that combined therapy can help overcome trastuzumab resistance. Related to lapatinib's small molecular size, research suggests that lapatinib may have activity for treating metastatic brain lesions by being able to cross the blood-brain barrier. However, preliminary studies have thus far produced mixed results (Lin et al., 2008, 2009).

Lapatinib is currently approved for use with capecitabine for patients with advanced or metastatic HER2-positive breast cancer and who have received prior therapy including an anthracycline, a taxane, and trastuzumab, and in conjunction with letrozole for postmenopausal women with hormone receptor–positive metastatic breast cancer (GlaxoSmithKline, 2010).

Because of the oral nature of TKIs, providing clear instructions with printed educational materials is useful for drug administration and management of side effects at home. Patients should take lapatinib one hour before or two hours after meals, as ingestion with food can slow absorption and increase plasma levels (Wilkes & Barton-Burke, 2010). Diarrhea is a prominent side effect of lapatinib, occurring in up to 65% of patients, and is worse when the drug is combined with other therapies (Frankel & Palmieri, 2010; Wilkes & Barton-Burke, 2010). Pretherapy bowel habits must be assessed, and the use of a diary can be beneficial for tracking severity. Dietary changes may be helpful for mild symptoms. Loperamide, starting with an initial dose of 4 mg and then 2 mg every four hours, can be used once infection has been ruled out (Mahon & Palmieri, 2009). Patients should be advised to increase fluid intake to prevent dehydration.

Dermatologic toxicities, ranging from dry, itching skin to an acneform rash, commonly occur with TKIs. Rashes can vary from mild grade 1 to severe grade 4. Detailed algorithms have been devised for EGFR-related skin toxicity. In general, for a mild to moderate rash, management goals focus on maintaining skin integrity while minimizing discomfort. Instruct patients to use a mild, nondrying soap. Products containing aloe may provide symptom relief. Topical steroids also may be ordered. Severe rashes can progress to infection. The physician may elect to hold the TKI and treat the rash with steroids and antibiotics, both topical and oral (Wilkes & Barton-Burke, 2010). Compliance with oral agents can be affected by severe side effects that have a significant impact on quality of life and self-image. Therefore, detailed patient education and follow-up is paramount.

### Dasatinib

Dasatinib is approved for the treatment of chronic myeloid leukemia. It is currently being studied for treatment of breast cancer because of its ability to block SRC-family kinases (SFKs), which have been strongly identified with oncogenesis. Dasatinib has been shown to inhibit growth of breast cancer cells in vitro, particularly basal type (triple negative) (Araujo & Logothetis, 2010). Blocking of SRC also may help decrease chemotherapy resistance, which has been associated with increased SRC (Araujo & Logothetis, 2010). Although no large-scale studies have been published, Pichot et al. (2009) demonstrated that dasatinib appears to sensitize breast cancer cell lines to doxorubicin in vitro. Further studies are ongoing.

## PARP Poly(Adenosine-Diphosphate-Ribose) Polymerase Inhibitors

Research continues in the area of targeted therapies, and a number of investigational agents are currently being trialed. Poly(adenosine-diphosphate-ribose) polymerase 1 (PARP-1) inhibitors can potentiate chemotherapy by preventing DNA repair and restoring chemosensitivity in previously unresponsive tumors (Jones & Buzdar, 2009). Overexpression of PARP-1 has been identified in many tumors, including breast. Two agents, BSI-201 and olaparib, currently are being studied (Andreetta et al., 2010).

## mTOR Inhibitors

mTOR is a protein kinase responsible for many cellular functions, including protein synthesis, proliferation, and cellular motility (Wong, 2009). The mTOR pathway is interrelated with other signaling pathways, including PI3K and AKT. Currently, everolimus is FDA approved for the treatment of

renal cell cancer. However, phase I studies for patients with breast cancer have demonstrated efficacy, and additional clinical trials currently are under way (Wong, 2009).

## Additional Pathways

Histone deacetylase inhibitors are being explored in phase I and phase II trials. Vorinostat is FDA approved for the treatment of cutaneous T-cell lymphoma. No results from large trials have been published for breast cancer treatment, but considerable interest exists in this novel agent and related compounds. Other targeted therapies, including heat shock protein 90 inhibitors and farnesyl transferase inhibitors, are being studied.

## Drug Resistance

Regardless of which systemic therapy is chosen for breast cancer treatment, resistance remains a troublesome issue. With the increasing use of taxanes and anthracyclines, resistance will become more common. Once it occurs with primary therapy, alternative (and potentially less efficacious) treatments are required.

Resistance can be primary—a genetic trait occurring in patients prior to treatment exposure—or acquired after repeated administration of agents (Toppmeyer & Goodin, 2009). Genetic mutations causing a loss of the cellular ability to detect DNA damage can lead to aberrations in the normal apoptotic sequence, resulting in mutated clonal cells that are resistant to chemotherapy. In addition, resistance to one class of medication (e.g., taxanes) can frequently lead to cross-resistance to other classes (e.g., anthracyclines). This multidrug resistance occurs irrespective of the drug class or mechanism of action and can severely limit treatment options.

Researchers continue to look at various mechanisms, including the role of signaling pathways. It has been established that the presence of p-glycoproteins on the surface of cancer cells act to pump chemotherapy out of the cell (Barton-Burke & Wilkes, 2006; Moreno-Aspitia & Perez, 2009). Interestingly, many patients will be drug resistant prior to therapy because of the overexpression of the multidrug resistance protein *MRP1* gene (Toppmeyer & Goodin, 2009). HER2 activation has been implicated in the proliferation of tumor cells resistant to tamoxifen, and the MAPK pathway may play a role in resistance seen in TNBC (Haagenson & Wu, 2010).

Malignant cells can readily adapt to anticancer treatment. In vivo studies showed that while letrozole initially decreased tumor growth, resistance eventually occurred as the tumor used alternate pathways to proliferate (Santen et al., 2009). Likewise, resistance to tamoxifen is due in part to modulation of transduction pathways affecting ER sensitivity (De Amicis et al., 2010; Haagenson & Wu, 2010). Anthracycline resistance can be caused by the breast cancer resistance protein or mutations in topoisomerase II enzyme, which is targeted by the chemotherapy (Moreno-Aspitia & Perez, 2009). Other mechanisms of resistance include impaired drug metabolism resulting from glutathione-S transferase and aldehyde-dehydrogenase production (Pronzato, 2008).

New agents such as ixabepilone may be effective in patients with drug resistance. It is also theorized that anti-EGFR agents may be able to partially remove resistance to tamoxifen in ER-positive patients (Di Cosimo & Baselga, 2010).

## Supportive Therapy: Bisphosphonates

Between 50%–75% of patients with advanced breast cancer will develop bone metastasis (Kohno et al., 2005; Winter & Coleman, 2009). Loss of BMD is a common consequence in both pre- and postmenopausal patients and is the result of accelerated osteoclastic activity from the secretion of interleukin-6, prostaglandin $E_2$, tumor necrosis factor, and, in particular, parathyroid hormone–related protein from the metastatic cells (Mehrotra, 2009; Mundy, 2002). Stimulation of the receptor activator of nuclear factor $\kappa\beta$ ligand (RANKL) also plays a pivotal role in this signaling pathway (Mehrotra, 2009; Winter & Coleman, 2009). Approximately 50% of patients who develop metastatic disease to the bone will also develop some type of skeletal-related event, such as fractures (Fitch et al., 2009). The anatomic location with the greatest loss of BMD is the lumbar spine region, although the hips also are commonly affected (Hershman et al., 2010).

As described previously, osteoporosis is a side effect of the AIs. The frequency of fractures varies depending on the trial, but it is consistently greater than with patients treated with tamoxifen (Howell et al., 2005; Perez et al., 2006; Thürlimann et al., 2005). In addition to the AIs, antineoplastic therapies such as cyclophosphamide, which produce chemical ovarian ablation, can cause premature menopause and resultant osteoporosis (Hadji et al., 2008; Yamamoto & Viale, 2009).

Other risk factors for the development of osteoporosis include low levels of endogenous vitamin D, caffeine consumption, history of cigarette use, low body mass index, age greater than 65, and inactivity (Hadji et al., 2008; Mortimer, 2010).

The IV bisphosphonates pamidronate and zoledronic acid (ZA) are potent inhibitors of osteoclastic activity. Both drugs have demonstrated efficacy in preventing or slowing bone loss in patients with breast cancer (Hortobagyi et al., 1996; Rosen et al., 2003). Of the two agents, ZA has been shown to be more effective (Pavlakis, Schmidt, & Stockler, 2005), with a correspondingly greater number of recent studies in patients with breast cancer.

In particular, investigators have looked at the efficacy of different scheduling strategies. A large study by Black et al. (2007) demonstrated a 70% reduction in fractures with an annual dose of ZA over a three-year period when compared to placebo. One double-blind study using ZA given every three months found that at 24 months, BMD remained stable compared to the placebo arm, which showed a decrease of 6.3% in the lumbar spine region (Hershman et al., 2010). The study also demonstrated that greatest loss of BMD occurs within the first year of treatment. In the Z-FAST study, it was noted that delaying the administration of ZA for 12 months after initiating AI therapy resulted in a 2.4% loss of lumbar spine BMD, validating the benefits of receiving ZA up front (Brufsky et al., 2007). In their phase III, four-arm study comparing goserelin to tamoxifen, with and without ZA, Gnant and colleagues (2007) demonstrated that ZA given every six months protected patients from loss of BMD (p = 0.0001). The NCCN guidelines recommend IV bisphosphonates along with vitamin D and calcium for women with metastatic disease (NCCN, 2011).

Limited data also have suggested that ZA may have antitumor effects. Gnant et al. (2009) concluded that the addition of ZA to patients randomized to receive goserelin in combination with either tamoxifen or anastrozole resulted in a 33% decrease in disease progression (HR = 0.64; 95% CI, 0.46–0.91; p = 0.01), although there was no difference in OS. In a neoadjuvant subset of the AZURE study (currently in progress), Coleman et al. (2010) looked at the effects of ZA on residual tumor size and reported a mean decrease of 12 mm (95% CI; p = 0.0059). In vitro analysis has led researchers to postulate that ZA can induce apoptosis, reduce cellular adhesion, and inhibit growth (Neville-Webbe, Coleman, & Holen, 2010). Further research regarding the antineoplastic role of ZA is warranted.

Pamidronate should be administered over two hours; ZA can safely be given in 15 minutes. Because both drugs can cause renal insufficiency, serum creatinine should be checked prior to administration (Yamamoto & Viale, 2009), and caution should be exercised when used in conjunction with renal-toxic medications. Although rare, osteonecrosis of the jaw also has been reported with these agents.

The oral bisphosphonates risedronate, alendronate, and ibandronate have obvious administration advantages over IV pamidronate or ZA, although long-term compliance and gastrointestinal side effects are potential concerns. Oral bisphosphonates currently are approved for the treatment of benign osteoporosis. Conflicting results have been seen with studies using risedronate in the setting of breast cancer. One study demonstrated efficacy when it was used with anastrozole for postmenopausal women (Van Poznak et al., 2010). However, in another study of premenopausal patients receiving chemotherapy and risedronate, no difference in BMD was noted (Hines et al., 2009).

Denosumab (Xgeva®, Amgen, Inc.) is a fully humanized MoAb that binds to RANKL and inhibits osteoclastic activation and has been shown to decrease skeletal-related events, particularly in patients no longer responsive to bisphosphonates (Amgen, Inc., 2010; Body et al., 2009; Michaud, 2010). FDA approval was based on a pivotal double-blinded study comparing denosumab to ZA in patients with metastatic breast cancer (Stopeck et al., 2010). Denosumab was shown to be superior to ZA in delaying onset of initial skeletal related events by 18% when compared to zoledronic acid (HR, 0.82; 95% CI, 0.71–0.95; p < 0.001 noninferiority; p = 0.01 superiority). Denosumab is administered subcutaneously every four weeks. Side effects include potentially severe hypocalcemia, and the manufacturer recommends adequate monitoring of serum calcium levels and correction of low levels prior to administration (Amgen, Inc., 2010). Concurrent use of calcium and vitamin D are also recommended. Other side effects include arthralgias, fatigue, bone pain, and nausea. Osteonecrosis of the jaw can occur, and patients should have an oral examination before initiating therapy. Denosumab should not be given to patients who are pregnant.

## Complementary and Integrative Medicine: Potential for Drug Interactions

The concurrent use of herbal remedies in patients with cancer raises serious potential consequences. Patients may turn to herbals in the belief that natural substance can mitigate the side effects of cancer treatment or strengthen the immune system. Unfortunately, relatively little is known about the interactions between most herbals and the dozens of therapies employed for breast cancer treatment. Herbal use is likely underreported, and interactions may not be well documented by clinicians (Engdal, Klepp, & Nilsen, 2009). Patients inclined to use herbal remedies frequently take combinations, thus increasing the likelihood of interactions and further complicating the ability to isolate an individual component. Supplements themselves are not FDA regulated; even the same herbal may be formulated differently depending on the manufacturer (Smith, 2005). Some herbals also may interfere with the absorption of oral agents, a particularly worrisome problem as more oral AIs and TKIs are developed.

Herbal supplements—even without concurrent systemic therapy—can lead to hepatic failure (Smith, 2005). However, the absence of obvious toxicities does not infer a lack of interaction. Indeed, side effects can mimic those anticipated with systemic therapy, making them impossible to distinguish. Furthermore, poor response to systemic treatment can be attributed to any number of resistance mechanisms, masking the potential role of herbals in treatment failure.

Limited studies exist for some herbals; other interactions are based on case studies or have been postulated based on the role of metabolic pathways. Engdal et al. (2009) conducted an in vitro study of the most commonly used herbals and found numerous interactions via the cytochrome P450 or P-glycoprotein pathways. Many anticancer medications utilize the CYP3A4 metabolic pathway.

Investigators have explored interactions with St. John's wort, a potent inducer of CYP3A4 and CYP2B6 (Zhou, Chan, Pan, Huang, & Lee, 2004). St. John's wort has been found to decrease the efficacy of exemestane (Pharmacia & Upjohn, 2011). It also can decrease the efficacy of benzodiazepines (e.g., lorazepam) and increase levels of some SSRIs (Di, Li, Xue, & Zhou, 2008; Izzo & Ernst, 2009). Although not commonly used in breast cancer treatment, irinotecan pharmacokinetic levels are decreased by this herbal (Zhou et al., 2004).

In view of the large number of potential drug-herbal combinations and the limited information available, the initial patient assessment should include a thorough assessment for use of herbals, with ongoing discussions throughout the duration of therapy.

## Conclusion

Systemic therapy for breast cancer requires the use of multiple types of agents, each with its own distinct properties and serious toxicities. Researchers continue to hone existing therapies while searching for better treatment options with fewer side effects. Nurses must remain current in their knowledge of these agents, exercise caution with their administration, be proactive in managing their side effects, and provide the necessary patient education.

## References

Aapro, M., Crawford, J., & Kamioner, D. (2010). Prophylaxis of chemotherapy-induced febrile neutropenia with granulocyte colony-stimulating factors: Where are we now? *Supportive Care in Cancer, 18,* 529–541. doi:10.1007/s00520-010-0816-y

Allegra, J.C., Lippman, M.E., Thompson, E.B., & Simon, R. (1978). An association between steroid hormone receptors and response to cytotoxic chemotherapy in patients with metastatic breast cancer. *Cancer Research, 38*(11, Pt. 2), 4299–4304.

Amgen, Inc. (2010). *Xgeva®* [Package insert]. Thousand Oaks, CA: Author.

Anders, C.J., & Kemp, N.H. (1961). Cyclophosphamide in treatment of disseminated malignant disease. *BMJ, 2,* 1516–1523.

Andreetta, C., Minisini, A.M., Miscoria, M., & Puglisi, F. (2010). First-line chemotherapy with or without biologic agents for metastatic breast cancer. *Critical Reviews in Oncology/Hematology, 76,* 99–111. doi:10.1016/j.critrevonc.2010.01.007

Aprile, G., Mazzer, M., Moroso, S., & Puglisi, F. (2009). Pharmacology and therapeutic efficacy of capecitabine: Focus on breast and colorectal cancer. *Anti-Cancer Drugs, 20,* 217–229. doi:10.1097/CAD.0b013e3283293fd4

Araujo, J., & Logothetis, C. (2010). Dasatinib: A potent SRC inhibitor in clinical development for the treatment of solid tumors. *Cancer Treatment Reviews, 36,* 492–500. doi:10.1016/j.ctrv.2010.02.015

Arimidex, Tamoxifen, Alone or in Combination Trialists' Group. (2008). Effect of anastrozole and tamoxifen as adjuvant treatment for early-stage breast cancer: 100-month analysis of the ATAC trial. *Lancet Oncology, 9,* 45–53. doi:10.1016/S1470-2045(07)70385-6

Arpino, G., Weiss, H., Lee, A.V., Schiff, R., De Placido, S., Osborne, C.K., & Elledge, R.M. (2005). Estrogen receptor-positive, progesterone receptor-negative breast cancer: Association with growth factor receptor expression and tamoxifen resistance. *Journal of the National Cancer Institute, 97,* 1254–1261. doi:10.1093/jnci/dji249

AstraZeneca Pharmaceuticals. (2004). *Faslodex®* [Package insert]. Wilmington, DE: Author.

AstraZeneca Pharmaceuticals. (2009a). *Arimidex®* [Package insert]. Wilmington, DE: Author.

AstraZeneca Pharmaceuticals. (2009b). *Zoladex®* [Package insert]. Retrieved from http://www.accessdata.fda.gov/drugsatfda_docs/label/2009/019726s050s051s052lbl.pdf

Barton-Burke, M., & Wilkes, G.M. (2006). *Cancer therapies*. Sudbury, MA: Jones and Bartlett.

Baselga, J., Gelmon, K.A., Verma, S., Wardley, A., Conte, P., Miles, D., … Gianni, L. (2010). Phase II trial of pertuzumab and trastuzumab in patients with human epidermal growth factor receptor 2-positive metastatic breast cancer that progressed during prior trastuzumab therapy. *Journal of Clinical Oncology, 28,* 1138–1144. doi:10.1200/JCO.2009.24.2024

BASF Corp. (2008). *Cremophor® EL* [Technical leaflet]. Retrieved from http://www.pharma-ingredients.basf.com/Statements/Technical%20Informations/EN/Pharma%20Solutions/EMP%20030711e_Cremophor%20EL.pdf

Bellmunt, J., Navarro, M., Hidalgo, R., & Solé, L.A. (1988). Palmar-plantar erythrodysesthesia syndrome associated with short-term continuous infusion (5 days) of 5-fluorouracil. *Tumori, 74,* 329–331.

Bernardi, D., Errante, D., Galligioni, E., Crivellari, D., Bianco, A., Salvagno, L., & Fentiman, I.S. (2008). Treatment of breast cancer in older women. *Acta Oncologica, 47,* 187–198. doi:10.1080/02841860701630234

Beslija, S., Bonneterre, J., Burstein, H.J., Cocquyt, V., Gnant, M., Heinemann, V., … Zwierzina, H. (2009). Third consensus on medical treatment of metastatic breast cancer. *Annals of Oncology, 20,* 1771–1785. doi:10.1093/annonc/mdp261

Bianchi, G., Loibl, S., Zamagni, C., Salvagni, S., Raab, G., Siena, S., … Gianni, L. (2009). Phase II multicenter, uncontrolled trial of sorafenib in patients with metastatic breast cancer. *Anti-Cancer Drugs, 20,* 616–624. doi:10.1097/CAD.0b013e32832b2ea0

Black, D.M., Delmas, P.D., Eastell, R., Reid, I.R., Boonen, S., Cauley, J.A., … Cummings, S.R. (2007). Once-yearly zoledronic acid for treatment of postmenopausal osteoporosis. *New England Journal of Medicine, 356,* 1809–1822. doi:10.1056/NEJMoa067312

Blackwell, K.L., Burstein, H.J., Storniolo, A.M., Rugo, H., Sledge, G., Koehler, M., … O'Shaughnessy, J. (2010). Randomized study of lapatinib alone or in combination with trastuzumab in women with ErbB2-positive, trastuzumab-refractory metastatic breast cancer. *Journal of Clinical Oncology, 28,* 1124–1130. doi:10.1200/JCO.2008.21.4437

Blum, R.H., & Carter, S.K. (1974). Adriamycin. A new anticancer drug with significant clinical activity. *Annals of Internal Medicine, 80,* 249–259.

Body, J.J., Lipton, A., Gralow, J., Steger, G.G., Gao, G., Yeh, H., & Fizazi, K. (2009). Effects of denosumab in patients with bone metastases, with and without previous bisphosphonate exposure. *Journal of Bone Mineral Research, 25,* 440–446. doi:10.1359/jbmr.090810

Bonadonna, G., Moliterni, A., Zambetti, M., Daidone, M.G., Pilotti, S., Gianni, L., & Valagussa, P. (2005). 30 years' follow up of randomised studies of adjuvant CMF in operable breast cancer: Cohort study. *BMJ, 330,* 217. doi:10.1136/bmj.38314.622095.8F

Bonadonna, G., Valagussa, P., Moliterni, A., Zambetti, M., & Brambilla, C. (1995). Adjuvant cyclophosphamide, methotrexate, and fluorouracil in node-positive breast cancer: The results of 20 years of follow-up. *New England Journal of Medicine, 332,* 901–906. doi:10.1056/NEJM199504063321401

Bose, D., Meric-Bernstam, F., Hofstetter, W., Reardon, D.A., Flaherty, K.T., & Ellis, L.M. (2010). Vascular endothelial growth factor targeted therapy in the perioperative setting: Implications for patient care. *Lancet Oncology, 11,* 373–382. doi:10.1016/S1470-2045(09)70341-9

Bramwell, V.H., Pritchard, K.I., Tu, D., Tonkin, K., Vachhrajani, H., Vandenberg, T.A., … Shepherd, L. (2010). A randomized placebo-controlled study of tamoxifen after adjuvant chemotherapy in premenopausal women with early breast cancer (National Cancer Institute of Canada–Clinical Trials Group Trial, MA.12). *Annals of Oncology, 21,* 283–290. doi:10.1093/annonc/mdp326

Bristol-Myers Squibb Co. (2000). *Taxol®* [Package insert]. Princeton, NJ: Author.

Bristol-Myers Squibb Co. (2010). *Ixempra®* [Package insert]. Princeton, NJ: Author.

Browder, T., Butterfield, C.E., Kräling, B.M., Shi, B., Marshall, B., O'Reilly, M.S., & Folkman, J. (2000). Antiangiogenic scheduling of chemotherapy improves efficacy against experimental drug-resistant cancer. *Cancer Research, 60,* 1878–1886.

Brufsky, A. (2010). Trastuzumab-based therapy for patients with HER2-positive breast cancer: From early scientific development to foundation of care. *American Journal of Clinical Oncology, 33,* 186–195. doi:10.1097/COC.0b013e318191bfb0

Brufsky, A., Harker, W.G., Beck, J.T., Carroll, R., Tan-Chiu, E., Seidler, C., … Perez, E.A. (2007). Zoledronic acid inhibits adjuvant letrozole-induced bone loss in postmenopausal women with early breast cancer. *Journal of Clinical Oncology, 25,* 829–836. doi:10.1200/JCO.2005.05.3744

Burness, M.L., Grushko, T.A., & Olopade, O.I. (2010). Epidermal growth factor receptor in triple-negative and basal-like breast cancer: Promising clinical target or only a marker? *Cancer Journal, 16,* 23–32. doi:10.1097/PPO.0b013e3181d24fc1

Canellos, G.P., Devita, V.T., Gold, G.L., Chabner, B.A., Schein, P.S., & Young, R.C. (1974). Cyclical combination chemotherapy for advanced breast carcinoma. *BMJ, 1,* 218–220.

Cheang, M.C., Chia, S.K., Voduc, D., Gao, D., Leung, S., Snider, J., … Nielsen, T.O. (2009). Ki67 index, HER2 status, and prognosis of patients with luminal B breast cancer. *Journal of the National Cancer Institute, 101,* 736–750. doi:10.1093/jnci/djp082

Chevallier, B., Fumoleau, P., Kerbrat, P., Dieras, V., Roche, H., Krakowski, I., … Van Glabbeke, M. (1995). Docetaxel is a major cytotoxic drug for the treatment of advanced breast cancer: A phase II trial of the Clinical Screening Cooperative Group of the European Organization for Research and Treatment of Cancer. *Journal of Clinical Oncology, 13,* 314–322.

Chia, S., Gradishar, W., Mauriac, L., Bines, J., Amant, F., Federico, M., … Piccart, M. (2008). Double-blind, randomized placebo controlled trial of fulvestrant compared with exemestane after prior nonsteroidal aromatase inhibitor therapy in postmenopausal women with hormone receptor-positive, advanced breast cancer: Results from EFECT. *Journal of Clinical Oncology, 26,* 1664–1670. doi:10.1200/JCO.2007.13.5822

Citron, M.L. (2004). Dose density in adjuvant chemotherapy for breast cancer. *Cancer Investigation, 22,* 555–568.

Citron, M.L., Berry, D.A., Cirrincione, C., Hudis, C., Winer, E.P., Gradishar, W.J., … Norton, L. (2003). Randomized trial of dose-dense versus conventionally scheduled and sequential versus concurrent combination chemotherapy as postoperative adjuvant treatment of node-positive primary breast cancer: First report of Intergroup Trial C9741/Cancer and Leukemia Group B Trial 9741. *Journal of Clinical Oncology, 21,* 1431–1439. doi:10.1200/JCO.2003.09.081

Coleman, R.E., Winter, M.C., Cameron, D., Bell, R., Dodwell, D., Keane, M.M., … Thorpe, H. (2010). The effects of adding zoledronic acid to neoadjuvant chemotherapy on tumour response: Exploratory evidence for direct anti-tumour activity in breast cancer. *British Journal of Cancer, 102,* 1099–1105. doi:10.1038/sj.bjc.6605604

Colleoni, M., Rocca, A., Sandri, M.T., Zorzino, L., Masci, G., Nolè, F., … Goldhirsch, A. (2002). Low-dose oral methotrexate and cyclophosphamide in metastatic breast cancer: Antitumor activity and correlation with vascular endothelial growth factor levels. *Annals of Oncology, 13,* 73–80. doi:10.1093/annonc/mdf013

Conzen, S.D., Grushko, T.A., & Olopade, O.I. (2008). The molecular biology of breast cancer. In V.T. DeVita Jr., T.S. Lawrence, & S.A. Rosenberg (Eds.), *Cancer: Principles and practice of oncology* (8th ed., pp. 1595–1605). Philadelphia, PA: Lippincott Williams & Wilkins.

Coombes, R.C., Kilburn, L.S., Snowdon, C.F., Paridaens, R., Coleman, R.E., Jones, S.E., … Bliss, J.M. (2007). Survival and safety of exemestane versus tamoxifen after 2–3 years' tamoxifen treatment (Intergroup Exemestane Study): A randomised controlled trial. *Lancet, 369,* 559–570. doi:10.1016/S0140-6736(07)60200-1

Crane-Okada, R., & Loney, M. (2007). Breast cancers. In M.E. Langhorne, J.S. Fulton, & S.E. Otto (Eds.), *Oncology nursing* (5th ed., pp. 101–124). St. Louis, MO: Elsevier Mosby.

Cristofanilli, M., Valero, V., Mangalik, A., Royce, M., Rabinowitz, I., Arena, F.P., … Magill, P.J. (2010). Phase II, randomized trial to compare anastrozole combined with gefitinib or placebo in postmenopausal women with hormone receptor-positive metastatic breast cancer. *Clinical Cancer Research, 16,* 1904–1914. doi:10.1158/1078-0432.CCR-09-2282

Crivellari, D., Aapro, M., Leonard, R., von Minckwitz, G., Brain, E., Goldhirsch, A., … Muss, H. (2007). Breast cancer in the elderly. *Journal of Clinical Oncology, 25,* 1882–1890. doi:10.1200/JCO.2006.10.2079

Dalenc, F., Doisneau-Sixou, S.F., Allal, B.C., Marsili, S., Lauwers-Cances, V., Chaoui, K., … Roché, H. (2010). Tipifarnib plus tamoxifen in tamoxifen-resistant metastatic breast cancer: A negative phase II and screening of potential therapeutic markers by proteomic analysis. *Clinical Cancer Research, 16,* 1264–1271. doi:10.1158/1078-0432.CCR-09-1192

De Amicis, F., Thirugnansampanthan, J., Cui, Y., Selever, J., Beyer, A., Parra, I., … Fuqua, S.A. (2010). Androgen receptor overexpression induces tamoxifen resistance in human breast cancer cells. *Breast Cancer Research and Treatment, 121,* 1–11. doi:10.1007/s10549-009-0436-8

Deeks, E.D., & Scott, L.J. (2009). Exemestane: A review of its use in postmenopausal women with breast cancer. *Drugs, 69,* 889–918. doi:10.2165/00003495-200969070-00007

De Grandis, D. (2007). Acetyl-L-carnitine for the treatment of chemotherapy-induced peripheral neuropathy: A short review. *CNS Drugs, 21*(Suppl. 1), 39–43.

Dellapasqua, S., Bertolini, F., Bagnardi, V., Campagnoli, E., Scarano, E., Torrisi, R., … Colleoni, M. (2008). Metronomic cyclophosphamide and capecitabine combined with bevacizumab in advanced breast cancer. *Journal of Clinical Oncology, 26,* 4899–4905. doi:10.1200/JCO.2008.17.4789

Di, Y.M., Li, C.G., Xue, C.C., & Zhou, S.F. (2008). Clinical drugs that interact with St. John's wort and implication in drug development. *Current Pharmaceutical Design, 14,* 1723–1742.

Di Cosimo, S., & Baselga, J. (2010). Management of breast cancer with targeted agents: Importance of heterogeneity. *Nature Reviews Clinical Oncology, 7,* 139–147. doi:10.1038/nrclinonc.2009.234

Donovan, D. (2009). Management of peripheral neuropathy caused by microtubule inhibitors. *Clinical Journal of Oncology Nursing, 13,* 686–694. doi:10.1188/09.CJON.686-694

Eisenberg, S. (2009). Safe handling and administration of antineoplastic chemotherapy. *Journal of Infusion Nursing, 32,* 23–32. doi:10.1097/NAN.0b013e31819246e0

Engdal, S., Klepp, O., & Nilsen, O.G. (2009). Identification and exploration of herb-drug combinations used by cancer patients. *Integrative Cancer Therapies, 8,* 29–36. doi:10.1177/1534735408330202

Ewer, S.M., & Ewer, M.S. (2008). Cardiotoxicity profile of trastuzumab. *Drug Safety, 31,* 459–467.

Fabian, C.J. (2007). The what, why and how of aromatase inhibitors: Hormonal agents for treatment and prevention of breast cancer. *International Journal of Clinical Practice, 61,* 2051–2063. doi:10.1111/j.1742-1241.2007.01587.x

Fisher, B., Brown, A.M., Dimitrov, N.V., Poisson, R., Redmond, C., Margolese, R.G., … Kardinal, C.G. (1990). Two months of doxorubicin-cyclophosphamide with and without interval reinduction therapy compared with 6 months of cyclophosphamide, methotrexate, and fluorouracil in positive-node breast cancer patients with tamoxifen-nonresponsive tumors: Results from the National Surgical Adjuvant Breast and Bowel Project B-15. *Journal of Clinical Oncology, 8,* 1483–1496.

Fitch, M., Maxwell, C., Ryan, C., Löthman, H., Drudge-Coates, L., & Costa, L. (2009). Bone metastases from advanced cancers: Clinical implications and treatment options. *Clinical Journal of Oncology Nursing, 13,* 701–710. doi:10.1188/09.CJON.701-710

Frankel, C., & Palmieri, F.M. (2010). Lapatinib side-effect management. *Clinical Journal of Oncology Nursing, 14,* 223–233. doi:10.1188/10.CJON.223-233

Frasor, J., Stossi, F., Danes, J.M., Komm, B., Lyttle, C.R., & Katzenellenbogen, B.S. (2004). Selective estrogen receptor modulators: Discrimination of agonistic versus antagonistic activities by gene expression profiling in breast cancer cells. *Cancer Research, 64,* 1522–1533. doi:10.1158/0008-5472.CAN-03-3326

Frye, D.K., Mahon, S.M., & Palmieri, F.M. (2009). New options for metastatic breast cancer. *Clinical Journal of Oncology Nursing, 13*(Suppl. 1), 11–18. doi:10.1188/09.CJON.S1.11-18

Geyer, C.E., Forster, J., Lindquist, D., Chan, S., Romieu, C.G., Pienkowski, T., … Cameron, D. (2006). Lapatinib plus capecitabine for HER2-positive advanced breast cancer. *New England Journal of Medicine, 355,* 2733–2743. doi:10.1056/NEJMoa064320

Giobbie-Hurder, A., Price, K.N., & Gelber, R.D. (2009). Design, conduct, and analyses of Breast International Group (BIG) 1-98: A randomized, double-blind, phase-III study comparing letrozole and tamoxifen as adjuvant endocrine therapy for postmenopausal women with receptor-positive, early breast cancer. *Clinical Trials, 6,* 272–287. doi:10.1177/1740774509105380

GlaxoSmithKline. (2010). *Tykerb®* [Package insert]. Collegeville, PA: Author.

Gnant, M.F., Mlineritsch, B., Luschin-Ebengreuth, G., Grampp, S., Kaessmann, H., Schmid, M., … Jakesz, R. (2007). Zoledronic acid prevents cancer treatment-induced bone loss in premenopausal women receiving adjuvant endocrine therapy for hormone-responsive breast cancer: A report from the Austrian Breast and Colorectal Cancer Study Group. *Journal of Clinical Oncology, 25,* 820–828. doi:10.1200/JCO.2005.02.7102

Gnant, M., Mlineritsch, B., Schippinger, W., Luschin-Ebengreuth, G., Pöstlberger, S., Menzel, C., … Greil, R. (2009). Endocrine therapy plus zoledronic acid in premenopausal breast cancer. *New England Journal of Medicine, 360,* 679–691. doi:10.1056/NEJMoa0806285

Goel, S., Sharma, R., Hamilton, A., & Beith, J. (2009). LHRH agonists for adjuvant therapy of early breast cancer in premenopausal women. *Cochrane Database of Systematic Reviews* 2009, Issue 4. Art. No.: CD004562. doi:10.1002/14651858.CD004562.pub4

Goss, P.E., Ingle, J.N., Pater, J.L., Martino, S., Robert, N.J., Muss, H.B., … Tu, D. (2008). Late extended adjuvant treatment with letrozole improves outcome in women with early-stage breast cancer who complete 5 years of tamoxifen. *Journal of Clinical Oncology, 26,* 1948–1955. doi:10.1200/JCO.2007.11.6798

Gossage, L., & Eisen, T. (2010). Targeting multiple kinase pathways: A change in paradigm. *Clinical Cancer Research, 16,* 1973–1978. doi:10.1158/1078-0432.CCR-09-3182

Gradishar, W.J., Krasnojon, D., Cheporov, S., Makhson, A.N., Manikhas, G.M., Clawson, A., & Bhar, P. (2009). Significantly longer progression-free survival with nab-paclitaxel compared with docetaxel as first-line therapy for metastatic breast cancer. *Journal of Clinical Oncology, 27,* 3611–3619. doi:10.1200/JCO.2008.18.5397

Gradishar, W.J., Tjulandin, S., Davidson, N., Shaw, H., Desai, N., Bhar, P., ... O'Shaughnessy, J. (2005). Phase III trial of nanoparticle albumin-bound paclitaxel compared with polyethylated castor oil-based paclitaxel in women with breast cancer. *Journal of Clinical Oncology, 23,* 7794–7803. doi:10.1200/JCO.2005.04.937

Greenberg, S., & Rugo, H.S. (2010). Triple-negative breast cancer: Role of antiangiogenic agents. *Cancer Journal, 16,* 33–38. doi:10.1097/PPO.0b013e3181d38514

Gressett, S.M., Stanford, B.L., & Hardwicke, F. (2006). Management of hand-foot syndrome induced by capecitabine. *Journal of Oncology Pharmacy Practice, 12,* 131–141. doi:10.1177/1078155206069242

Grevelman, E.G., & Breed, W.P. (2005). Prevention of chemotherapy-induced hair loss by scalp cooling. *Annals of Oncology, 16,* 352–358. doi:10.1093/annonc/mdi088

Gucalp, A., & Traina, T.A. (2010). Triple-negative breast cancer: Role of the androgen receptor. *Cancer Journal, 16,* 62–65. doi:10.1097/PPO.0b013e3181ce4ae1

Haagenson, K.K., & Wu, G.S. (2010). The role of MAP kinases and MAP kinase phosphatase-1 in resistance to breast cancer treatment. *Cancer Metastasis Reviews, 29,* 143–149. doi:10.1007/s10555-010-9208-5

Hackshaw, A., Baum, M., Fornander, T., Nordenskjold, B., Nicolucci, A., Monson, K., ... Sainsbury, R. (2009). Long-term effectiveness of adjuvant goserelin in premenopausal women with early breast cancer. *Journal of the National Cancer Institute, 101,* 341–349. doi:10.1093/jnci/djn498

Hadji, P., Body, J.J., Aapro, M.S., Brufsky, A., Coleman, R.E., Guise, T., ... Tubiana-Hulin, M. (2008). Practical guidance for the management of aromatase inhibitor-associated bone loss. *Annals of Oncology, 19,* 1407–1416. doi:10.1093/annonc/mdn164

Henderson, I.C., Berry, D.A., Demetri, G.D., Cirrincione, C.T., Goldstein, L.J., Martino, S., ... Norton, L. (2003). Improved outcomes from adding sequential paclitaxel but not from escalating doxorubicin dose in an adjuvant chemotherapy regimen for patients with node-positive primary breast cancer. *Journal of Clinical Oncology, 21,* 976–983. doi:10.1200/JCO.2003.02.063

Hershman, D.L., McMahon, D.J., Crew, K.D., Shao, T., Cremers, S., Brafman, L., ... Shane, E. (2010). Prevention of bone loss by zoledronic acid in premenopausal women undergoing adjuvant chemotherapy persist up to one year following discontinuing treatment. *Journal of Clinical Endocrinology and Metabolism, 95,* 559–566. doi:10.1210/jc.2009-1366

Hesketh, P.J., Batchelor, D., Golant, M., Lyman, G.H., Rhodes, N., & Yardley, D. (2004). Chemotherapy-induced alopecia: Psychosocial impact and therapeutic approaches. *Supportive Care in Cancer, 12,* 543–549. doi:10.1007/s00520-003-0562-5

Hines, S.L., Mincey, B.A., Sloan, J.A., Thomas, S.P., Chottiner, E., Loprinzi, C.L., ... Perez, E.A. (2009). Phase III randomized, placebo-controlled, double-blind trial of risedronate for the prevention of bone loss in premenopausal women undergoing chemotherapy for primary breast cancer. *Journal of Clinical Oncology, 27,* 1047–1053. doi:10.1200/JCO.2008.19.1783

Hortobagyi, G.N., Theriault, R.L., Porter, L., Blayney, D., Lipton, A., Sinoff, C., ... Knight, R.D. (1996). Efficacy of pamidronate in reducing skeletal complications in patients with breast cancer and lytic bone metastases. Protocol 19 Aredia Breast Cancer Study Group. *New England Journal of Medicine, 335,* 1785–1791. doi:10.1056/NEJM199612123352401

Howell, A. (2006). Pure oestrogen antagonists for the treatment of advanced breast cancer. *Endocrine-Related Cancer, 13,* 689–706. doi:10.1677/erc.1.00846

Howell, A., Cuzick, J., Buzdar, A., Dowsett, M., Forbes, J.F., Hoctin-Boes, G., ... Tobias, J.S. (2005). Results of the ATAC (Arimidex, Tamoxifen, Alone or in Combination) trial after completion of 5 years' adjuvant treatment for breast cancer. *Lancet, 365,* 60–62. doi:10.1016/S0140-6736(04)17666-6

Howell, A., Robertson, J.F., Abram, P., Lichinitser, M.R., Elledge, R., Bajetta, E., ... Osborne, C.K. (2004). Comparison of fulvestrant versus tamoxifen for the treatment of advanced breast cancer in postmenopausal women previously untreated with endocrine therapy: A multinational, double-blind, randomized trial. *Journal of Clinical Oncology, 22,* 1605–1613. doi:10.1200/JCO.2004.02.112

International Breast Cancer Study Group. (2003). Adjuvant chemotherapy followed by goserelin versus either modality alone for premenopausal lymph node-negative breast cancer: A randomized trial. *Journal of the National Cancer Institute, 95,* 1833–1846. doi:10.1093/jnci/djg119

ICI Americas, Inc. (2006). *Tween® 80* [Package insert]. Retrieved from http://www.sigmaaldrich.com/etc/medialib/docs/Sigma-Aldrich/Product_Information_Sheet/p8074pis.Par.0001.File.tmp/p8074pis.pdf

Isakoff, S.J. (2010). Triple-negative breast cancer: Role of specific chemotherapy agents. *Cancer Journal, 16,* 53–61. doi:10.1097/PPO.0b013e3181d24ff7

Izzo, A.A., & Ernst, E. (2009). Interactions between herbal medicines and prescribed drugs: An updated systematic review. *Drugs, 69,* 1777–1798. doi:10.2165/11317010-000000000-00000

Janni, W., & Hepp, P. (2010). Adjuvant aromatase inhibitor therapy: Outcomes and safety. *Cancer Treatment Reviews, 36,* 249–261. doi:10.1016/j.ctrv.2009.12.010

Jin, H.W., Flatters, S.J., Xiao, W.H., Mulhern, H.L., & Bennett, G.J. (2008). Prevention of paclitaxel-evoked painful peripheral neuropathy by acetyl-L-carnitine: Effects on axonal mitochondria, sensory nerve fiber terminal arbors, and cutaneous Langerhans cells. *Experimental Neurology, 210,* 229–237. doi:10.1016/j.expneurol.2007.11.001

Johnston, S.R. (2010). New strategies in estrogen receptor-positive breast cancer. *Clinical Cancer Research, 16,* 1979–1987. doi:10.1158/1078-0432.CCR-09-1823

Jones, K.L., & Buzdar, A.U. (2009). Evolving novel anti-HER2 strategies. *Lancet Oncology, 10,* 1179–1187. doi:10.1016/S1470-2045(09)70315-8

Katz, A. (2007). *Breaking the silence on cancer and sexuality.* Pittsburgh, PA: Oncology Nursing Society.

Kaufman, B., Mackey, J.R., Clemens, M.R., Bapsy, P.P., Vaid, A., Wardley, A., ... Jones, A. (2009). Trastuzumab plus anastrozole versus anastrozole alone for the treatment of postmenopausal women with human epidermal growth factor receptor 2-positive, hormone receptor-positive metastatic breast cancer: Results from the randomized phase III TAnDEM study. *Journal of Clinical Oncology, 27,* 5529–5537. doi:10.1200/JCO.2008.20.6847

Kearney, N., & Friese, C. (2008). Clinical practice guidelines for the use of colony-stimulating factors in cancer treatment: Implications for oncology nurses. *European Journal of Oncology Nursing, 12,* 14–25. doi:10.1016/j.ejon.2007.10.001

Kelly, C.M., Juurlink, D.N., Gomes, T., Duong-Hua, M., Pritchard, K.I., Austin, P.C., & Paszat, L.F. (2010). Selective serotonin reuptake inhibitors and breast cancer mortality in women receiving tamoxifen: A population based cohort study. *BMJ, 340,* c693. doi:10.1136/bmj.c693

Kerbel, R.S. (2009). Issues regarding improving the impact of antiangiogenic drugs for the treatment of breast cancer. *Breast, 18*(Suppl. 3), S41–S47. doi:10.1016/S0960-9776(09)70271-1

Kerbel, R.S., & Kamen, B.A. (2004). The anti-angiogenic basis of metronomic chemotherapy. *Nature Reviews Cancer, 4*, 423–436. doi:10.1038/nrc1369

Kohno, N., Aogi, K., Minami, H., Nakamura, S., Asaga, T., Iino, Y., ... Takashima, S. (2005). Zoledronic acid significantly reduces skeletal complications compared with placebo in Japanese women with bone metastases from breast cancer: A randomized, placebo-controlled trial. *Journal of Clinical Oncology, 23*, 3314–3321. doi:10.1200/JCO.2005.05.116

Konecny, G.E., Pegram, M.D., Venkatesan, N., Finn, R., Yang, G., Rahmeh, M., ... Slamon, D.J. (2006). Activity of the dual kinase inhibitor lapatinib (GW572016) against HER-2-overexpressing and trastuzumab-treated breast cancer cells. *Cancer Research, 66*, 1630–1639. doi:10.1158/0008-5472.CAN-05-1182

Kossoff, E. (2010). Alternative dosing schedules and administration updates for ixabepilone. *Journal of Oncology Pharmacy Practice.* Advance online publication. doi:10.1177/1078155210364273

Langer, S.W., Sehested, M., & Jensen, P.B. (2000). Treatment of anthracycline extravasation with dexrazoxane. *Clinical Cancer Research, 6*, 3680–3686.

Laxmi, Y.R., Liu, X., Suzuki, N., Kim, S.Y., Okamoto, K., Kim, H.J., ... Shibutani, S. (2010). Anti-breast cancer potential of SS1020, a novel antiestrogen lacking estrogenic and genotoxic actions. *International Journal of Cancer, 127*, 1718–1726. doi:10.1002/ijc.25167

Legha, S.S., Davis, H.L., & Muggia, F.M. (1978). Hormonal therapy of breast cancer: New approaches and concepts. *Annals of Internal Medicine, 88*, 69–77.

Lemieux, J., Amireault, C., Provencher, L., & Maunsell, E. (2009). Incidence of scalp metastases in breast cancer: A retrospective cohort study in women who were offered scalp cooling. *Breast Cancer Research and Treatment, 118*, 547–552. doi:10.1007/s10549-009-0342-0

Lin, N.U., Carey, L.A., Liu, M.C., Younger, J., Come, S.E., Ewend, M., ... Winer, E.P. (2008). Phase II trial of lapatinib for brain metastases in patients with human epidermal growth factor receptor 2-positive breast cancer. *Journal of Clinical Oncology, 26*, 1993–1999. doi:10.1200/JCO.2007.12.3588

Lin, N.U., Diéras, V., Paul, D., Lossignol, D., Christodoulou, C., Stemmler, H.J., ... Winer, E.P. (2009). Multicenter phase II study of lapatinib in patients with brain metastases from HER2-positive breast cancer. *Clinical Cancer Research, 15*, 1452–1459. doi:10.1158/1078-0432.CCR-08-1080

Loprinzi, C.L., Sloan, J., Stearns, V., Slack, R., Iyengar, M., Diekmann, B., ... Novotny, P. (2009). Newer antidepressants and gabapentin for hot flashes: An individual patient pooled analysis. *Journal of Clinical Oncology, 27*, 2831–2837. doi:10.1200/JCO.2008.19.6253

Loven, D., Levavi, H., Sabach, G., Zart, R., Andras, M., Fishman, A., ... Gadoth, N. (2009). Long-term glutamate supplementation failed to protect against peripheral neurotoxicity of paclitaxel. *European Journal of Cancer Care, 18*, 78–83. doi:10.1111/j.1365-2354.2008.00996.x

Lurje, G., & Lenz, H.J. (2009). EGFR signaling and drug discovery. *Oncology, 77*, 400–410. doi:10.1159/000279388

Ma, A.M., Barone, J., Wallis, A.E., Wu, N.J., Garcia, L.B., Estabrook, A., ... Tartter, P.I. (2008). Noncompliance with adjuvant radiation, chemotherapy, or hormonal therapy in breast cancer patients. *American Journal of Surgery, 196*, 500–504. doi:10.1016/j.amjsurg.2008.06.027

Mahon, S.M., & Palmieri, F.M. (2009). Metastatic breast cancer: The individualization of therapy. *Clinical Journal of Oncology Nursing, 13*(Suppl. 1), 19–28. doi:10.1188/09.CJON.S1.19-28

Mamounas, E.P., Bryant, J., Lembersky, B., Fehrenbacher, L., Sedlacek, S.M., Fisher, B., ... Wolmark, N. (2005). Paclitaxel after doxorubicin plus cyclophosphamide as adjuvant chemotherapy for node-positive breast cancer: Results from NSABP B-28. *Journal of Clinical Oncology, 23*, 3686–3696. doi:10.1200/JCO.2005.10.517

Martin, M., Welch, J., Luo, J., Ellis, M.J., Graubert, T.A., & Walter, M.J. (2009). Therapy related acute myeloid leukemia in breast cancer survivors, a population-based study. *Breast Cancer Research and Treatment, 118*, 593–598. doi:10.1007/s10549-009-0376-3

Martin, S. (2005, April-May). *Chemotherapy handling and effects among nurses and their offspring.* Paper presented at the Oncology Nursing Society 30th Annual Congress, Orlando, FL.

Mathew, J., Asgeirsson, K.S., Jackson, L.R., Cheung, K.L., & Robertson, J.F. (2009). Neoadjuvant endocrine treatment in primary breast cancer—Review of literature. *Breast, 18*, 339–344. doi:10.1016/j.breast.2009.09.012

Mauri, D., Kamposioras, K., Tsali, L., Bristianou, M., Valachis, A., Karathanasi, I., ... Polyzos, N.P. (2010). Overall survival benefit for weekly vs. three-weekly taxanes regimens in advanced breast cancer: A meta-analysis. *Cancer Treatment Reviews, 36*, 69–74. doi:10.1016/j.ctrv.2009.10.006

Mayers, C., Panzarella, T., & Tannock, I.F. (2001). Analysis of the prognostic effects of inclusion in a clinical trial and of myelosuppression on survival after adjuvant chemotherapy for breast carcinoma. *Cancer, 91*, 2246–2257. doi:10.1002/1097-0142(20010615)91:12<2246::AID-CNCR1255>3.0.CO;2-4

McArthur, H.L., & Hudis, C.A. (2007a). Adjuvant chemotherapy for early-stage breast cancer. *Hematology/Oncology Clinics of North America, 21*, 207–222. doi:10.1016/j.hoc.2007.03.008

McArthur, H.L., & Hudis, C.A. (2007b). Breast cancer chemotherapy. *Cancer Journal, 13*, 141–147. doi:10.1097/PPO.0b013e318074dc6f

Mehrotra, B. (2009). Bisphosphonates—Role in cancer therapies. *Journal of Oral and Maxillofacial Surgery, 67*(Suppl. 5), 19–26. doi:10.1016/j.joms.2009.01.012

Michaud, L.B. (2010). Managing cancer treatment-induced bone loss and osteoporosis in patients with breast or prostate cancer. *American Journal of Health-System Pharmacy, 67*(7, Suppl. 3), S20–S30. doi:10.2146/ajhp100078

Miller, K., Wang, M., Gralow, J., Dickler, M., Cobleigh, M., Perez, E.A., ... Davidson, N.E. (2007). Paclitaxel plus bevacizumab versus paclitaxel alone for metastatic breast cancer. *New England Journal of Medicine, 357*, 2666–2676. doi:10.1056/NEJMoa072113

Montemurro, F., & Aglietta, M. (2009). Hormone receptor-positive early breast cancer: Controversies in the use of adjuvant chemotherapy. *Endocrine-Related Cancer, 16*, 1091–1102. doi:10.1677/ERC-09-0033

Moreno-Aspitia, A., & Perez, E.A. (2009). Treatment options for breast cancer resistant to anthracycline and taxane. *Mayo Clinic Proceedings, 84*, 533–545. doi:10.4065/84.6.533

Mortimer, J. (2010). Managing the toxicities of the aromatase inhibitors. *Current Opinion in Obstetrics and Gynecology, 22*, 56–60. doi:10.1097/GCO.0b013e328334e44e

Mortimer, J.E., Lauman, M.K., Tan, B., Dempsey, C.L., Shillington, A.C., & Hutchins, K.S. (2003). Pyridoxine treatment and prevention of hand-and-foot syndrome in patients receiving capecitabine. *Journal of Oncology Pharmacy Practice, 9*, 161–166. doi:10.1191/1078155203jp116oa

Moss, L.S., Starbuck, M.F., Mayer, D.K., Harwood, E.B., & Glotzer, J. (2009). Trastuzumab-induced cardiotoxicity. *Oncology Nursing Forum, 36*, 676–685. doi:10.1188/09.ONF.676-685

Moulder, S.L., Holmes, F.A., Tolcher, A.W., Thall, P., Broglio, K., Valero, V., ... Hortobagyi, G.N. (2010). A randomized phase 2 trial comparing 3-hour versus 96-hour infusion schedules of paclitaxel for the treatment of metastatic breast cancer. *Cancer, 116*, 814–821. doi:10.1002/cncr.24870

Mouridsen, H.T., Langer, S.W., Buter, J., Eidtmann, H., Rosti, G., de Wit, M., ... Giaccone, G. (2007). Treatment of anthracycline extravasation with Savene (dexrazoxane): Results from two prospective clinical multicentre studies. *Annals of Oncology, 18,* 546–550. doi:10.1093/annonc/mdl413

Mouridsen, H.T., Rose, C., Brodie, A.H., & Smith, I.E. (2003). Challenges in the endocrine management of breast cancer. *Breast, 12*(Suppl. 2), S2–S19. doi:10.1016/S0960-9776(03)80158-3

Mundy, G.R. (2002). Metastasis to bone: Causes, consequences and therapeutic opportunities. *Nature Reviews Cancer, 2,* 584–593. doi:10.1038/nrc867

Murphy, C.G., & Fornier, M. (2010). HER2-positive breast cancer: Beyond trastuzumab. *Oncology, 24,* 410–414.

Muss, H.B., Berry, D.A., Cirrincione, C.T., Theodoulou, M., Mauer, A.M., Kornblith, A.B., … Winer, E.P. (2009). Adjuvant chemotherapy in older women with early-stage breast cancer. *New England Journal of Medicine, 360,* 2055–2065. doi:10.1056/NEJMoa0810266

Nabholtz, J.-M.A. (2008). Long-term safety of aromatase inhibitors in the treatment of breast cancer. *Therapeutics and Clinical Risk Management, 4,* 189–204. doi:10.2147/TCRM.S1566

Nabholtz, J.M., Bonneterre, J., Buzdar, A., Robertson, J.F., & Thürlimann, B. (2003). Anastrozole (Arimidex) versus tamoxifen as first-line therapy for advanced breast cancer in postmenopausal women: Survival analysis and updated safety results. *European Journal of Cancer, 39,* 1684–1689. doi:10.1016/S0959-8049(03)00326-5

National Comprehensive Cancer Network. (2010, June). *NCCN Clinical Practice Guidelines in Oncology™: Myeloid growth factors* [v.1.2010]. Retrieved from http://www.nccn.org/professionals/physician_gls/PDF/myeloid_growth.pdf

National Comprehensive Cancer Network. (2011, January). *NCCN Clinical Practice Guidelines in Oncology™: Breast cancer* [v.2.2011]. Retrieved from http://www.nccn.org/professionals/physician_gls/PDF/breast.pdf

Neville-Webbe, H.L., Coleman, R.E., & Holen, I. (2010). Combined effects of the bisphosphonate, zoledronic acid and the aromatase inhibitor letrozole on breast cancer cells in vitro: Evidence of synergistic interaction. *British Journal of Cancer, 102,* 1010–1017. doi:10.1038/sj.bjc.6605579

Novartis Pharmaceuticals Corp. (2010). *Femara®* [Package insert]. East Hanover, NJ: Author.

O'Shaughnessy, J., Miles, D., Vukelja, S., Moiseyenko, V., Ayoub, J.P., Cervantes, G., … Leonard, R. (2002). Superior survival with capecitabine plus docetaxel combination therapy in anthracycline-pretreated patients with advanced breast cancer: Phase III trial results. *Journal of Clinical Oncology, 20,* 2812–2823. doi:10.1200/JCO.2002.09.002

Paice, J.A. (2009). Clinical challenges: Chemotherapy-induced peripheral neuropathy. *Seminars in Oncology Nursing, 25*(2, Suppl. 1), S8–S19. doi:10.1016/j.soncn.2009.03.013

Palmieri, F.M., Frye, D.K., & Mahon, S.M. (2009). Current clinical issues in systemic therapy for metastatic breast cancer. *Clinical Journal of Oncology Nursing, 13*(Suppl. 1), 4–10. doi:10.1188/09.CJON.S1.4-10

Patani, N., & Mokbel, K. (2010). Herceptin and breast cancer: An overview for surgeons. *Surgical Oncology, 19,* e11–e21. doi:10.1016/j.suronc.2008.11.001

Pavlakis, N., Schmidt, R.L., & Stockler, M.R. (2005). Bisphosphonates for breast cancer. *Cochrane Database of Systematic Reviews* 2005, Issue 3. Art. No.: CD003474. doi:10.1002/14651858.CD003474.pub2

Perez, E.A., Josse, R.G., Pritchard, K.I., Ingle, J.N., Martino, S., Findlay, B.P., … Goss, P.E. (2006). Effect of letrozole versus placebo on bone mineral density in women with primary breast cancer completing 5 or more years of adjuvant tamoxifen: A companion study to NCIC CTG MA.17. *Journal of Clinical Oncology, 24,* 3629–3635. doi:10.1200/JCO.2005.05.4882

Perez, E.A., Lerzo, G., Pivot, X., Thomas, E., Vahdat, L., Bosserman, L., … Hortobagyi, G.N. (2007). Efficacy and safety of ixabepilone (BMS-247550) in a phase II study of patients with advanced breast cancer resistant to an anthracycline, a taxane, and capecitabine. *Journal of Clinical Oncology, 25,* 3407–3414. doi:10.1200/JCO.2006.09.3849

Perez, E.A., Moreno-Aspitia, A., Thompson, E.A., & Andorfer, C.A. (2010). Adjuvant therapy of triple negative breast cancer. *Breast Cancer Research and Treatment, 120,* 285–291. doi:10.1007/s10549-010-0736-z

Perez, E.A., Patel, T., & Moreno-Aspitia, A. (2010). Efficacy of ixabepilone in ER/PR/HER2-negative (triple-negative) breast cancer. *Breast Cancer Research and Treatment, 121,* 261–271. doi:10.1007/s10549-010-0824-0

Petrakis, I.E., & Paraskakis, S. (2010). Breast cancer in the elderly. *Archives of Gerontology and Geriatrics, 50,* 179–184. doi:10.1016/j.archger.2009.03.007

Pharmacia & Upjohn. (2011). *Aromasin®* [Package insert]. New York, NY: Author.

Pichot, C.S., Hartig, S.M., Xia, L., Arvanitis, C., Monisvais, D., Lee, F.Y., … Corey, S.J. (2009). Dasatinib synergizes with doxorubicin to block growth, migration, and invasion of breast cancer cells. *British Journal of Cancer, 101,* 38–47. doi:10.1038/sj.bjc.6605101

Polovich, M., Whitford, J., & Olsen, M. (Eds.). (2009). *Chemotherapy and biotherapy guidelines and recommendations for practice* (3rd ed.). Pittsburgh, PA: Oncology Nursing Society.

Portera, C.C., Walshe, J.M., Rosing, D.R., Denduluri, N., Berman, A.W., Vatas, U., … Swain, S.M. (2008). Cardiac toxicity and efficacy of trastuzumab combined with pertuzumab in patients with trastuzumab-insensitive human epidermal growth factor receptor 2-positive metastatic breast cancer. *Clinical Cancer Research, 14,* 2710–2716. doi:10.1158/1078-0432.CCR-07-4636

Pronzato, P. (2008). New therapeutic options for chemotherapy-resistant metastatic breast cancer: The epothilones. *Drugs, 68,* 139–146.

Pusztai, L. (2009). Gene expression profiling of breast cancer. *Breast Cancer Research, 11*(Suppl. 3), S11. doi:10.1186/bcr2430

Quirion, E. (2009). Filgrastim and pegfilgrastim use in patients with neutropenia. *Clinical Journal of Oncology Nursing, 13,* 324–328. doi:10.1188/09.CJON.324-328

Renwick, W., Pettengell, R., & Green, M. (2009). Use of filgrastim and pegfilgrastim to support delivery of chemotherapy: Twenty years of clinical experience. *BioDrugs, 23,* 175–186. doi:10.2165/00063030-200923030-00004.

Ring, A. (2010). The influences of age and co-morbidities on treatment decisions for patients with HER2-positive early breast cancer. *Critical Reviews in Oncology/Hematology, 76,* 127–132. doi:10.1016/j.critrevonc.2010.01.002

Robert, N., Leyland-Jones, B., Asmar, L., Belt, R., Ilegbodu, D., Loesch, D., … Slamon, D. (2006). Randomized phase III study of trastuzumab, paclitaxel, and carboplatin compared with trastuzumab and paclitaxel in women with HER-2-overexpressing metastatic breast cancer. *Journal of Clinical Oncology, 24,* 2786–2792. doi:10.1200/JCO.2005.04.1764

Roche Pharmaceuticals. (2005). *Xeloda®* [Package insert]. Nutley, NJ: Author.

Rosen, L.S., Ashurst, H.L., & Chap, L. (2010). Targeting signal transduction pathways in metastatic breast cancer: A comprehensive review. *Oncologist, 15,* 216–235. doi:10.1634/theoncologist.2009-0145

Rosen, L.S., Gordon, D., Kaminski, M., Howell, A., Belch, A., Mackey, J., … Seaman, J.J. (2003). Long-term efficacy and safety of zoledronic acid compared with pamidronate disodium in the treatment of skeletal complications in patients with advanced multiple myeloma or breast carcinoma: A randomized, double-blind, multicenter, comparative trial. *Cancer, 98,* 1735–1744. doi:10.1002/cncr.11701

Roy, V., LaPlant, B.R., Gross, G.G., Bane, C.L., & Palmieri, F.M. (2009). Phase II trial of weekly nab (nanoparticle albumin-bound)-paclitaxel (nab-paclitaxel) (Abraxane) in combination with gemcitabine in patients with metastatic breast cancer (N0531). *Annals of Oncology, 20,* 449–453. doi:10.1093/annonc/mdn661

sanofi-aventis. (2010). *Taxotere®* [Package insert]. Bridgewater, NJ: Author.

Santen, R.J., Brodie, H., Simpson, E.R., Siiteri, P.K., & Brodie, A. (2009). History of aromatase: Saga of an important biological mediator and therapeutic target. *Endocrine Reviews, 30,* 343–375. doi:10.1210/er.2008-0016

Schmid, P., Untch, M., Kossé, V., Bondar, G., Vassiljev, L., Tarutinov, V., … Possinger, K. (2007). Leuprorelin acetate every-3-months depot versus cyclophosphamide, methotrexate, and fluorouracil as adjuvant treatment in premenopausal patients with node-positive breast cancer: The TABLE study. *Journal of Clinical Oncology, 25,* 2509–2515. doi:10.1200/JCO.2006.08.8534

Schulmeister, L. (2007). Infiltration and extravasation [Comment]. *American Journal of Nursing, 107*(10), 16. doi:10.1097/01.NAJ.0000292181.28549.99

Schulmeister, L. (2009). Vesicant chemotherapy extravasation antidotes and treatments. *Clinical Journal of Oncology Nursing, 13,* 395–398. doi:10.1188/09.CJON.395-398

Schwenkglenks, M., Pettengell, R., Jackisch, C., Paridaens, R., Constenla, M., Bosly, A., … Leonard, R. (2010). Risk factors for chemotherapy-induced neutropenia occurrence in breast cancer patients: Data from the INC-EU Prospective Observational European Neutropenia Study. *Supportive Care in Cancer.* Advance online publication. doi:10.1007/s00520-010-0840-y

Scotté, F., Banu, E., Medioni, J., Levy, E., Ebenezer, C., Marsan, S., … Oudard, S. (2008). Matched case-control phase 2 study to evaluate the use of a frozen sock to prevent docetaxel-induced onycholysis and cutaneous toxicity of the foot. *Cancer, 112,* 1625–1631. doi:10.1002/cncr.23333

Scotté, F., Tourani, J.M., Banu, E., Peyromaure, M., Levy, E., Marsan, S., … Oudard, S. (2005). Multicenter study of a frozen glove to prevent docetaxel-induced onycholysis and cutaneous toxicity of the hand. *Journal of Clinical Oncology, 23,* 4424–4429. doi:10.1200/JCO.2005.15.651

Seidman, A.D., Reichman, B.S., Crown, J.P., Yao, T.J., Currie, V., Hakes, T.B., … Forsythe, P. (1995). Paclitaxel as second and subsequent therapy for metastatic breast cancer: Activity independent of prior anthracycline response. *Journal of Clinical Oncology, 13,* 1152–1159.

Seidman, A.D., Tiersten, A., Hudis, C., Gollub, M., Barrett, S., Yao, T.J., … Crown, J. (1995). Phase II trial of paclitaxel by 3-hour infusion as initial and salvage chemotherapy for metastatic breast cancer. *Journal of Clinical Oncology, 13,* 2575–2581.

Serra, V., Markman, B., Scaltriti, M., Eichhorn, P.J., Valero, V., Guzman, M., … Baselga, J. (2008). NVP-BEZ235, a dual PI3K/mTOR inhibitor, prevents PI3K signaling and inhibits the growth of cancer cells with activating PI3K mutations. *Cancer Research, 68,* 8022–8030. doi:10.1158/0008-5472.CAN-08-1385

Shenoy, H.G., Peter, M.B., Masannat, Y.A., Dall, B.J., Dodwell, D., & Horgan, K. (2009). Practical advice on clinical decision making during neoadjuvant chemotherapy for primary breast cancer. *Surgical Oncology, 18,* 65–71. doi:10.1016/j.suronc.2008.07.005

Shih, V., Wan, H.S., & Chan, A. (2009). Clinical predictors of chemotherapy-induced nausea and vomiting in breast cancer patients receiving adjuvant doxorubicin and cyclophosphamide. *Annals of Pharmacotherapy, 43,* 444–452. doi:10.1345/aph.1L437

Slamon, D.J., Leyland-Jones, B., Shak, S., Fuchs, H., Paton, V., Bajamonde, A., … Norton, L. (2001). Use of chemotherapy plus a monoclonal antibody against HER2 for metastatic breast cancer that overexpresses HER2. *New England Journal of Medicine, 344,* 783–792. doi:10.1056/NEJM200103153441101

Slichenmyer, W.J., & Von Hoff, D.D. (1991). Taxol: A new and effective anti-cancer drug. *Anti-Cancer Drugs, 2,* 519–530.

Smalley, R.V., Murphy, S., Huguley, C.M., Jr., & Bartolucci, A.A. (1976). Combination versus sequential five-drug chemotherapy in metastatic carcinoma of the breast. *Cancer Research, 36*(11, Pt. 1), 3911–3916.

Smith, A.M. (2005). Opening the dialogue: Herbal supplementation and chemotherapy. *Clinical Journal of Oncology Nursing, 9,* 447–450. doi:10.1188/05.CJON.447-450

Sotiriou, C., & Pusztai, L. (2009). Gene-expression signatures in breast cancer. *New England Journal of Medicine, 360,* 790–800. doi:10.1056/NEJMra0801289

Sparano, J.A., Wang, M., Martino, S., Jones, V., Perez, E.A., Saphner, T., … Davidson, N.E. (2008). Weekly paclitaxel in the adjuvant treatment of breast cancer. *New England Journal of Medicine, 358,* 1663–1671. doi:10.1056/NEJMoa0707056

Stein, A. (2010). Ixabepilone. *Clinical Journal of Oncology Nursing, 14,* 65–71. doi:10.1188/10.CJON.65-71

Stopeck, A.T., Lipton, A., Body, J.-J., Steger, G.G., Tonkin, K., de Boer, R.H., … Braun, A. (2010). Denosumab compared with zoledronic acid for the treatment of bone metastases in patients with advanced breast cancer: A randomized, double-blind study. *Journal of Clinical Oncology, 28,* 5132–5139. doi:10.1200/JCO.2010.29.7101

Sugarman, S., Wasserheit, C., Hodgman, E., Coglianese, M., D'Alassandro, A., Fornier, M., … Hudis, C. (2009). A pilot study of dose-dense adjuvant paclitaxel without growth factor support for women with early breast carcinoma. *Breast Cancer Research and Treatment, 115,* 609–612. doi:10.1007/s10549-008-0152-9 [Erratum at doi:10.1007/s10549-009-0482-2]

Tan-Chiu, E., Yothers, G., Romond, E., Geyer, C.E., Jr., Ewer, M., Keefe, D., … Bryant, J. (2005). Assessment of cardiac dysfunction in a randomized trial comparing doxorubicin and cyclophosphamide followed by paclitaxel, with or without trastuzumab as adjuvant therapy in node-positive, human epidermal growth factor receptor 2-overexpressing breast cancer: NSABP B-31. *Journal of Clinical Oncology, 23,* 7811–7819. doi:10.1200/JCO.2005.02.4091

Tanaka, M., Takamatsu, Y., Anan, K., Ohno, S., Nishimura, R., Yamamoto, Y., … Tamura, K. (2010). Oral combination chemotherapy with capecitabine and cyclophosphamide in patients with metastatic breast cancer: A phase II study. *Anti-Cancer Drugs, 21,* 453–458. doi:10.1097/CAD.0b013e328336acb1

Thomas, E., Tabernero, J., Fornier, M., Conté, P., Fumoleau, P., Lluch, A., … Martin, M. (2007). Phase II clinical trial of ixabepilone (BMS-247550), an epothilone B analog, in patients with taxane-resistant metastatic breast cancer. *Journal of Clinical Oncology, 25,* 3399–3406. doi:10.1200/JCO.2006.08.9102

Thomas, E.S., Gomez, H.L., Li, R.K., Chung, H.C., Fein, L.E., Chan, V.F., … Roché, H.H. (2007). Ixabepilone plus capecitabine for metastatic breast cancer progressing after anthracycline and taxane treatment. *Journal of Clinical Oncology, 25,* 5210–5217. doi:10.1200/JCO.2007.12.6557

Thürlimann, B., Keshaviah, A., Coates, A.S., Mouridsen, H., Mauriac, L., Forbes, J.F., … Goldhirsch, A. (2005). A comparison of letrozole and tamoxifen in postmenopausal women with early breast cancer. *New England Journal of Medicine, 353,* 2747–2757. doi:10.1056/NEJMoa052258 [Erratum at doi:10.1056/NEJMx060026]

Tkaczuk, K.H. (2009). Review of the contemporary cytotoxic and biologic combinations available for the treatment of metastatic breast cancer. *Clinical Therapeutics, 31*(Pt. 2), 2273–2289. doi:10.1016/j.clinthera.2009.11.011

Toppmeyer, D.L., & Goodin, S. (2009). Ixabepilone, a new treatment option for metastatic breast cancer. *American Journal of Clinical Oncology, 33,* 516–521. doi:10.1097/COC.0b013e3181b9cd52

Trüeb, R.M. (2009). Chemotherapy-induced alopecia. *Seminars in Cutaneous Medicine and Surgery, 28,* 11–14. doi:10.1016/j.sder.2008.12.001

Untch, M., Muscholl, M., Tjulandin, S., Jonat, W., Meerpohl, H.G., Lichinitser, M., ... Lück, H.J. (2010). First-line trastuzumab plus epirubicin and cyclophosphamide therapy in patients with human epidermal growth factor receptor 2-positive metastatic breast cancer: Cardiac safety and efficacy data from the Herceptin, Cyclophosphamide, and Epirubicin (HERCULES) trial. *Journal of Clinical Oncology, 28,* 1473–1480. doi:10.1200/JCO.2009.21.9709

U.S. Food and Drug Administration Center for Drug Evaluation and Research. (2010, December 15). Memorandum to the file BLA 125085 Avastin (bevacizumab). Retrieved from http://www.fda.gov/downloads/Drugs/DrugSafety/PostmarketDrugSafetyInformationforPatientsandProviders/UCM237171.pdf

Valachis, A., Mauri, D., Polyzos, N.P., Mavroudis, D., Georgoulias, V., & Casazza, G. (2010). Fulvestrant in the treatment of advanced breast cancer: A systematic review and meta-analysis of randomized controlled trials. *Critical Reviews in Oncology/Hematology, 73,* 220–227. doi:10.1016/j.critrevonc.2009.03.006

Valachis, A., Polyzos, N.P., Patsopoulos, N.A., Georgoulias, V., Mavroudis, D., & Mauri, D. (2010). Bevacizumab in metastatic breast cancer: A meta-analysis of randomized controlled trials. *Breast Cancer Research and Treatment, 122,* 1–7. doi:10.1007/s10549-009-0727-0

Valero, V., Holmes, F.A., Walters, R.S., Theriault, R.L., Esparza, L., Fraschini, G., ... Hortobagyi, G.N. (1995). Phase II trial of docetaxel: A new, highly effective antineoplastic agent in the management of patients with anthracycline-resistant metastatic breast cancer. *Journal of Clinical Oncology, 13,* 2886–2894.

van de Velde, C.J., Verma, S., van Nes, J.G., Masterman, C., & Pritchard, K.I. (2010). Switching from tamoxifen to aromatase inhibitors for adjuvant endocrine therapy in postmenopausal patients with early breast cancer. *Cancer Treatment Reviews, 36,* 54–62. doi:10.1016/j.ctrv.2009.10.003

van den Hurk, C.J., Mols, F., Vingerhoets, A.J., & Breed, W.P. (2009). Impact of alopecia and scalp cooling on the well-being of breast cancer patients. *Psycho-Oncology, 19,* 701–709. doi:10.1002/pon.1615

Van Poznak, C., Hannon, R.A., Mackey, J.R., Campone, M., Apffelstaedt, J.P., Clack, G., ... Eastell, R. (2010). Prevention of aromatase inhibitor-induced bone loss using risedronate: The SABRE trial. *Journal of Clinical Oncology, 28,* 967–975. doi:10.1200/JCO.2009.24.5902

Venturini, M., Del Mastro, L., Aitini, E., Baldini, E., Caroti, C., Contu, A., ... Bruzzi, P. (2005). Dose-dense adjuvant chemotherapy in early breast cancer patients: Results from a randomized trial. *Journal of the National Cancer Institute, 97,* 1724–1733. doi:10.1093/jnci/dji398

Venturini, M., Paridaens, R., Rossner, D., Vaslamatzis, M.M., Nortier, J.W., Salzberg, M., ... Bell, R. (2007). An open-label, multicenter study of outpatient capecitabine monotherapy in 631 patients with pretreated advanced breast cancer. *Oncology, 72,* 51–57. doi:10.1159/000111094

Visvanathan, K., Lippman, S.M., Hurley, P., & Temin, S. (2009). American Society of Clinical Oncology clinical practice guideline update on the use of pharmacologic interventions including tamoxifen, raloxifene, and aromatase inhibition for breast cancer risk reduction. *Gynecologic Oncology, 115,* 132–134. doi:10.1016/j.ygyno.2009.06.006

Vogel, V.G. (2009). The NSABP Study of Tamoxifen and Raloxifene (STAR) trial. *Expert Review of Anticancer Therapy, 9,* 51–60. doi:10.1586/14737140.9.1.51 [Erratum at doi:10.1586/14737140.9.3.388]

Vogel, V.G., Costantino, J.P., Wickerham, D.L., Cronin, W.M., Cecchini, R.S., Atkins, J.N., ... Wolmark, N. (2010). Update of the National Surgical Adjuvant Breast and Bowel Project Study of Tamoxifen and Raloxifene (STAR) P-2 Trial: Preventing breast cancer. *Cancer Prevention and Research, 3,* 696–706. doi:10.1158/1940-6207.CAPR-10-0076

von Minckwitz, G., Rezai, M., Loibl, S., Fasching, P.A., Huober, J., Tesch, H., ... Untch, M. (2010). Capecitabine in addition to anthracycline- and taxane-based neoadjuvant treatment in patients with primary breast cancer: Phase III GeparQuattro study. *Journal of Clinical Oncology, 28,* 2015–2023. doi:10.1200/JCO.2009.23.8303

Ward, J.H. (2010). Duration of adjuvant endocrine therapy of breast cancer: How much is enough? *Current Opinion in Obstetrics and Gynecology, 22,* 51–55. doi:10.1097/GCO.0b013e328334ff40

Wardley, A.M., Pivot, X., Morales-Vasquez, F., Zetina, L.M., de Fátima Dias Gaui, M., Reyes, D.O., ... Torres, A.A. (2010). Randomized phase II trial of first-line trastuzumab plus docetaxel and capecitabine compared with trastuzumab plus docetaxel in HER2-positive metastatic breast cancer. *Journal of Clinical Oncology, 28,* 976–983. doi:10.1200/JCO.2008.21.6531

Wilkes, G.M., & Barton-Burke, M. (2010). *2010 oncology nursing drug handbook.* Sudbury, MA: Jones and Bartlett.

Winter, M.C., & Coleman, R.E. (2009). Bisphosphonates in breast cancer: Teaching an old dog new tricks. *Current Opinion in Oncology, 21,* 499–506. doi:10.1097/CCO.0b013e328331c794

Wong, S.T. (2009). Emerging treatment combinations: Integrating therapy into clinical practice. *American Journal of Health-System Pharmacy, 66*(23, Suppl. 6), S9–S14. doi:10.2146/ajhp090439

Yamamoto, D.S., & Viale, P.H. (2009). Update on identifying and managing osteoporosis in women with breast cancer [Online exclusive]. *Clinical Journal of Oncology Nursing, 13*(5), E18–E29. doi:10.1188/09.CJON.E18-E29

Zauderer, M., Patil, S., & Hurria, A. (2009). Feasibility and toxicity of dose-dense adjuvant chemotherapy in older women with breast cancer. *Breast Cancer Research and Treatment, 117,* 205–210. doi:10.1007/s10549-008-0116-0

Zhou, S., Chan, E., Pan, S.Q., Huang, M., & Lee, E.J. (2004). Pharmacokinetic interactions of drugs with St John's wort. *Journal of Psychopharmacology, 18,* 262–276. doi:10.1177/0269881104042632

# CHAPTER 9

# Symptom Management

Carole H. Martz, RN, MS, AOCN®, CBCN®, and Katina Kirby, MS, OTR/L, CLT-LANA

## Introduction

More than 2.6 million women in the United States were survivors of breat cancer in 2008 (Howlander et al., 2011) because of improved early detection and multimodal therapy. However, the potential to cure or prolong the lives of these women has not come without a price. Treatment-related side effects can range from minor to life altering. Some are self-limiting, and some are long term in nature. Some can contribute to a decrease in quality of life (QOL) and psychological well-being. Recent studies also have shown that symptom severity can be affected by age, ethnicity, treatment, anxiety, and socioeconomic status (Eversley et al., 2005; Royer, Phelan, & Heidrich, 2009). This chapter will review the most common side effects associated with breast cancer treatment along with symptom management strategies.

## Surgical Complications

The most common long-term side effects from breast cancer surgery are pain, numbness, limited shoulder and arm range of motion (ROM), and lymphedema (Baron et al., 2007; Bosompra, Ashikaga, O'Brien, Nelson, & Skelly, 2002; Kärki, Simonen, Mälkiä, & Selfe, 2005; Swenson et al., 2002). The incidence of these side effects varies by the length of follow-up, measurement techniques used, and patient- and treatment-related factors (Gärtner et al., 2009). The severity of symptoms can range from mild to severe and can affect QOL months to years later (Gärtner et al., 2009; Lee, Kilbreath, Sullivan, Refshauge, & Beith, 2010; Rietman et al., 2003).

Studies comparing the frequency of side effects from axillary lymph node dissection (ALND) to sentinel lymph node (SLN) biopsy indicate more favorable outcomes with the latter procedure (Baron et al., 2007; Gärtner et al., 2009; Langer et al., 2007; Sener et al., 2001; Swenson et al., 2002). These studies include both retrospective and prospective studies, many of which are based on patient reports of symptoms.

## Surgery-Related Pain and Limitation of Movement

The incidence of postsurgery pain has been noted to range from 12% to 51% (Gärtner et al., 2009; Rietman et al., 2003). The type of breast pain experienced has been described as tightness in the breast scar and axilla, tenderness at the incision, and nerve entrapment symptoms (burning and stabbing), which are sometimes referred to as *postmastectomy pain syndrome*. However, pain is not always limited to the breast area (Bosompra et al., 2002; Jud et al., 2010; Kärki et al., 2005; Swenson et al., 2002). Patients in the Jud et al. (2010) study utilized a visual pain mapping device, which illustrated that patients' pain was noted in a variety of areas, including across the upper trunk, axilla, and inner-upper arm, with a predominance of chest wall symptoms noted in mastectomy patients. Patients in the Bosompra et al. (2002) study who underwent modified radical mastectomy were more likely to complain of problems with scar tightness than patients undergoing breast-conserving surgery. Wallace, Wallace, Lee, and Dobke (1996) noted, in one of the first studies of its kind, that patients undergoing reconstruction experienced similar incidences of pain, especially with movement. The Baron et al. (2007) study found that tenderness at the incision site was the most common patient-related symptom at baseline for those who had SLN surgery and that tenderness and soreness persisted for at least five years after breast cancer surgery yet decreased in prevalence from baseline to three months in patients having both SLN and ALND. Breast cancer survivors also used the terms *twinges* and *soreness or tenderness* to describe their symptoms. In patients undergoing ALND, more patients complained of tightness, numbness, and pain at baseline, and tightness, numbness, pulling, and tingling at 48 months. Numbness was the most distressing symptom in the ALND group at baseline and at 48 months. For those patients undergoing immediate breast reconstruction, Dell, Weaver, Kozempel, and Barsevick (2008) found that pain in the reconstructed breast, along with numbness, may be expected along with donor site pain for those undergoing autologous tissue procedures. Women with preexisting back pain also experienced more back pain following transverse rectus abdominis myocutaneous (TRAM) flap reconstruction, and those having a free TRAM flap experienced more postoperative abdominal pain in their study. Both of these bodily pains may persist beyond eight weeks after surgery. According to Wallace et al. (1996), women who underwent tissue expander procedures are more likely to report pectoralis muscle spasms with stretching of this muscle and an increased incidence of chronic pain compared to women who received a mastectomy without implants. The use of botulinum toxin at the time of mastectomy has been investigated as a means to reduce the incidence of postoperative pain with subpectoral implant reconstruction by some plastic surgeons, and Layeeque et al. (2004) described this technique. Radiation therapy was associated with breast and chest wall pain in patients undergoing accelerated partial-breast intensity-modulated radiotherapy in whom the planning target chest wall volume was greater than 35 gray (Gy) (Reeder et al., 2009).

Stiffness was the only sensation that was significant in patients who had both a total mastectomy and SLN surgery in the Baron et al. (2007) study, and it likely had some impact on shoulder and arm ROM. Fifty-six percent of patients undergoing mastectomy were found to experience phantom breast sensations at least one time during the 24-month evaluation period. Overall, the level of severity and distress for these symptoms was low. The study by Gärtner et al. (2009) found a 47% incidence of pain in postsurgical patients, 13% of whom rated their pain as severe. Rowland et al. (2000) found that women undergoing mastectomy with or without reconstruction had more physical symptoms, particularly discomfort at the surgical site, than women undergoing breast-conserving procedures. Symptoms described included pins and needles (26% incidence in mastectomy-alone patients) and numbness occurring in 52% of patients undergoing reconstruction. Baron et al. (2007) found that at five years, 40% of their study subjects continued to experience phantom sensations; however, those experiencing it at five years were not always the same patients who experienced it at the first time point, showing variability in onset. Most studies find that although women report a high prevalence of numbness following surgery, it does not affect their daily lives and activities after the first year. Most breast cancer survivors learn to adjust to these sensation changes.

Altered sensations likely result from injury or resection of specific nerves in the operative field. The intercostobrachial cutaneous nerve innervates the axilla and medial upper arm. This nerve is directly in the path of surgeons as they perform ALND and often is sacrificed to gain wider access to the axillary lymph nodes during SLN surgery. Even when preserved, it can be injured. A recent literature search by Kim et al. (2005) looked at SLN technique and the risk of increased postoperative sensory changes. A lower rate of changes occurred when lymphoscintigraphy was used to assist in localization of the SLN compared to when lymphoscintigraphy was not used. Numbness was more frequent when blue dye or an intraoperative handheld probe without lymphoscintigraphy or skin markings was used, suggesting that a change in surgical technique could affect the development of postmastectomy pain.

Injury to motor nerves is a very rare occurrence in the hands of a skilled surgeon. However, the brachial plexus may be injured as a result of hyperabduction of the arm on the operative side during surgery. Women who receive radiation therapy to the brachial plexus region also can develop chronic pain in the ipsilateral arm. Neuroma formation has also been implicated in causing similar pain. Becker et al. (2008) described the results of a microsurgical lymph node transplantation technique performed on six patients with intolerable pain and upper-extremity lymphedema (LE) following level II ALND and axillary, supraclavicular, and sternal regional radiation (mastectomy and lumpectomy patients included in sample). Debilitating pain disappeared immediately following surgery and persisted up to 38 months after surgery in these patients. Resection of local fibrotic tissue in the axilla performed to access the lymph node graft was thought to have contributed to some of the pain relief experienced in these patients.

Nonpharmacologic measures for treating mild pain include resting the operative arm on a pillow, limiting movement, applying heat (may be contraindicated in patients at risk for LE), or icing the painful area and protecting the skin from thermal injury. Over-the-counter nonsteroidal anti-inflammatory drugs (NSAIDs), acetaminophen, and short-term use of prescription cyclooxygenase-2 inhibitors may be helpful for pain that is caused by inflammation. Cognitive modalities such as distraction, relaxation, and imagery also are suggested as possible nonpharmacologic measures in the National Comprehensive Cancer Network (NCCN) *Adult Cancer Pain* guidelines (NCCN, 2010a).

A study by Katz et al. (2005) found that more severe acute postoperative pain increased the risk of chronic pain following breast cancer surgery. Attempts to minimize postsurgical pain have focused on the use of adjunctive aids such as paravertebral block (Boughey et al., 2009; Kairaluoma, Bachmann, Rosenberg, & Pere, 2006; Moller, Nikolajsen, Rodt, Ronning, & Carlsson, 2007) and wound infiltration with local anesthetics such as ropivacaine (Sidiropoulou et al., 2008). Reuben, Makari-Judson, and Lurie (2004) examined the effect of venlafaxine starting the night before partial or radical mastectomy and continuing for two weeks afterward with surgeries that included ALND. A significant decrease occurred in the incidence of chest wall, arm, and axillary pain at follow-up and six months after surgery. Postsurgical complications such as the development of a seroma, hematoma, or infection also have been shown to increase the risk of developing chronic pain. Most chronic pain syndromes associated with surgery are related to dysesthesias. Dysesthesias are defined as unpleasant, abnormal sensations often described as burning, tingling, or numbness ("Dysesthesia," n.d.). The treatment of dysesthesias depends on the severity of the symptoms and their impact on the patient's QOL. Both pharmacologic and nonpharmacologic strategies have been employed. Randomized clinical trials have looked at topical capsaicin and EMLA® (eutectic mixture of local anesthetics [lidocaine and prilocaine], AstraZeneca Pharmaceuticals) application for the prevention of postmastectomy pain at varying dosages and administration times. All achieved a good to excellent response, with the main side effect of the medications being a burning sensation (Fassoulaki, Sarantopoulos, Melemeni, & Hogan, 2000). Other pharmaceutical options include NSAIDs, tricyclic antidepressants, and anticonvulsants. Kalso, Tasmuth, and Neuvonen (1996) found that amitriptyline 50 mg significantly relieved neuropathic pain in the arm and around the breast scar. However, the drug's side effects affected patients' willingness to take the drug. Venlafaxine (Effexor®, Wyeth Pharmaceuticals) also has been shown to be effective in the management of neuropathic pain associated with breast surgery. Fassoulaki, Triga, Melemeni, and Sarantopoulos (2005) evaluated the effect of multimodal analgesia on acute and chronic pain after breast cancer surgery using gabapentin, EMLA, and ropivacaine in the wound, each of which reduced acute and chronic pain compared to controls. Morrison and Jacobs (2003) demonstrated a reduction or elimination of postoperative pain medication after mastectomy through the use of a temporarily placed local anesthetic pump as compared with a control group 72 hours after mastectomy. In a follow-up study, Kairaluoma et al. (2006) found that patients in whom preincisional paravertebral block was performed, the prevalence and severity of motion-related chronic pain after breast surgery, independent as to whether axillary surgery was performed, were reduced in the operative area one year following the procedure. They also found that the use of radiotherapy was related to pain at rest 12 months after surgery. Other strategies advocated by the NCCN (2010a) treatment guidelines include the use of topical agents such as lidocaine patch (5%) daily, topical diclofenac gel 1% applied four times daily, or diclofinac patch 180 mg applied once or twice daily.

For patients whose pain persists or is not relieved by the previous measures, a weak opioid such as codeine or hydrocodone should be added, followed by a more potent narcotic or referral to a pain clinic for consideration of nerve blocks (NCCN, 2010a). Kudel et al. (2007) noted that different types of postmastectomy pain are related to one another and possess potentially additive effects on the patient's overall functioning even years after the initial surgical procedure. This study clearly exemplifies the need to address all aspects of the pain experience in order to control patient symptoms.

Shoulder and arm ROM difficulties at one year after surgery range from 1.5% to 23% and are more commonly seen in women who have undergone ALND, mastectomy, and radiation therapy (Duff et al., 2001; Kärki et al., 2005; McCredie et al., 2001; Swenson et al., 2002). Most ROM limitations improved during follow-up (Knobf & Sun, 2005; Yang et al.,

2010). However, restrictions in shoulder and arm movement can persist for up to 12 years after surgery in both SLN and ALND groups (Ghazinouri, Levy, Ben-Porat, & Stubblefield, 2005; Macdonald, Bruce, Scott, Smith, & Chambers, 2005) and can be a disturbing factor for woman undergoing surgery for breast cancer. In a randomized trial of 127 patients, patients with SLN biopsy alone versus those with ALND experienced significantly less severe morbidity (arm strength, arm mobility, LE, and sensitivity) (Helms, Kühn, Moser, Remmel, & Kreienberg, 2009). Radiation therapy can contribute to scarring, adding additional restrictions, so continuing arm and shoulder exercises during radiation therapy should be advised (Hwang et al., 2008). However, newer radiation therapy techniques that spare the axilla result in a lower risk of ROM limitations (Deutsch & Flickinger, 2001). Now that more patients are receiving adjuvant chemotherapy, the start of radiation treatments may be delayed following surgery. Fortunately, protocols allow for the concurrent administration of trastuzumab and radiation therapy. Patients should be advised that ROM limitations might recur during radiation therapy. A study on upper-limb dysfunction in breast cancer survivors found that patients experiencing pectoralis tightness at 3 and 6 months postoperatively showed a higher prevalence of rotator cuff disease at 12 months, as well as with LE at any stage of evaluation (Yang et al., 2010). As such, patient reports of symptoms should continue to be taken seriously and further evaluation recommended if symptoms are worsening. Identification of people with preexisting mobility difficulties or significant early postoperative ROM problems should lead to earlier intervention.

All patients undergoing axillary surgery should be advised about the possibility of ROM limitations and should be provided with exercises to decrease long-term restrictions. However, a cross-sectional survey of patients with breast cancer performed by Lee et al. (2010) indicated that patients were dissatisfied with the amount of information provided on postoperative exercises and felt they were given inconsistent advice on exercises and arm care.

Postoperative physical therapy can help to restore motion and strength and reduce pain following breast cancer surgery (Beurskens, van Uden, Strobbe, Oostendorp, & Wobbes, 2007). The timing of postoperative exercises is controversial, with randomized clinical trials showing mixed results. Some researchers suggest delaying exercises until one week after surgery in order to reduce seroma formation (Bendz, & Olsén, 2002; Box, Reul-Hirche, Bullock-Saxton, & Furnival, 2002; Petrek et al., 1990; Shamley, Barker, Simonite, & Beardshaw, 2005). The recommended timing of initiation of shoulder and arm exercises may be different for patients undergoing reconstruction depending on the type of reconstruction done so as to avoid damage to microvascular anastomoses. Patients who exhibit limited ROM four to six weeks after surgery will benefit from referral to a physical medicine specialist (McAnaw & Harris, 2002). Very detailed examples of exercises to be performed after breast surgery can be downloaded and printed for patients from the American Cancer Society Web site at www.cancer.org/Cancer/BreastCancer/MoreInformation/index. Nurses need to familiarize themselves with these exercises and the proper technique in order to reinforce the instructions and to determine whether the patient is performing them properly. These guidelines have been recently updated with assistance of the Oncology Section of the American Physical Therapy Association. According to the authors, patients should perform these exercises following a warm shower and should do the exercises until they feel a slow stretch. Patients are advised to hold the stretch for a count of five and to repeat the set five to seven times. The entire routine is to be repeated twice a day until normal flexibility and strength are regained. Patients must be advised that the stretch may cause some discomfort. The use of pain medication 30–45 minutes prior to beginning these exercises can limit the degree of discomfort. Patients are advised to inform their healthcare professionals if they have worsening pain, new heaviness, or swelling in the arm or develop weakness, dizziness, or other concerning symptoms while exercising (ACS, 2010).

A rarely reported axillary web syndrome, termed *banding* or *cording*, can result in pain along a cord leading from the axilla to the elbow (and occasionally extending to the wrist) with associated limitation in ROM. This syndrome can develop in the immediate postoperative period or months later. Therapy can relieve symptoms (Lacomba et al., 2009).

Exercise programs are aimed at preventing joint ROM limitation, LE, and postural alterations. Box et al. (2002) found that LE after ALND was decreased with the use of a monitoring, counseling, and early physiotherapy intervention. Studies by Bendz and Olsén (2002), Cinar et al. (2008), and Morimoto et al. (2003) showed that early intervention physiotherapy did not worsen postoperative complications and led to improved shoulder mobility and functional capacity compared to patient-led home or delayed exercise programs, and the effect persisted for up to two years. These authors did identify that preexisting shoulder ROM difficulty, older age, and a lower level of education resulted in poorer outcomes and suggested that these patients may require closer follow-up and reinforcement of instructions. The visual aids provided on the ACS Web site can be especially helpful for these individuals.

Acupuncture was found to improve ROM in individuals diagnosed with LE in a small study by Alem and Gurgel (2008). Thomas-MacLean et al. (2008) found that a significant percentage of patients one year after axillary surgery (both ALND and SLN) continued to experience some form of pain and limited ROM that affected their ability to perform more difficult tasks and certain leisure activities.

Side effects from the surgical treatment of breast cancer are varied and are summarized in Table 9-1. Patients must be aware of the expected side effects (mild discomfort, tightness, numbness) and which side effects will require intervention (limited ROM, pain that disrupts daily activities). This information should be discussed during preoperative teaching and reviewed postoperatively. Additional evaluations should be performed during follow-up examinations to alleviate patient concerns when symptoms develop and allow for prompt referral for ongoing issues. Reassuringly, the severity of most surgical-related symptoms lessens over time (Sagen, Kåresen, Sandvik, & Risberg, 2009).

## Lymphedema

Perhaps one of the most life-altering surgical breast cancer treatment–related side effects is upper-extremity or chest wall LE. It can develop in the immediate postoperative period or years later. LE occurs when the lymph load (volume) exceeds the lymph transport capacity, thus causing impaired lymphatic function (Lerner, 2000; Smoot, Wampler, & Topp, 2009). It can cause discomfort, swelling, and a decrease in function and may affect QOL.

Two types of LE exist: primary and secondary. Primary LE is caused by a failure in the lymphatic system itself, and secondary LE is caused by a known insult to the lymphatic system, such as removal of lymph nodes or radiation therapy for the treatment of cancer (Browse, Burnard, & Mortimer, 2003; Casley-Smith & Casley-Smith, 1997). See Figure 9-1 for an example of a patient experiencing LE following breast surgery.

Unfortunately, no accepted definition of clinically significant LE exists, so an actual report of the incidence is hard to identify. Therefore, there is confusion as to the percentage of people with LE following breast cancer surgeries (Koul et al., 2007). Stanton, Levick, and Mortimer (1996) suggested that the percentage of women who develop LE following full ALND varies from 8% to 63%. Two studies reported a LE rate of 3%–3.5% in women after SLN procedures in the first two years following surgery (Sener et al., 2001; Swenson et al., 2002). Sener et al. (2001) determined that ipsilateral upper-extremity LE was more common when tumors were located in the upper outer quadrant of the breast, regardless of the type of surgery. No follow-up studies have been reported on this cohort of patients. In a 30-month study, Armer, Stewart, and Shook (2009) found that, after breast cancer surgery, 41% of the women they studied reported heaviness and swelling and 45% had a 10% lymph volume increase.

The two main functions of the lymphatic system are drainage and transport (Földi, M., & Földi, E., 2006; Weissleder & Schuchhardt, 2001). The lymphatics are responsible for transporting proteins and large particulate matter away from the tissue spaces, as neither of these substances can be removed by absorption directly into the blood capillaries (Guyton, 1997). The lymphatic system relies on active and passive muscle contractions, arterial pulsation, respiration, and lymphangions, valve segments within the lymph collectors, to transport fluid (Földi, M., & Földi, E., 2006). A Starling's law equilibrium is responsible for the creation of lymph fluid (Casley-Smith &

| Table 9-1. Complications of Breast Cancer Surgery and Nursing Interventions | | | |
|---|---|---|---|
| **Complication** | **Symptoms** | **Nursing Interventions** | **Refer for Treatment** |
| Pain (breast, axilla, chest wall, upper arm) | Scar tightness<br>Incision tenderness<br>Soreness<br>Muscle spasms | Application of heat or ice<br>Resting arm on pillow<br>Limiting movement<br>Distraction<br>Relaxation<br>Guided imagery<br>Nonsteroidal anti-inflammatory drugs (NSAIDs) or acetaminophen<br>Obtain order for narcotic analgesics. | Pain that is not well controlled with conservative measures and disrupts activities of daily living |
| Numbness and dysesthesias | Twinges<br>Tingling<br>Pins and needles<br>Burning<br>Stabbing | Keeping soft clothing close to skin<br>Avoiding heavy prosthesis<br>Application of ice<br>NSAIDs or acetaminophen<br>Obtain order for topical anesthetics.<br>Obtain order for oral antidepressants or anticonvulsants. | Pain that is not controlled by conservative measures and disrupts activities of daily living<br>Any signs of motor nerve injury (muscle weakness) |
| Range-of-motion (ROM) limitations | Stiffness<br>Pain with arm, shoulder, elbow, or wrist movement<br>Cording<br>Pulling sensation | Evaluate for preexisting ROM difficulties and refer for evaluation early.<br>Instruct patients in proper technique of postoperative exercise.<br>Advise patients to take a warm shower before doing exercises.<br>Advise patients to take pain medication 30–45 minutes before performing exercises.<br>Remind patients to continue exercises during radiation therapy. | Limitation of ROM that predated surgery<br>Limitation of ROM that persists beyond 4–6 weeks postoperatively<br>Worsening of pain with ROM exercises despite conservative measures |
| Lymphedema (LE) | Feeling of heaviness, fullness, or aching in operative limb<br>Swelling in hand, arm, chest wall, breast, or posterior trunk on side of surgery<br>Increase in arm circumference or volumetric measurements | Identify patients at higher risk for LE development (higher body mass index, tumor in upper outer quadrant, axillary lymph node dissection).<br>Educate patients on risk reduction strategies before and after surgery.<br>Measure both arms preoperatively in order to make postoperative comparisons.<br>Encourage exercise in the postoperative period.<br>Assess all areas at risk for signs of infection. | Any signs of swelling in at-risk areas or increase in arm measurements |

*Note.* Based on information from Alem & Gurgel, 2008; Armer et al., 2003; Cheville & Gergich, 2004; Fassoulaki et al., 2000; Lacomba et al., 2009; National Comprehensive Cancer Network, 2010a; National Lymphedema Network Medical Advisory Committee, 2008a.

Casley-Smith, 1997; Földi, M., & Földi, E., 2006; Simon & Cody, 1992). As Simon and Cody (1992) explained, "Under normal physiologic conditions, tissue fluid is in balance with outflow from the arterial side of the capillary bed, inflow on the venous side, and lymph drainage removing excess fluids and protein" (p. 545). In essence, when homeostasis becomes disrupted, LE may occur as a result of a "mechanical failure" in the lymph.

LE can be measured circumferentially (through the use of a tape measure), volumetrically (by water displacement or calculated through circumference measures), or by weight. An example of a therapist performing a circumferential arm measurement is shown in Figure 9-2. However, no agreed-upon quantitative definition currently is available for LE following breast cancer surgery (Browse et al., 2003; Stanton et al., 1996). As a result, no universally accepted measure exists that would articulate at what level of increase in circumference or at what increase in volume a diagnosis of LE is warranted. Most physicians use a range scale and rely on patient symptoms to make a diagnosis. Symptoms may include fullness, tightness, loss of mobility, or heaviness (Kelly, 2002). These symptoms and sensations may be experienced in any at-risk area, which include the ipsilateral upper extremity, the chest wall (including but not limited to the breast), and the

## Figure 9-1. Secondary Lymphedema Following Mastectomy With Axillary Dissection

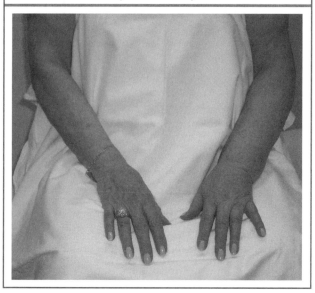

## Figure 9-2. Measurement of Lymphedema

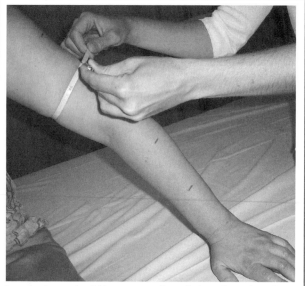

Lymphedema should be measured regularly and consistently to assess the effectiveness of therapy.

should consist of skin care, manual lymphatic drainage (sometimes called manual lymphatic treatment), compression bandaging, compression garments, and possibly a compression pump (Casley-Smith & Casley-Smith, 1997). For treatment of LE, the National Lymphedema Network (NLN) position statement recommends that a therapist meet a minimum of 135 hours of CDT coursework from one LE training program to provide care (NLN Medical Advisory Committee, 2005). This recommendation is also consistent with the Lymphology Association of North America (LANA) standards, which allow a person to take the LANA national examination after completing the aforementioned requirements and one year of training (LANA, 2005). CDT should be administered by a therapist (i.e., occupational therapist, physical therapist, massage therapist, RN) who specializes in LE. LANA (2005) has developed a national certifying examination for competency standards in LE therapy. Lymphologists, physicians who specialize in the treatment of LE, are not numerous in the United States. As a result, the physician referring the patient for treatment is frequently the primary care physician or oncologist, thus making the skill level of the therapist critical.

Skin care is an essential component of LE care. The skin should be screened for incidental lesions and breaks in skin integrity (Cheville & Gergich, 2004). The body has a more difficult time clearing bacteria in lymphedematous tissue, and therefore the risk of developing a localized infection is greater (Muscari, 2004). A study performed by Simon and Cody (1992) demonstrated that cellulitis was more likely to occur in the first year after surgery in women who underwent lumpectomy with radiation, and that women who underwent more radical surgical procedures, generally without radiation, had cellulitis after a longer time frame. Individuals with re-

| Table 9-2. International Society of Lymphology Lymphedema Staging | |
|---|---|
| Lymphedema Stage | Definition |
| 0 | Latent or subclinical condition where swelling is not evident despite impaired lymph transport |
| 1 | Early accumulation of fluid relatively high in protein content, which subsides with limb elevation (pitting may occur) |
| 2 | May or may not pit as tissue fibrosis supervenes |
| 3 | Lymphostatic elephantiasis where pitting is absent and trophic skin changes such as acanthosis, fat deposits, and warty overgrowths develop |

*Note.* Based on information from International Society of Lymphology, 2003.

upper back quadrant. It is important that the assessment for LE includes all of these areas. The International Society of Lymphology (2003) developed consensus guidelines with a new staging schema for LE (see Table 9-2).

Once LE is suspected, the patient should be evaluated by an experienced physician and LE therapist. If LE is identified, a treatment protocol including complete decongestive therapy (CDT), also known as complex physical therapy or complete decongestive physiotherapy, can be developed. Treatment peated cellulitis may require prophylactic antibiotic therapy (Feldman, 2005).

Manual lymphatic drainage "is a massage technique that stimulates lymph vessels to contract more frequently and to channel lymphatic fluid towards adjacent, functioning lymph systems" (Ko, Lerner, Klose, & Cosimi, 1998, p. 454). Specific gentle movements begin on the contralateral quadrant of the body, working from proximal to distal yet always directing the fluid proximally (Browse et al., 2003). Ideally, the therapist performs this treatment daily and then teaches the patient the technique as a home program.

Compression bandaging consists of many layers (i.e., protective stockinet, padding, elastic bandage) (Asmussen & Strössenreuther, 2006; Browse et al., 2003; Casley-Smith & Casley-Smith, 1997). The bandages used are low-stretch elastic that have a low resting pressure and high working pressure placed in a gradient manner (more pressure distally than proximally) (Casley-Smith & Casley-Smith, 1997). An example of LE bandaging can be seen in Figure 9-3. It is important to note that use of an Ace® (Becton, Dickinson and Co.) wrap bandage is **contraindicated** for patients with LE.

A patient with LE should wear a compression bandage throughout therapy until measures have stabilized. The individual's circumferential and volumetric measurements should steadily decrease and then remain fairly constant. At this point, the individual should be fitted for a compression garment. Afterward, the individual will use the compression bandage as a source of reduction and the compression garment as a form of maintenance. Patients are instructed to wear the garment continuously during the day and remove the garment at night (Casley-Smith & Casley-Smith, 1997). Garments

should be checked every six months for proper fit (Weissleder & Schuchhardt, 2001). Studies by Ko et al. (1998) and Boris, Weindorf, and Lasinski (1997) showed that patients demonstrated a significantly increased rate of maintenance and decreased LE because of the use of CDT. Figure 9-4 shows a patient who has been fitted with a compression sleeve and detachable gauntlet.

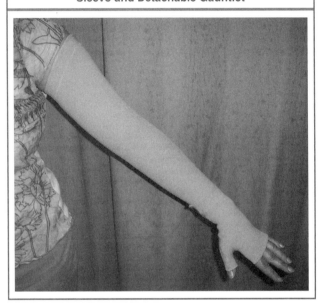

**Figure 9-4. Example of Patient Wearing a Compression Sleeve and Detachable Gauntlet**

The use of compression pumps for LE therapy remains controversial (Casley-Smith, Casley-Smith, Lasinski, & Boris, 1996). However, the use of compression pumps may be applicable for "the patient who cannot or will not tolerate LE bandaging, for the patient with minimal fibrotic changes to subcutaneous tissues, and the patient who cannot come for daily treatment" (Kelly, 2002, p. 103). No official indications for pump therapy exist. A major concern regarding compression pumps is the inability to move fluid beyond the extremity itself. A new pump that compresses the abdominal region along with the affected extremity may have some effect if used along with CDT, but more studies need to be completed to validate its effectiveness.

No medications are currently approved in the United States to treat LE. Surgical procedures have never shown a durable response and are rarely attempted, except for the treatment of persistent pain as described in the Becker et al. (2008) article discussed earlier.

LE may occur immediately or many years after a person completes treatment for breast cancer. Therefore, the patient could initially present with LE to a nurse, a physician, or a therapist. The limb and trunk area that is at risk should be inspected at each visit. Inspection should include color, warmth, tex-

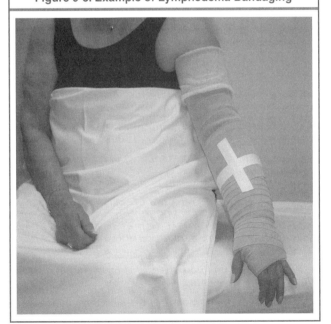

**Figure 9-3. Example of Lymphedema Bandaging**

ture, and skin changes such as injuries and scars. Simple circumferential measurements using a tape measure also should be taken and compared with the unaffected extremity (Marrs, 2007). Most commonly, a difference of 2 cm between the two extremities is used as a defining factor of whether a person should be sent for evaluation or therapy (Muscari, 2004). If LE is suspected, then referral should be made to a physician or a certified LE therapist.

Research has shown that some symptoms may be predictors of LE related to breast cancer (Armer, Radina, Porock, & Culbertson, 2003). These prodromal symptoms include heaviness, swelling, and numbness. Early identification of patients experiencing these symptoms may enable healthcare professionals to target women who may benefit from early referral for LE evaluation and review of precautions and to establish the criteria for the use of compression garments.

It is important to educate women about the risk of LE and how to potentially decrease the risk of developing it. The literature does not report a direct correlation between education and either a reduction in LE development or a delay in onset. Anecdotal case reports have driven the development of most of the guidelines for risk reduction. It is assumed that risk is decreased if an individual avoids triggers that can further decrease the lymph vessels' transport capacity or unnecessarily increase the fluid and protein load of the lymphatic system in the affected region (Kelly, 2002). The NLN Medical Advisory Committee (2008c) has published a concise list of triggers in *Lymphedema Risk Reduction Practices*. Triggers include trauma to the skin, infection, sunburn, weight gain, intense upper-body activities, limb constriction, ill-fitting compression garments, and temperature extremes (e.g., saunas, hot tubs). A complete copy of this position statement is available on the NLN Web site at www.lymphnet.org/pdfDocs/nlnriskreduction .pdf. Table 9-3 summarizes LE triggers, pathophysiology, and risk-reduction strategies.

Exercise is important for an individual with or at risk for LE. Exercise produces muscle contraction, which is believed to increase the pressure in the interstitium, increase uptake of initial lymphatics, promote muscle strengthening, and mobilize the joints (Browse et al., 2003; Casley-Smith & Casley-Smith, 1997; Kelly, 2002; NLN Medical Advisory Committee, 2008b; Strössenreuther, 2006). Discussions regarding the kind of exercise one engages in and resulting decreases or increases in the risk of developing LE have taken place. Researchers have conducted studies to determine whether isometric exercise, exercises following drainage pathways, or simply any exercise that an individual performs has a higher impact over another in preventing or prolonging the onset of LE. An article in the *New England Journal of Medicine* (Schmitz et al., 2009) described a weight-lifting study titled Physical Activity and Lymphedema. This report initiated a flurry of opinions on exercise and LE. The lead investigator, Kathryn Schmitz, wrote an article to clarify

| Table 9-3. Lymphedema Triggers, Pathophysiology, and Risk-Reduction Examples | | |
|---|---|---|
| **Trigger** | **Pathophysiologic Basis** | **Risk Reduction** |
| Air travel | Pressure may decrease in cabin, changing interstitial pressures in the body (National Lymphedema Network [NLN] Medical Advisory Committee, 2008a). | Wear a form of compression while traveling. (External pressure may decrease potential of fluid accumulation in tissue.) |
| Constriction | Constriction may slow or stop lymphatic flow (Kelly, 2002). | Avoid wearing tight-fitting clothing (e.g., bra straps/bands). Avoid taking blood pressure readings on arm at risk. |
| Cuts/scrapes to at-risk area | Bacteria may enter through cracks, causing a cellulitic infection (Cheville & Gergich, 2004; Kelly, 2002; Okhuma, 1990; Simon & Cody, 1992). | Wear gloves while washing dishes or gardening. Keep skin pliable and well lubricated. Avoid needle punctures on area at risk. |
| Exercise | More lymph fluid may be produced secondary to (a) increased pulse leading to increased arterial blood flow and (b) overuse syndrome (NLN Medical Advisory Committee, 2008b). | Wear a form of compression while exercising, and monitor for signs of edema. |

any misconceptions that may have been created by the media hype (Schmitz, 2010). The exercises performed in this study, specifically weight lifting, were done in a controlled environment in which the participants wore a well-fitted compression garment throughout the exercise and the day, only removing it for stretches and showering (Schmitz, 2010). The NLN position statement on exercise suggests that a person with LE wear compression bandages or garments while exercising. However, its position on a person "at risk" for LE has changed. The NLN's position for at-risk individuals is that it *may* be helpful to wear a compression garment, but it may not be necessary (NLN Medical Advisory Committee, 2008b). The introduction of any exercise, including weight training, must be done slowly, with the patient monitoring the at-risk area before, during, and after exercise.

The NLN Medical Advisory Committee (2008a) recommends that people *with* LE wear a compression garment or compression bandages while traveling by air. Patients are advised to don the compression garment or bandage prior to the flight and remove it once the final destination is reached.

People at risk for LE must make a decision about sleeve use with the guidance of their physician. The rationale for compression during airplane travel is that changes in cabin pressure can affect the interstitial pressures in the limb, causing increased swelling (NLN Medical Advisory Committee, 2008a). External pressure (i.e., compression) on the limb may decrease the potential of fluid accumulation in the tissue. The lack of activity (i.e., walking) while on an airplane lends itself to edema development because muscles pump less to propel the fluid than when ambulatory. Therefore, people with or at risk for LE are encouraged to ambulate or perform frequent, simple upper-extremity ROM exercises while on an airplane (NLN Medical Advisory Committee, 2008a). Additionally, patients need to keep in mind that traveling usually involves carrying or pulling luggage—recognized triggers for LE development. Although no research is documented to support this recommendation, patients should consider what precautions to take based on the length and mode (i.e., car, train, or bus) of travel.

The risk of infection is another consideration with LE. As explained by Simon and Cody (1992), "Lymphatic impairment favors development of infection due to impaired host response, and the stagnated lymph fluid provides an ideal medium for bacterial growth" (p. 546). The surgery decreases the number of lymph nodes, reducing function and creating stasis of fluid, which increases the risk for infection (Smoot et al., 2009). *Cellulitis*, *erysipelas*, and *dermatolymphangioadenitis* are terms often used synonymously for a lymphatic infection (Földi, E., & Földi, M., 2006). Most breast and arm infections are caused by *Staphylococcus aureus*, penicillin-sensitive *Streptococcus*, or fungus (Chikly, 2001). Symptoms include redness, warmth, fever, chills, generalized malaise, pain, and edema (Browse et al., 2003; Casley-Smith & Casley-Smith, 1997). Treatment of infection consists of rest, elevation of the affected limb, and oral or IV antibiotics. In some cases, prophylactic antibiotics are prescribed for patients with recurrent infections (Browse et al., 2003). CDT can decrease the incidence of infection in women who currently have LE (Browse et al., 2003; Casley-Smith & Casley-Smith, 1997; Földi, E., & Földi, M., 2006).

Although LE is not life threatening, it does pose a substantial threat to QOL for breast cancer survivors. It can affect the person's relationships with family and friends, ability to perform activities of daily living, and body image and self-esteem (Armer et al., 2003). Even an updated review of the current literature demonstrates a continued need for research to better understand the true incidence, prevalence, and severity of LE, whether preventive interventions are valid, and whether less-invasive lymph node sampling will result in long-term decreases in LE development. Moreover, although much has been learned about LE, work on the development of a quantification system to produce comparable data is still sorely needed.

## Radiation Skin Changes

The majority of patients with breast cancer receiving radiation therapy will develop some skin and tissue toxicity. Skin damage is caused by the effect of radiation on the rapidly dividing cells of the basal layer of the epidermis and the dermis (Williams et al., 1996). Sekine et al. (2000) suggested that sweat gland damage also might play a role. The intensity of side effects depends on the fractionation, total dose, anatomic area, radiation type, and patient characteristics (Perera, Chisela, Stitt, Engel, & Venkatesan, 2005; Póti et al., 2004; Whelan et al., 2010). Treatment delays may be required for severe skin reactions. Acute skin reactions can occur during radiation treatment and for as long as six months after therapy. Newer radiation techniques treating smaller volumes of tissue with different doses and fractionations recently have gained favor (Baglan et al., 2003; Whelan et al., 2010), and long-term data regarding side effects with these newer techniques are just starting to be reported. Most follow-up studies are 2–10 years post-therapy.

Conventional breast cancer radiotherapy involves the use of external beam whole-breast radiation using a linear accelerator with daily fractions over the course of five to six weeks, with or without skin bolus or boost. More recently, whole-breast hypofractionated and accelerated partial-breast irradiation treatments (interstitial and intracavitary brachytherapy, intraoperative, intensity-modulated radiation therapy) have come into vogue. In addition, the use of three-dimensional conformal radiation techniques and those using intensity-modulated radiation therapy (or IMRT) have been developed with the intention of delivering a more accurate and homogeneous dose throughout the breast and minimizing acute and late toxicity (Pignol et al., 2008).

The most commonly identified acute radiation skin changes are erythema, increased pigmentation, pruritus, dry desquamation (peeling), and moist desquamation. Other symptoms include breast heaviness, mild discomfort, and shooting pains. The degree of skin toxicity is variable and is related to concurrent chemotherapy, concurrent tamoxifen use, larger breast size, smoking history, body mass index (BMI), boost or bolus skin fields, treatment of the chest wall, and African American ancestry (Deutsch & Flickinger, 2003; Heggie et al., 2002; Okumura et al., 2003; Pignol et al., 2008; Wells et al., 2004). Supraclavicular fields can result in skin reactions on the upper back along with the anterior chest. Transient erythema can occur with the first treatment. More intense erythema and hyperpigmentation generally occur after two to three weeks of treatment (Knobf & Sun, 2005). Destruction of the basal layer of the skin can result in dry desquamation. Higher doses of radiation can cause moist desquamation characterized by a bright erythema, clear serous exudate, and pain, which usually occurs toward the end of the longer treatment courses. Skin folds within the treatment field (axilla and inframammary crease) are at greater risk for developing skin toxicity because of the movement of skin on skin, warmth, and moisture buildup with development of moist desquamation (Pignol et al., 2008).

The most commonly cited radiation-related breast symptoms reported in a prospective longitudinal study of external beam radiation therapy by Knobf and Sun (2005) were skin changes in 36%–100% of patients, sensation changes in 28%–79%, and breast swelling in 11%–28%. Severity ratings were mild to moderate but were higher by the end of the treatment, with gradual improvement over the following three months. One hundred percent of the patients developed skin changes by week 5 or 6. The ratings of symptom severity were higher in the final three weeks of treatment yet still rated as mild. Skin irritation was described as red, itchy, and sensitive. However, the sensation of heaviness persisted over the next three months. Studies by Pignol et al. (2008) and Wengström, Häggmark, Strander, and Forsberg (2000) have reported similar findings. The Pignol study was done via a multicenter, double-blind, randomized fashion and found that the use of intensity-modulated radiation therapy reduced the incidence of moist desquamation compared with standard whole-breast radiation.

Skin care recommendations vary and are based on individual practice patterns rather than empirically based in centers. A review of radiation skin care studies (Bieck & Phillips, 2010; McQuestion, 2006) provides overviews on washing techniques, use of lotions and potions, trolamine (Biafine®, Ortho Dermatologics), hyaluronic acid cream, corticosteroids, sucralfate, barrier films, antimicrobials, and hydrophilic and silver dressings. Only the use of *Calendula officinalis* with trolamine (Pommier et al., 2004), hyaluronic cream (Liguori, Guillemin, Pesce, Mirimanoff, & Bernier, 1997), and Cavilon™ no-sting barrier film (3M Health Care) (Graham et al., 2004) showed positive effects. Several randomized clinical trials involving patients with breast cancer found trends favoring the use of sucralfate (Maiche, Isokangas, & Gröhn, 1994) and mometasone furoate (Boström, Lindman, Swartling, Berne, & Bergh, 2001) in preventing radiation skin effects. Aloe vera was found to have a protective effect when higher doses of radiation were used (Olsen et al., 2001). Tegaderm™ (3M Health Care) and Vigilon® (C.R. Bard, Inc.) wound dressings and Biafine topical emulsions were found to promote patient comfort (Fisher et al., 2000; Strunk & Maher, 1993). Masferrer et al. (2010) found that intensive use of a lotion containing urea, polidocanol, and hyaluronic acid prevented the development of radiodermatitis of grade 2 or higher based on standard toxicity scales. Heggie et al. (2002) showed that an aqueous cream of aloe vera was useful in reducing dry desquamation and pain. Enomoto et al. (2005) showed that the use of RayGel™ (ITI Wellness), a combination of glutathione and anthocyanins, promoted patient comfort and protection compared with standard skin care therapies. The Oncology Nursing Society (ONS) Putting Evidence Into Practice (PEP) resource on radiodermatitis by Baney et al. (2011) rated calendula, hyaluronic acid, and sodium hyal-

uronate as skin care products that were likely to be effective in the prevention of radiation skin changes. Use of aloe vera, anionic polar phospholipid cream, dexpanthenol (Bepanthen), chamomile cream, almond ointment, glutathione, anthocyanin, Lipiderm® (International Veterinary Sciences), sodium sucrose octasulfate, steroids, sucralfate, theta cream, topical vitamin C, urea lotions, XClair™ (Align Pharmaceuticals), honey, hydrocolloid dressings, proteolytic enzymes, red wine, and zinc were categorized as treatments whose effectiveness had not been established. Baney et al. (2011) also listed trolamine and Biafine® (Ortho Dermatologics) as products unlikely to be effective based on their review of the literature.

Table 9-4 lists commonly recommended self-care strategies to promote skin integrity during radiation therapy. Many recommendations remain based on anecdotal information and the radiotherapist's preference. In an attempt to standardize radiation skin care practices in British Columbia, Nystedt et al. (2005) described their difficulties in this process. A study by Théberge, Harel, and Dagnault (2009) showed that no evidence existed to prohibit the use of deodorant (except for the use of aluminum-containing products) during radiation therapy for breast cancer.

**Table 9-4. Skin Care Instructions for Patients Undergoing Breast Irradiation**

| Precautions | Skin Care |
|---|---|
| Avoid temperature extremes in the treatment field. | Do not use hot water bottles, hot soaks, heating pads, or ice packs in the area of treatment.<br>Do not expose treatment field to cold wind or intense sunlight. Skin in the area will remain sun-sensitive for years to come.<br>Do not take cold or hot baths or use a sauna during treatment. Lukewarm water is preferred. |
| Avoid trauma to the skin in the treatment field. | Gentle washing of the skin with a mild soap and water is allowed.<br>Do not scrub the skin. Pat skin dry.<br>Use mild soap, and avoid rubbing off any skin markings (tattoos).<br>Wear soft, loose, cotton clothing.<br>Do not scratch or rub skin in the treatment area.<br>Do not shave in the treatment area. Hair loss may be permanent. |
| Avoid application of topical agents to skin in the treatment field. | Do not apply powder, deodorant, perfume, or lotions to the treatment area.<br>Cornstarch may be used to control itching.<br>Use only radiation therapy–approved lotions or creams. Apply two hours prior to treatment. |

*Note.* Based on information from McQuestion, 2010; National Cancer Institute, 2007.

Breast edema, mild hyperpigmentation, fibrosis, and telangiectasia are some of the late side effects following breast irradiation as seen in a number of small, single-institution studies using a variety of dose schedules (Perera et al., 2005; Póti et al., 2004; Vicini et al., 2007). Acute skin reactions predict the incidence of skin pigmentation and telangiectasia. They are related to boost doses and higher skin doses (Perera et al., 2005). Edema and fibrosis incidence peaked at three years after treatment with three-dimensional conformal external beam radiation with accelerated partial-breast irradiation in the Vicini et al. (2007) study. Severe fibrosis, seen in a small number of patients, is related to older age, clinical tumor size, surgical complications, use of chemotherapy, and high boost dose and may result in patient dissatisfaction with cosmetic outcome in the more common standard external beam therapy (Borger et al., 1994; Taylor et al., 1995). Breast edema is more commonly seen in women with ALND. Breast erythema in an edematous breast following radiation must be viewed as a possible infection, and inflammatory breast cancer recurrence must be included in the differential diagnosis. However, a syndrome of lymphangitis or cellulitis of the breast following breast-conserving therapy has been recognized (Indelicato et al., 2006). In addition, the phenomenon of radiation recall—namely, erythema of the skin in the treatment field—can occur with the administration of chemotherapy at a later time. Fat necrosis was found to occur in the short term with patients undergoing multicatheter interstitial brachytherapy in a small institutional study by Kaufman, DiPetrillo, Price, Midle, and Wazer (2007) and developed in some subjects after five years of follow-up. However, most patients in the study (89%) felt that cosmesis, including skin toxicity, improved over time.

A retrospective review of patients' subjective evaluation of early and late sequelae (described as after six months) of treatment with short fractionation radiation (44 Gy in 16 fractions over 22 days) with breast conservation found that compared to whole-breast regular fractionation (50 Gy in 25 fractions over 35 days), the shorter course resulted in more breast hardness (Inomata et al., 2008). However, no difference in acute side effects (erythema, heat sensation, discomfort) was reported. The location of the tumor in the breast and the volume of tissue removed at surgery may also affect reported cosmetic outcomes (Reeder et al., 2009).

Patient education regarding the expected side effects of breast irradiation can promote comfort, reduce the severity of reactions, and allay anxiety. Reinforcement that acute skin reactions will heal is extremely important for patients experiencing moist desquamation. Long-term cosmetic changes are more difficult to predict and generally are not modifiable by the patient and type of skin care used. As radiation therapy techniques evolve, cutaneous and cosmetic outcomes may become more or less apparent. Patients should be aware of late changes that they should report to their healthcare provider, namely breast erythema, breast swelling, and changes noticed during self-examination. Prompt evaluation can al-leviate patient concerns or enable timely treatment of infection, LE, and potential ipsilateral breast cancer recurrences.

## Chemotherapy-Induced Nausea and Vomiting

Despite medical advances in the treatment of chemotherapy-induced nausea and vomiting (CINV), they continue to be a concern for women undergoing moderately and highly emetic chemotherapy for breast cancer (Schnell, 2003). CINV can lead to poor QOL, electrolyte imbalances, dehydration, poor nutrition, and diminished ability to work. Patient factors such as prior nausea and vomiting during pregnancy, history of motion sickness, and lack of exposure to alcohol often affect the development of CINV. In addition, uncontrolled CINV can lead to some patients withdrawing from further therapy (Wickham, 2004), thereby compromising their care.

The most commonly used drugs to treat breast cancer in the adjuvant setting are a combination of two or more of the following medications: cyclophosphamide, methotrexate, 5-fluorouracil, paclitaxel, docetaxel, doxorubicin, epirubicin, and the monoclonal antibody trastuzumab. Cyclophosphamide, methotrexate, 5-fluorouracil, and doxorubicin are considered moderately emetic at the doses commonly used to treat breast cancer. Moderately emetic chemotherapy is defined as chemotherapy that produces vomiting in 30%–60% of patients who do not receive effective nausea and vomiting treatment (NCCN, 2011). Doxorubicin or epirubicin in combination with cyclophosphamide is considered highly emetic, whereby at least 90% of patients will develop CINV without treatment (NCCN, 2011).

Patients frequently use the terms *queasiness*, *upset stomach*, and *throwing up* to describe their symptoms. CINV can be categorized as anticipatory, acute, delayed, refractory, or breakthrough (see Table 9-5). Each process seems to be caused by different mechanisms, as drugs designed to manage acute CINV are not as effective in managing the other types of CINV. The primary mediators of acute nausea and vomiting result from direct or indirect stimulation of the chemoreceptor trigger zone and vomiting center, or emetic zone. Olfactory, emotional, and peripheral stimuli from the gastrointestinal tract also can affect the development of nausea and trigger emesis. Key brain and gastrointestinal receptors involved in this process are serotonin (5-HT$_3$), dopamine, and neurokinin (NK-1) (Bender et al., 2002). However, a final common pathway has yet to be identified, so no single agent can be expected to provide complete control. Other conditions that can cause nausea in the breast cancer population include concurrent use of opiates or antibiotics, constipation, hypercalcemia, progressive disease, brain metastasis, hyperglycemia, hyponatremia, vestibular dysfunction, and renal or hepatic failure (NCCN, 2011).

Patient-related risk factors for CINV include female gender; history of vomiting with prior exposure to chemotherapy;

## Table 9-5. Definitions of Chemotherapy-Induced Nausea and Vomiting

| Type | Definition |
| --- | --- |
| Anticipatory | Occurs days before the administration of chemotherapy and is likely a conditioned response; more common in patients who had poorly controlled chemotherapy-induced nausea and vomiting. Nausea is more common than vomiting. |
| Acute | Occurs within the first minutes to first 24 hours after drug administration; peak incidence of vomiting at 5–6 hours after dose |
| Delayed | Occurs 24 hours after chemotherapy, peaking at 48–72 hours after administration; can last as long as 6–7 days |
| Breakthrough | Emesis that is unresponsive to medication and may require the addition of less commonly used or higher-level antiemetics to control symptoms |
| Refractory | Emesis that occurs during subsequent treatment cycles having failed prophylactic and rescue medications |

*Note.* Based on information from Eckert, 2001; National Comprehensive Cancer Network, 2011.

poor performance status; emetogenicity of the drugs; younger age; preexisting fatigue; low level of social functioning; low alcohol consumption; and a history of anxiety, motion sickness, or nausea and vomiting during pregnancy (Dibble, Israel, Nussey, Casey, & Luce, 2003). Studies by Roscoe et al. (2004) and Booth et al. (2007) have shown that patient expectations of nausea are a strong predictor of subsequent nausea but not emesis. However, this observation is not documented as a risk factor in antiemetic guidelines or taken into account when prescribing medications. An interesting finding by Dibble et al. (2003) was that women with a higher BMI had worse CINV than their smaller counterparts. This may be associated with a potential underdosing of antiemetics. African American women also seem to be at greater risk, suggesting genetic differences in drug metabolism.

Acute nausea and acute emesis in patients undergoing moderately emetic chemotherapy for breast cancer continue to be problematic as illustrated in studies by Dibble, Casey, Nussey, Israel, and Luce (2004) and Grunberg et al. (2004). The prevalence of delayed nausea was high as well. Since then, the addition of aprepitant, an NK-1 receptor antagonist, to treatment guidelines has led to improvements in the management of both acute and delayed nausea and vomiting, but there is still room for improvement (Booth et al., 2007; Grunberg et al., 2004; Herrstedt et al., 2005; Warr et al., 2005). Other commonly used and frequently effective 5-HT$_3$ antagonists include ondansetron, granisetron, palonosetron, and dolasetron. The

NCCN consensus panel recently revised its decision tree to assist clinicians in CINV management. It is available online at www.nccn.org/professionals/physician_gls/PDF/antiemesis.pdf (NCCN, 2011).

Most chemotherapy protocols for breast cancer use highly and moderately emetic drugs given in combination. Practitioners must be cognizant that the risk for emesis with these protocols extends for at least four days and should prescribe antiemetics accordingly. If nausea or vomiting occurs after the first cycle of chemotherapy, a change in the antiemetic protocol is recommended. For breakthrough nausea, a change in 5-HT$_3$ receptor antagonist is suggested, with the addition of one of the following medications in a scheduled rather than PRN basis: prochlorperazine, metoclopramide with or without diphenhydramine, lorazepam, haloperidol, dronabinol, dexamethasone, promethazine, nabilone, or olanzapine. For patients who develop indigestion during treatment, the addition of antacids (H$_2$ blockers and proton pump inhibitors) can be helpful (NCCN, 2011). Booth et al. (2007) showed a lower incidence of severe CINV (less than 10%) when the evidence-based antiemetic protocols were strictly followed and preemptive pretreatment patient education was given. They noted, however, a 70% incidence of delayed nausea. Clearly, more work still needs to be done in this area of symptom management.

According to experts, as many as 1 in 3 patients undergoing chemotherapy experiences anticipatory nausea, and 1 in 10 has anticipatory emesis. This is thought to be a conditioned response. Sensory stimuli associated with chemotherapy administration are the triggers. After repeated exposures, any associated stimuli can elicit the symptoms (King, 1997). The most significant risk factors for anticipatory emesis appear to be the occurrence, magnitude, and duration of previously experienced CINV. Treatment for patients who develop anticipatory emesis includes behavioral therapy and medications. Nonpharmacologic interventions under study include acupuncture, foot massage, progressive muscle relaxation, acupressure, and music therapy. Eckert (2001) and Bender et al. (2002) provide a thorough overview of these techniques. Most of these interventions, however, are based on pilot studies with small sample sizes. Behavioral interventions can assist patients in gaining a sense of control over their symptoms, are easy to use, and can be self-administered. A recent randomized clinical trial of 160 women undergoing breast cancer chemotherapy showed that the use of acupressure at the P6 point was a value-added technique when used in conjunction with guideline-recommended antiemetics over a 10-day period following chemotherapy (Dibble et al., 2007). Of interest, this prolonged follow-up of symptoms after chemotherapy found that 30% of patients continued to have nausea at post-treatment day 11. Antianxiety medications taken the night prior to the following chemotherapy cycle and on the morning of treatment also may be useful in reducing CINV. Some practitioners also start antinausea medications prior to chemotherapy in an attempt to avert anticipatory nausea (NCCN, 2011).

As another intervention strategy to counteract nausea, patients often are encouraged to use dietary measures that they found helpful during pregnancy, illness, or stressful periods. Altering food preparation and freezing meals for later can help to avoid exposure to strong odors during cooking at times of heightened sensitivity. Other helpful hints include eating smaller, more frequent meals; keeping the mouth clean and moist; eating cold or room-temperature foods, which give off fewer odors than hot foods; eating sour foods; eating crackers, breadsticks, and toast; sitting up while eating; and sucking on hard candies, such as peppermints or lemon drops. Most clinicians recommend that patients avoid their favorite foods on the day of chemotherapy administration and during periods of potential nausea so that they do not develop food aversions. Other foods to avoid include fatty foods, which delay gastric emptying, and spicy, salty, and sweet foods (Wickham, 2004). Herbal teas such as peppermint, cinnamon, or chamomile may help to soothe dyspepsia, as well as lessen nausea and vomiting (Deng, Cassileth, & Yeung, 2004). Booth et al. (2007) found that eating a small meal the day of chemotherapy administration actually minimized the occurrence of nausea. A recent abstract presented at the American Society of Clinical Oncology (ASCO) conference reported on a phase II/III randomized, placebo-controlled, double-blind trial that assessed the efficacy of ginger for the prevention or treatment of CINV (Ryan et al., 2009). A total of 644 patients with breast, alimentary, and lung cancer (90% female) were randomized to different doses of ginger or placebo given in conjunction with standard antiemetic therapy. All doses of ginger significantly reduced nausea with a linear decrease over 24 hours, with the largest reduction in nausea occurring in those who were given 0.5–1 g of ginger twice daily for six days starting three days before the first day of the next two cycles after having experienced nausea with their first cycle.

A less commonly advocated strategy to control nausea in patients undergoing chemotherapy for breast cancer is exercise. Lee, Dodd, Dibble, and Abrams (2008) found that moderate levels of exercise during treatment were related to less intense nausea at the completion of adjuvant therapy in patients who exercised compared to controls. Participants were considered to be exercisers if their actual exercise corresponded to a minimum of moderate-intensity exercise 20 minutes per session three times a week. Exercise as simple as a 2–10 minute walk is an inexpensive and effective way to help patients manage a variety of treatment-related symptoms, including nausea. See Figure 9-5 for an overview of nonpharmacologic and complementary measures to prevent or lessen CINV. The ONS PEP resource on chemotherapy-induced nausea and vomiting (Friend et al., 2009) listed interventions for nausea and vomiting that are supported by adequate empirical evidence to include benzodiazepines,

---

**Figure 9-5. Nonpharmacologic and Complementary Strategies to Manage Chemotherapy-Induced Nausea and Vomiting in Breast Cancer Survivors**

**Dietary**
- Alter food preparation techniques.
- Reduce food aromas and other stimuli with strong odors.
- Avoid greasy, spicy, and overly sweet foods.
- Drink herbal teas (peppermint, cinnamon, chamomile).
- Eat a small meal on the day of treatment.
- Eat small, frequent meals on nontreatment days.
- Keep mouth moist and clean.
- Eat foods cold or at room temperature.
- Eat crackers, bread, or rice to settle stomach.
- Suck on sugar-free hard candies (peppermint, lemon).
- Avoid favorite foods on the day of treatment.
- Take a ginger supplement.

**Complementary**
- Acupuncture
- Foot massage
- Progressive muscle relaxation
- Music therapy
- Daily moderate exercise

*Note.* Based on information from Booth et al., 2007; Deng et al., 2004; Dibble et al., 2007; Lee et al., 2008; Polovich et al., 2009; Ryan et al., 2009; Wickham, 2004.

---

5-$HT_3$ receptor antagonists, NK1 receptor antagonists, corticosteroids, metoclopramide, phenothiazine, butyrophenones, cannabinoids, olanzapine, promethazine, acupuncture, acupressure, guided imagery, music therapy, and progressive muscle relaxation (for anticipatory nausea). At the time of the review, hypnosis, acustimulation with wristband device, Chinese herbal medicine, ginger, massage therapy, yoga, and hypnosis were not found to have established efficacy.

In the present era of cost containment, the use of expensive antiemetics as first-line therapy has been slow to gain acceptance. In addition, insurance coverage of outpatient oral medications remains variable. Letters of medical necessity may be needed to petition insurance carriers to authorize their use. Patients with limited financial means should be assisted in accessing a variety of pharmaceutical and philanthropic organizations for financial assistance. Because of the profound impact of CINV on the QOL of patients with breast cancer, research into more gender-effective antiemetics, complementary and behavioral adjunct measures, and chemoprotective agents must continue. Patients should be encouraged to report distressing symptoms to their healthcare providers so that effective treatment can be planned. Healthcare providers must be aware of the significant impact that unrecognized delayed nausea and vomiting has on their patients and act proactively.

## Cancer-Related Fatigue

The definition of cancer-related fatigue (CRF) is "a distressing persistent, subjective sense of physical, emotional and/or cognitive tiredness or exhaustion related to cancer or cancer treatment that is not proportional to recent activity and interferes with usual functioning" (NCCN, 2010d, p. FT-1). CRF is different from fatigue in healthy individuals and adversely affects the QOL of cancer survivors (Curt et al., 2000). It is less likely to be relieved by rest. CRF is one of the most distressing symptoms experienced by patients with cancer. Furthermore, 21%–75% of cancer survivors studied reported experiencing fatigue months to years after the end of treatment (Bower et al., 2006; Gélinas & Fillion, 2004; Jacobsen et al., 2007).

The cause of CRF is multifactorial and has physical, psychological, and situational elements (Curt et al., 2000). It has been associated with insomnia, sleep disturbances, hot flashes, and pain, suggesting a symptom cluster effect. A study by Beck, Dudley, and Barsevick (2005) showed that relieving pain was an important strategy in improving sleep and reducing fatigue. A longitudinal study by Von Ah, Kang, and Carpenter (2008) showed that mood disturbance was the most significant predictor of CRF in a sample of 44 postsurgical patients. Also, interleukin-1 beta predicted CRF levels before adjuvant therapy, and morning cortisol levels before adjuvant therapy predicted CRF during and after adjuvant therapy (Von Ah et al., 2008). A longitudinal study by Nieboer et al. (2005) found that joint and muscle pain and poor mental health were more commonly associated with fatigue over time. The study by Bower et al. (2006) showed that predictors of fatigue included depression, cardiovascular problems, and the type of treatments received in their sample of 763 long-term survivors at 5–10 years after diagnosis. So et al. (2009) evaluated the impact of the symptom cluster of fatigue, pain, anxiety, and depression on the QOL of women receiving treatment for breast cancer in China and found significant correlations. Woo, Dibble, Piper, Keating, and Weiss (1998) reported that the younger the woman with breast cancer, the more likely she was to perceive cancer stressors in her life, and the more fatigued she was, the less likely she was to use active coping skills. A study by Winters-Stone, Bennett, Nail, and Schwartz (2008) identified that older breast cancer survivors' fatigue was linked to lower physical activity and muscle strength, suggesting that exercise may be protective in older cancer survivors. Clearly, the cause of CRF is multifactorial and, as such, may be difficult to treat with one standardized approach. Therefore, patients should be screened for multiple symptoms that may vary according to the patient's type of treatment and stage of disease.

Trends toward the use of regimens with higher doses and dose densities in patients receiving breast cancer chemotherapy may result in an increased incidence of CRF. A study by Wu, Dodd, and Cho (2008) showed worse fatigue in women undergoing treatment with doxorubicin and cyclophospha-mide regimens compared to other regimens. Berger, Lockhart, and Agrawal (2009) found that fatigue was a common problem associated with lower QOL in all types of chemotherapy treatment regimens and that patterns of fatigue did not change based on the type of regimens used. They did note, however, that taxane-containing regimens were more associated with what they termed *physical fatigue*. They suggested that patients with lower physical functioning prior to starting taxane chemotherapy might benefit from an early exercise intervention. Fatigue also is a commonly reported and distressing side effect of radiation therapy (Knobf & Sun, 2005; Magnan & Mood, 2003). Figure 9-6 summarizes potential contributing factors for fatigue in breast cancer survivors.

The NCCN (2010d) guidelines for the screening, assessment, and management of CRF can be accessed online at www.nccn.org. The consensus guidelines recommend that all patients with cancer be screened for CRF at their initial oncology visit and at regular intervals thereafter. Although many sophisticated assessment tools exist, most clinicians assess fatigue by using a 0–10 scale or by allowing patients to categorize their fatigue as mild, moderate, or severe. If mild fatigue is identified at the initial visit, it should be monitored for an increase in severity at follow-up visits. This assessment also provides a teachable moment to educate patients about fatigue patterns during and after treatment. This approach prevents patients from assuming that increasing fatigue indicates disease progression. Patients experiencing fatigue at a level of 4 or greater should receive a more detailed assessment, including a history and physical examination evaluating whether disease progression or recurrence is a factor. More detailed questioning about the frequency and duration of fatigue; when it is noted; whether it affects the patient's ability to perform

---

**Figure 9-6. Potential Contributing Factors to Fatigue in Breast Cancer Survivors**

- Pretreatment and ongoing sleep disturbances
- Persistent pain
- Sedentary lifestyle with little daytime activity
- Nutritional deficiencies (iron, vitamin $B_1$, $B_6$, $B_{12}$)
- Electrolyte imbalances (calcium, magnesium, phosphate)
- Cancer treatment (surgery, radiation, chemotherapy)
- Menopausal symptoms that affect sleep (joint pain, vasomotor symptoms)
- Stress
- Medical conditions (anemia, electrolyte imbalances, hypothyroidism, adrenal insufficiency, hypogonadism)
- Comorbidities (heart disease, pulmonary disease, hepatic and renal dysfunction)
- Psychological distress (anxiety, depression)
- Medication side effects (narcotics, anxiolytics, antiemetics, antidepressants)
- Caffeine withdrawal

*Note.* Based on information from Berger et al., 2003; Mock & Olsen, 2003; Nail, 2002; National Comprehensive Cancer Network, 2010d.

activities of daily living, mood, or relationships with other people; what makes it better; and determining whether other symptoms contribute to it, such as nausea, pain, sleep disturbance, difficulty moving around, and shortness of breath, also can assist the nurse in making treatment recommendations. Having this information at hand will enable the nurse to better communicate with the advanced practice nurse or the oncologist to treat or mitigate these concerns (Mitchell, 2009; Mota & Pimenta, 2006).

Monitoring of laboratory values to detect anemia, electrolyte imbalances, or nutritional deficiencies also is critical. Additional clinical conditions that can contribute to CRF include comorbidities such as heart disease and hypothyroidism. If fatigue remains unrelieved after implementing interventions directed at these conditions, a more detailed medical workup by the patient's physician or advanced practice nurse should be pursued (Berger et al., 2003; Mock & Olsen, 2003; Nail, 2002; NCCN, 2010d).

Magnan and Mood (2003) found that women who experienced CRF while undergoing traditional five- to six-week radiation therapy developed it during the second week of treatment, and it worsened by the fifth week. Earlier onset may occur because of preexisting treatment such as recent surgery or chemotherapy, lower hemoglobin levels, and symptom and mood distress. Most studies of radiation therapy for breast cancer have found a return to baseline level by three months after treatment. Gélinas and Fillion (2004) found that in a group of women who had completed radiation therapy 3–24 months prior to the study, menopausal symptoms, pain, and stress were related to persistent fatigue.

Self-care interventions that might be useful for women experiencing CRF include practicing energy conservation, pacing activities, requesting help with household tasks, getting daily exercise, using distraction, taking short naps, eating balanced meals, receiving massage therapy, delegating activities, and managing stress (Barsevick, Whitmer, Sweeney, & Nail, 2002; NCCN, 2010d). Dietary counseling also may be useful if nutritional deficiencies are contributory. Patients should be provided with a list of these self-care strategies at the initiation of treatment to enable greater control of their symptoms and assist in planning activities.

Of all the coping strategies, exercise appears to be the most credible and validated (Ahlberg, Ekman, Gaston-Johansson, & Mock, 2003; Stricker, Drake, Hoyer, & Mock, 2004). It is important for patients to know how to balance rest and activity to prevent deconditioning. Mock et al. (2001) evaluated the effectiveness of a walking program in adult patients with breast cancer undergoing radiation treatment or chemotherapy and found that women experienced lower levels of fatigue, increased ability to perform daily tasks, less psychological distress, and greater QOL while participating in the exercise intervention. This walking program was 20–30 minutes in length, occurred five to six times a week, and was moderately intensive, causing an increase in resting heart rate.

A study by Payne, Held, Thorpe, and Shaw (2008) substantiated the use of a prescribed home-based walking intervention in older breast cancer survivors on hormonal therapy to reduce the incidence of fatigue, sleep disturbances, and depressive symptoms. Overall, recent studies have shown that moderate-intensity, individualized exercise programs can reduce fatigue during and after cancer treatment (Schneider, Hsieh, Sprod, Carter, & Hayward, 2007; Wu et al., 2008). A randomized controlled trial of 87 women treated for breast cancer in Quebec by Fillion et al. (2008) showed greater improvements in fatigue, energy level, and emotional distress at a three-month follow-up in women who underwent an exercise and mood intervention compared with controls, suggesting that this type of combined approach may be beneficial. Hanna, Avila, Meteer, Nicholas, and Kaminsky (2008) found that a comprehensive exercise program consisting of low- to moderate-intensity aerobic, resistance exercise education and support, twice a week for eight weeks, resulted in significant improvements in physical functioning, fatigue, and mood in patients undergoing active cancer treatment (one-third of the participants were breast cancer survivors). Headley, Ownby, and John (2004) reported that even seated exercise was effective in reducing fatigue in women with advanced breast cancer.

For exercise to be a successful intervention, barriers to its use must be identified (see Figure 9-7). Huberty et al. (2009) developed an instrument to measure adherence to strength training in postmenopausal breast cancer survivors who had experienced bone loss after treatment for breast cancer. They found that barriers to exercising included not prioritizing time for oneself and less self-efficacy. Having an exercise partner and having a breast cancer role model were positively correlated with physical activity in this group. Healthcare providers must educate patients about the importance of exercise. Providing a prescription for moderate exercise with explicit instructions regarding limitations that might be necessary is a simple way to provide motivation (Mustian et al., 2009).

---

**Figure 9-7. Potential Barriers to Exercise as an Intervention for Fatigue**

- Not prioritizing time for oneself
- Having less self-efficacy (feel one can make a difference)
- Being unaware of the benefits of exercise on management of cancer-related fatigue
- Lack of social support and encouragement to exercise
- Not being confident in one's ability to exercise safely or not being aware of what exercises would be beneficial
- Lack of access to a fitness center
- Perception of exercise as being boring
- Lack of an exercise partner
- Side effects from treatment

*Note.* Based on information from Huberty et al., 2009; Mustian et al., 2009; Rogers et al., 2005.

Referral to a qualified exercise specialist may be beneficial. The American College of Sports Medicine (ACSM) and ACS have recently partnered to establish a credentialing program for cancer exercise specialists. Local certified cancer exercise trainers can be located through the ACSM Web site at http://forms.acsm.org/_frm/crt/online_locator.asp. The current exercise literature provides consistent support for the efficacy of exercise interventions in managing cancer-related symptoms and improving QOL. Small sample sizes of studies and lack of consistency in the type, amounts, and intensity of exercise regimens make it difficult to generalize recommendations but does give the healthcare community incentive to encourage patients to move. Moderately intensive exercise can include activities such as walking, resistance training, aerobic exercise, biking, and swimming, as well as mindfulness-based exercise, such as Tai Chi and yoga.

A study comparing breast cancer survivors to healthy controls found that CRF had a significant effect on QOL and mood, and some evidence showed that fatigue was related to sleep disturbance (Alexander, Minton, Andrews, & Stone, 2009). A study by Palesh et al. (2010) documented that those breast cancer survivors with insomnia (n = 362) had significantly more depression and fatigue. A randomized controlled trial of cognitive-behavioral therapy for insomnia in breast cancer survivors by Espie et al. (2008), which included stimulus control, sleep restriction, and cognitive therapy strategies, was able to reduce wakefulness per night, and the outcome was sustained for six months following treatment. The patients noted positive effects on complaints of difficulty initiating sleep and waking from sleep during the night and for sleep efficiency (percentage of time in bed spent asleep). Wielgus, Berger, and Hertzog (2009) showed that one predictor of fatigue 30 days after completing doxorubicin plus taxane therapy was less total sleep time prior to treatment and that a sleep intervention that began at treatment initiation combined with physical activity resulted in less fatigue. This suggests that identifying individuals with fatigue and poorer sleep quality at the onset of therapy and applying appropriate interventions can reduce subsequent CRF.

Behavioral therapy interventions in a study by Berger, Kuhn, et al. (2009) were shown to improve sleep quality in patients one year after the first intervention and following all phases of cancer therapy. However, by one year after the intervention, fatigue levels were mild in both the intervention and control groups, suggesting that most patients have a diminution or resolution of fatigue in the months following treatment. Berger's (2009) updated review of the state of science on sleep-wake disturbances in adults with cancer discusses the various limitations of studies but promotes continued evaluation of the use of cognitive-behavioral interventions, exercise, education on sleep hygiene, and relaxation therapies in the management of CRF.

The most common cause of CRF is anemia. It can occur as a result of bone marrow suppression from treatment, poor dietary intake, or disease progression. The symptoms of mild anemia can easily go unrecognized. However, symptoms of severe anemia, such as shortness of breath, weakness, tachycardia, and decreased exercise and activity tolerance, generally are easier to recognize. Options in the management of anemia-related CRF include erythropoiesis-stimulating agents (epoetin alfa, darbepoetin alfa) or transfusion, depending on how rapidly a correction is needed. Several randomized clinical trials have shown a benefit in QOL and functional status with this type of drug therapy (Boccia et al., 2006; Cella, Dobrez, & Glaspy, 2003; Waltzman et al., 2005). However, increased mortality, thrombotic events, and disease progression seen in patients with cancer treated with erythropoiesis-stimulating agents has led to a recommendation that their use should be limited to patients with cancer **not** being treated with curative intent (NCCN, 2010c).

Other medications that may help to relieve fatigue include thyroid replacement hormone for women with hypothyroidism, iron supplementation for those experiencing iron-deficiency anemia, vitamin therapy ($B_{12}$) for patients experiencing deficiency, psychostimulants (i.e., modafinil, dexmethylphenidate), corticosteroids, and antidepressants (NCCN, 2010d). A randomized, double-blind, placebo-controlled, parallel-group study evaluating the potential therapeutic effect and safety of dexmethylphenidate for the treatment of CRF found significant improvement in those treated with an individualized dosing schedule. However, use of this drug caused a higher rate of study withdrawal because of side effects, which included headache, nausea, and dry mouth (Lower et al., 2009). A pilot study using modafinil in 82 breast cancer survivors with prolonged fatigue found that 83% experienced a reduction in their fatigue (Morrow, Ryan, & Kohli, 2006). Figure 9-8 lists some of the pharmacologic interventions for the treatment of fatigue in people with breast cancer. The ONS PEP resource on fatigue (Mitchell, Beck, Hood, Moore, & Tanner, 2009) identified exercise as a proven intervention and listed the following interventions as likely to be effective: screening for other etiologies that may factor into fatigue, energy conservation with activity management, provision of education and infor-

---

### Figure 9-8. Pharmacologic Treatments for Fatigue in Select Breast Cancer Survivors

- Thyroid hormone replacement for people with hypothyroidism
- Iron (for people with iron-deficiency anemia)
- $B_{12}$ injections or vitamin B supplements (for patients who are deficient in these vitamins)
- Psychostimulants (modafinil, dexmethylphenidate)
- Corticosteroids
- Antidepressants (for people with depression)
- Erythropoiesis-stimulating agents* (for people with anemia)
- Transfusions (for people with anemia)

*Currently used only in those patients receiving palliative treatment

*Note.* Based on information from Lower et al., 2009; Morrow et al., 2006; National Comprehensive Cancer Network, 2010d.

mation, measures to optimize sleep quality, relaxation, massage, healing touch therapy, polarity therapy, and haptotherapy, the latter three of which are not discussed in this chapter.

Persistent CRF at the completion of breast cancer treatment has a negative impact on patients' return to normal functioning, especially given the variety of roles women play in society. Healthcare providers should focus on instituting prompt interventions when fatigue is noted regardless of whether it occurs before, during, or after therapy. Early communication to patients and their significant others that CRF may occur is essential to enable them to prepare for alterations in family equilibrium. Survivors should be advised that fatigue may continue months to years after treatment and does not necessarily mean that their cancer has recurred.

## Cognitive Dysfunction

The incidence of cognitive dysfunction (CD), often described as "chemo brain" or "chemo fog," by women who are undergoing breast cancer treatment is variable, ranging from 16% to 83% (Jenkins et al., 2006; Tannock, Ahles, Ganz, & van Dam, 2004). Some patients also refer to it as mental fatigue or cloudiness. CD is a multidimensional concept. Defects following chemotherapy have been observed up to 10 years after treatment (Ahles et al., 2002), yet most studies find these cognitive effects to be transitory following completion of chemotherapy, particularly by one year after treatment (Collins, Mackenzie, Stewart, Bielajew, & Verma, 2009; Schagen et al., 2002). A study by Wefel, Lenzi, Theriault, Davis, and Meyers (2004) found that 61% of patients with breast cancer experienced a change in cognitive functioning. Yamada, Denburg, Beglinger, and Schultz (2010) found that the 30 breast cancer survivors enrolled in their study who were older than age 65 and had received chemotherapy in mid-life continued to score significantly lower in the cognitive domains of executive functioning, working memory, and divided attention compared to healthy controls, suggesting a potential augmentation of treatment-related CD on age-related cognitive changes. Of note, many women demonstrate impaired cognitive functioning before the initiation of adjuvant chemotherapy, thus making a baseline assessment imperative (Wefel, Lenzi, Theriault, Buzdar, et al., 2004). It cannot be overemphasized, however, that changes in cognitive functioning also may be related to other cancer-related conditions (brain metastasis, anemia, electrolyte imbalances, brain radiotherapy), other comorbidities (dementia, Alzheimer disease), medication use (pain, antianxiety, and antiemetic medications), and other symptom clusters (pain, fatigue, sleep disturbance, depression, anxiety). These conditions should be ruled out as potential causes in this high-risk population (Wagner, 2010).

CD adversely affects patients' QOL and may reduce their ability to transition back into a "normal" life after treatment. A study by Von Ah, Russell, Storniolo, and Carpenter (2009)

found that in a group of 134 breast cancer survivors with a mean of 6.4 years since diagnosis, self-reported CD, particularly inability to direct attention, was negatively related to psychological and physical well-being, resulting in more depression and fatigue. The changes seen are subtle and cross a variety of cognitive domains (Bender, Paraska, Sereika, Ryan, & Berga, 2001; Jim et al., 2009; Quesnel, Savard, & Ivers, 2009). Symptoms often reported include deficits in attention; difficulty in comprehension or understanding; inability to follow instruction; being easily distracted; slower processing of information; difficulty with numbers and financing (e.g., balancing checkbook); difficulty with dates, details, and names; gait and dexterity disturbances; inability to recognize familiar objects; inability to perform multiple concurrent tasks; and complaints of increasing memory difficulties, behavioral changes, and socially inappropriate behavior (Jansen, Miaskowski, Dodd, Dowling, & Kramer, 2005). An in-depth qualitative study of a breast cancer survivor focus group (consisting of both Caucasian and African American women) reported that most participants asserted that changes in their cognitive functioning was their most troublesome post-treatment symptom affecting their ability to function effectively at work (Boykoff, Moieni, & Subramanian, 2009).

The assessment of CD in breast cancer survivors is limited by the lack of consistent evaluation tools, the length of many of the currently available assessment tools, and lack of the patient commitment required to complete testing, thereby discouraging patient evaluation. A thorough review article by Jansen, Miaskowski, Dodd, and Dowling (2005) describes the types of testing needed to assess the various cognitive functioning domains. Most of the current neuropsychological tests do not seem sensitive enough to detect the subtle changes that women report. To address this issue, the Functional Assessment of Cancer Therapy–Cognitive scale was developed to allow for a self-report measure that evaluates mental acuity, attention and concentration, memory, verbal fluency, functional interference, deficits observed by others, change from previous function, and impact on QOL (Rugo & Ahles, 2003; Tannock et al., 2004).

The causes of cancer treatment–related CD have yet to be fully identified. It is hypothesized that direct injury to the cerebral gray and white matter occurs with adjuvant chemotherapy, that microvascular injury may occur, and that immune-mediated inflammatory responses may predispose some patients to develop CD (Inagaki et al., 2006; Saykin, Ahles, & McDonald, 2003). Persistent brain changes compared to controls have been documented 5–10 years after chemotherapy. An additional risk factor for CD may be a genetic predisposition caused by a variant of the apolipoprotein E gene, which has been associated with an increased risk of early Alzheimer disease and preclinical cognitive decline (Ahles et al., 2003).

Comparison of the research studies documenting the incidence of CD in patients with breast cancer has been limited because of differences in the assessment tools, definitions of dysfunction, types of chemotherapy agents used, menopausal status, and frequency of evaluation; the use of cross-sectional design; and the lack of baseline assessments in some studies. A review of studies on CD in patients receiving chemotherapy showed a trend toward greater dysfunction when compared to controls (Phillips & Bernhard, 2003). However, a study of 187 patients found that patients who received chemotherapy with radiation and those who received radiation alone experienced cognitive deficits six months after diagnosis, suggesting that subtle cognitive deficits may be due to the general effects of a cancer diagnosis rather than systemic treatment (Jim et al., 2009).

Longitudinal studies have shown that the dose and type of chemotherapy may influence cognitive impairment, showing a worse effect in higher-dose protocols (van Dam et al., 1998) and in regimens that include cyclophosphamide compared to doxorubicin (Schagen et al., 2002). No data are currently available on the role of taxanes in the development of CD (Rugo & Ahles, 2003). Concurrent medications such as steroids and analgesics during treatment may have an additive effect (Shilling, Jenkins, Morris, Deutsch, & Bloomfield, 2005). Wefel, Lenzi, Theriault, Davis, et al. (2004) found that women who had more invasive surgery, were menopausal, and had not previously used hormone replacement therapy appeared to be more likely to present with greater cognitive impairment. Age, IQ, and pretest levels of CD must be taken into consideration. Normal age-related changes at the beginning of chemotherapy may cause older patients to have less capacity to overcome the cognitive effects of chemotherapy. Most studies have shown an associated increase in levels of fatigue and endocrine symptoms in patients experiencing CD. Patients who indicated that they were experiencing cognitive problems were more likely to have emotional distress related to their symptoms than women who were found to have limitations noted on sequential evaluation only (Shilling et al., 2005).

More recently, researchers have begun to study the influence of breast cancer hormonal therapy on the development of CD. Recent studies of women receiving hormonal therapy with tamoxifen and aromatase inhibitors showed variable effects on cognitive functioning when compared with age-matched controls. A longitudinal study of 101 patients who were given a battery of tests at baseline, toward the end of neoadjuvant therapy, and one year after baseline showed no adverse effects on CD in patients receiving tamoxifen or aromatase inhibitors. However, the authors admit that the time the patients were on these agents was likely too short to best assess the development of impairment effects (Hermelink et al., 2008). A multinational study by Schilder et al. (2010) was performed on postmenopausal breast cancer survivors who did not receive chemotherapy but were treated with either tamoxifen or exemestane. The researchers found that after one year of therapy, verbal memory, executive functioning, and information processing speed were worse in the tamoxifen users than the exemestane users and matched controls. The addition of tamoxifen to chemotherapy regimens showed a worsening of CD in a study by Castellon et al. (2004). In a study by Collins et al. (2009), both tamoxifen and anastrozole (Arimidex®, AstraZeneca Pharmaceuticals) were found to exert subtle negative cognitive effects in postmenopausal patients compared with controls. Patients must be advised about the potential for cognitive changes while on these medications.

The lack of solitary causal mechanisms and the variability in the cognitive domains affected have hampered treatment for CD. A longitudinal study of patients with anemia associated with chemotherapy administration showed increases in fatigue and CD in control subjects. Those patients who received epoetin alfa prior to the beginning of chemotherapy and weekly thereafter were found to experience fewer changes in hemoglobin levels, improved energy levels, improved overall QOL, and less deterioration in cognitive function than controls (Shilling et al., 2005). However, no difference in cognitive function was noted among patients at six months after completion of chemotherapy. Epoetin alfa is believed to have neuroprotective effects (O'Shaughnessy et al., 2005; Shilling et al., 2005), but its use is currently limited in the adjuvant treatment setting because of concerns about long-term safety effects as noted earlier.

A study of raloxifene for osteoporosis prevention found a trend toward lower declines in verbal memory and attention in the women taking it as a secondary end point of a study in healthy women. This finding may hold promise for patients with breast cancer in the future (Yaffe et al., 2001), as raloxifene is now included as a chemoprevention option for women at high risk for breast cancer development. However, its use should be discouraged in women who have received or are currently receiving breast cancer hormonal therapy, specifically tamoxifen and aromatase inhibitors, as part of their treatment. In the QOL portion of the randomized trial comparing letrozole to megestrol acetate in women with advanced breast cancer, patients taking letrozole experienced improvement in subjective cognitive function (Weinfurt, Wait, Boyko, & Schulman, 1998).

The only medications currently being explored for the treatment of persistent CD are methylphenidate and modafinil. A randomized, placebo-controlled trial by Mar Fan et al. (2008) did not show any benefit of methylphenidate in preventing CD in women undergoing adjuvant chemotherapy for breast cancer. However, on secondary analysis, a randomized clinical trial by Kohli et al. (2009) found a benefit of modafinil on cognitive function in breast cancer survivors. It was postulated that the drug enhanced memory and attention skills.

Interventions to assist patients in overcoming CD continue to be explored. A central tenet of cognitive-behavioral therapy is that how people think affects how they feel (Wagner, 2010). As such, symptom reframing may be helpful. Barton and Loprinzi (2002) outlined two interventional approaches that include behavioral and pharmacologic interventions for chemotherapy-induced cognitive changes. Ferguson and Ahles

(2003) formulated an intervention that involved stress management techniques for long-term survivors of breast cancer who continued to experience CD. Self-care strategies that often are recommended to improve memory include avoiding distraction, asking people to repeat information, practicing activities like crossword puzzles, writing down events in daily organizers, keeping a journal, posting reminders, managing stress, getting enough sleep, exercising regularly, maintaining routines, and using mnemonic devices (Mulrooney, 2008; Wagner, 2010). Cancer*Care* has developed two guides to help patients manage the effects of CD: "Combating Chemobrain: Keeping Your Memory Sharp" and "Improving Your Concentration: Three Key Steps," both of which can be downloaded free of charge at www.cancercare.org/pdf/fact_sheets/fs_chemobrain_memory.pdf and www.cancercare.org/pdf/fact_sheets/fs_chemobrain_concentration.pdf, respectively. Table 9-6 summarizes these strategies.

Recently, researchers have begun to explore the utility of exercise interventions in the treatment of CD. Hsieh et al. (2008) found that a supervised individualized exercise program resulted in improved fatigue and mood, as well as cognitive functioning, in all patients who underwent multimodal therapy. Once again, the benefits of exercise for breast cancer survivors cannot be overlooked. A recent exploration of the literature rating the effectiveness of the previously discussed interventions for cognitive impairment performed by Allen et al. (2011) reported that none demonstrate strong enough evidence to be recommended for routine practice.

Some researchers are studying brain function in breast cancer survivors at baseline and during chemotherapy to assess changes that might explain CD using magnetic resonance imaging and positron-emission tomography scanning changes (Saykin et al., 2003). Other researchers are working to develop easier assessment tools to identify patients who are at risk, as

| Table 9-6. Self-Care Strategies for the Management of Cognitive Changes in Breast Cancer Survivors | |
| --- | --- |
| **Overall Strategies** | **Examples** |
| Do not multitask. | Make lists of things to do. Prioritize tasks. Concentrate on one task at a time. Minimize distractions. Tune out thoughts on other tasks. Stay present and focused. If off track, stop and refocus. Guide yourself verbally through a task. |
| Use compensatory tools. | Keep a memory notebook and write down everything you feel is important to remember. Keep these notes in a central place so they are easy to retrieve. Use a daily planner and keep it with you at all times. Write in appointments immediately. Use a wall calendar at home to keep track of family activities. Create a daily routine and stick to it. Pace yourself. Prepare for tomorrow the night before. Review your calendar at the beginning, middle, and end of the day. Rehearse an activity or task you have to remember—visualize where you put something, verbally rehearse information you need to remember, use notes as a cue. Use memory tricks such as word associations, rhyming, or grouping numbers to help remember important details. Always bring someone else with you to remember important details. Request to tape record important conversations. Leave yourself a voice message or send yourself an e-mail reminder to do something. Use a timer so you do not lose track of time. Minimize distractions; use earplugs if you are in a noisy environment, or close the door to your office. Repeat information that you must remember out loud to help you remember details. Enlist your family or friends in helping you remember important steps or events. Proofread your work before submitting. |
| Organize your environment. | Keep your desk and workspace uncluttered. "A place for everything, and everything in its place" is a good motto to adopt. Have a central message place where you and the rest of your family can keep track of daily activities and upcoming appointments. Use a time-of-day pill box to facilitate taking medications properly. |

*(Continued on next page)*

**Table 9-6. Self-Care Strategies for the Management of Cognitive Changes in Breast Cancer Survivors** *(Continued)*

| Overall Strategies | Examples |
|---|---|
| Exercise your brain. | Continue to learn—take a class of interest to you.<br>Read a book that requires some concentration.<br>Balance your checkbook.<br>Join a book club.<br>Do crossword puzzles, word games, or Sudoku.<br>Play computer games that have been designed to build memory.<br>Play games that require you to strategize.<br>Keep your mind active. |
| Improve your concentration | Use a pencil or highlighter to emphasize important points.<br>Divide tasks into manageable parts.<br>Plan breaks according to your concentration span.<br>Take quick stretching breaks to reorient yourself to your task at hand.<br>Determine what time of day is your best time for concentration, and maximize your use of this time for important tasks.<br>Figure out what environment or conditions enable you to get your best work done.<br>Play soothing music that can calm you.<br>De-stress by exercising, doing yoga, or meditating. |

*Note.* Based on information from CancerCare, 2008a, 2008b; Mitchell, 2009; Mulrooney, 2008.

well as those with worsening symptoms, with the goal of discovering ways to prevent and treat cognitive changes. Ferguson et al. (2007) developed a Memory and Attention Adaptation Training (MAAT) program. MAAT is a cognitive-behavioral treatment aimed at helping patients to manage CD. The researchers found some success in their pilot study. The tool is lengthy and requires prolonged patient commitment. Clearly, further research is advised.

Even without compelling evidence to explain the causes of or effective interventions for cognitive changes after cancer treatment, healthcare providers must prepare women and their families for the potential development of CD so that adjustments to their lives can be anticipated. Special precautions may be needed for people with preexisting CD. Nurses should be certain to repeat self-care instructions and provide written home care instructions to assure that proper self-care is maintained. Because of the association of CD with other symptom clusters, assessment and treatment of concurrent issues is critical (Barsevick, 2007).

## Menopausal Effects of Breast Cancer Treatment

Management of estrogen deficiency states in breast cancer survivors is complicated by concerns related to the use of hormone replacement therapy to counteract the two most prevalent hormone-related side effects of adjuvant therapy— hot flashes (or hot flushes) and bone loss. Although other menopausal symptoms such as weight gain, vaginal dryness, sexual dysfunction, sleep disturbances, and depres-

sion are also of clinical importance, they will not be discussed in this chapter.

## Hot Flashes

Hot flashes, or vasomotor symptoms, are problematic in breast cancer survivors because many women are diagnosed around the time of natural menopause, and acute menopause may result from treatment. Hot flashes have been defined as sudden episodes of flushing, sweating, and a sensation of heat often preceded or followed by chills (Kronenberg, 1990) and are estimated to occur in 65% of breast cancer survivors (Carpenter et al., 1998; Couzi, Helzlsouer, & Fetting, 1995).

The physiology of hot flashes (or flushes) is associated with reduced hormone levels that are believed to affect the thermoregulatory system of the body, resulting in the sensation of heat (Stearns & Hayes, 2002). In addition, the expanding indications for the use of chemotherapy, increased use of antiestrogen agents, and acceptance of prophylactic oophorectomy in *BRCA1* and *BRCA2* gene mutation carriers have resulted in more breast cancer survivors being at risk for menopausal symptom development. Other risk factors found to have an impact on hot flashes in healthy women include smoking, higher BMI, lack of exercise, African American ancestry, and lower socioeconomic status (Avis et al., 2001; Whiteman et al., 2003). A cross-sectional study of postmenopausal women taking an aromatase inhibitor showed that women who had gained more than 10 pounds since their breast cancer diagnosis were two times more likely to experience hot flashes than those who had maintained or lost weight (Su et al., 2010). In a longitudinal study by Savard, Savard, Quesnel, and Ivers

(2009) to evaluate the severity of hot flashes in women treated with chemotherapy or radiation therapy, chemotherapy and hormonal therapy were both associated with increased severity of hot flashes. In this group, past use of hormone replacement therapy and lower BMI were associated with more severe hot flashes. How women adapt to menopausal symptoms is influenced by their level of uncertainty about the symptoms, the severity of the symptoms, the degree to which symptoms interfere with daily activities, and their preparation with information on what to expect (Knobf, 2002). Studies evaluating the incidence and severity of hot flashes in women undergoing a natural menopause compared to women undergoing menopause as a result of cancer therapy have shown worse symptomatology in the breast cancer survivors (Benshushan et al., 2009; Mar Fan et al., 2009).

Hot flashes have become recognized as a frequent, severe, and bothersome side effect among survivors (Carpenter, Johnson, Wagner, & Andrykowski, 2002). Women who discontinue hormone replacement therapy at the time of diagnosis are more likely to experience hot flashes if they had them in the past or were having them at the time of discontinuation of therapy. The effects of chemotherapy on the ovaries vary depending on the patient's age and the dose and type of chemotherapy or hormonal therapy. Younger women are better able to tolerate higher doses of chemotherapy and are less likely to undergo permanent menopause. However, younger premenopausal women have more hot flashes during endocrine therapy than older postmenopausal women and also may experience more distress related to this and other menopausal symptoms related to the earliness and abruptness of their menopause (Ganz, Greendale, Petersen, Kahn, & Bower, 2003; Knobf, 2002). Nonadherence to endocrine therapy has been reported to range from 25% to 55%, with the development of adverse effects being the primary reason for noncompliance (Cella & Fallowfield, 2008). Clearly, management of symptoms must be a priority to promote patient compliance with the use of these lifesaving medications.

Carpenter et al. (2002) compared healthy controls to breast cancer survivors and found that survivors experienced greater hot flash severity and bother and had more daily hot flashes with a longer duration of symptoms compared to healthy controls. Emotional factors were more commonly noted in breast cancer survivors, and hot flashes caused greater interference with daily activities and QOL—affecting sleep, concentration, mood, and sexuality. They found that compared to healthy women, the breast cancer survivors had a significantly different menopause experience than the natural menopause experience. Recent studies of women taking tamoxifen have indicated that the experience of hot flashes may have a predictive value in documenting drug effectiveness, but they caution that it should not be used as the only evidence (Henry et al., 2009). A similar outcome evaluating the onset of vasomotor and joint symptoms of women participating in the ATAC (Arimidex, Tamoxifen, Alone or in Combination) tri-

al indicated that the presence of these symptoms within the first three months of therapy was associated with a greater response and reduced risk for breast cancer recurrence (Cuzick, Sestak, Cella, & Fallowfield, 2008). The results of an open-label, prospective, crossover study of 184 postmenopausal women experiencing intolerant hot flashes on adjuvant tamoxifen showed that switching to an aromatase inhibitor resulted in an improvement in their QOL (Thomas, Williams, Marshall, & Walker, 2008), suggesting this may be an acceptable alternative in similar breast cancer survivors.

According to Carpenter et al. (2002), the most common self-care behaviors used by breast cancer survivors to ameliorate hot flashes were fanning, removing clothing, and moving to a cooler environment. In addition, exercise, vitamin therapy, and diet often are used to ameliorate symptoms, although these interventions lack empirical evidence supporting their use. Treatment should match the severity of the symptoms reported by the patient.

Mild to moderate hot flashes that do not seem to interfere with the patient's sleep patterns or ability to work can be managed with behavioral and nonprescription methods. Vitamin E 400–800 IU was tested in a randomized, placebo-controlled clinical trial and was found to decrease hot flash frequency and severity by 30% without toxicity (Barton et al., 1998). In a study comparing the efficacy of vitamin E to gabapentin, vitamin E demonstrated a marginal impact on vasomotor symptoms (Biglia et al., 2009). In addition, taking measures to keep cool may be useful, such as dressing in cotton layers, using fans, or drinking cold drinks. Avoidance of potential triggers, such as alcohol and spicy foods, also may be helpful. Stress management using paced respiration and relaxation techniques also has been shown to be beneficial (Carpenter et al., 2002). Yoga, acupuncture, and hypnosis for the treatment of hot flashes in breast cancer survivors have recently shown benefit, particularly in women undergoing hormonal therapy for their cancer (Carson, Carson, Porter, Keefe, & Seewaldt, 2009; Hervik & Mjåland, 2009; Wyon, Wijma, Nedstrand, & Hammar, 2004). The limitations of these studies include their small size and lack of reliable or placebo control groups. Elkins et al. (2008) found that in a randomized trial of 60 female breast cancer survivors, using a hypnosis intervention for treatment of hot flashes resulted in a 68% decrease in hot flash scores (frequency × average severity) from baseline to end point in the hypnosis arm. They also found that self-reported anxiety, depression, and interference of hot flashes on daily activities and sleep were improved compared to those in the control group, lending credence to the addition of hypnosis to the options available for women who experience breast cancer treatment–related hot flashes. Self-paced respirations and relaxation have shown some promise as effective interventions for hot flashes in small group studies (Nedstrand, Wyon, Hammar, & Wijman, 2006). A study in which breast cancer survivors were randomly assigned to receive applied relaxation or electroacupuncture found a significant decrease in hot flashes in both groups, but this study lacked a control group (Nedstrand, Wijman, Wyon, & Hammar, 2005). One of the largest combined interventional studies performed in breast cancer survivors assigned women to a tailored intervention that included pharmacologic therapy and paced respiration as appropriate or usual care (Ganz et al., 2000). Patients who received the tailored intervention showed a statistically significant improvement in menopausal symptoms over usual care, but the study had no control group. All of the previously described mind-body and behavioral interventions are attractive to survivors and their healthcare team because they are associated with minimal risk. Reimbursement for these forms of interventions is lacking in many healthcare insurance plans, however. Complementary medicinal products that have undergone clinical trial evaluation and were found *not* to be better than placebo in controlling hot flashes include soy, black cohosh, red clover, dong quai, evening primrose oil, kava kava, and Chinese herbs (Kronenberg & Fugh-Berman, 2002). Even so, many women continue to use these products despite their lack of efficacy and proven safety.

For women with moderate to severe hot flashes that have a greater impact on their QOL, additional interventions may be necessary. Several selective serotonin and norepinephrine reuptake inhibitors and antidepressant medications have been tested in clinical trials and found to be effective in reducing the number and severity of hot flashes in breast cancer survivors. They include venlafaxine, paroxetine, fluoxetine, citalopram, and gabapentin (Biglia et al., 2009; Boekhout, Beijnen, & Schellens, 2006; Buijs et al., 2009; Carpenter, 2005; Loprinzi, Barton, et al., 2002; Loprinzi et al., 2000; Loprinzi, Sloan, et al., 2002; Stearns & Loprinzi, 2003; Stearns et al., 2005). Transdermal clonidine also has been shown to moderately reduce hot flashes compared to placebo (Goldberg et al., 1994). Mirtazapine, a newer antidepressant that is categorized as a noradrenergic and specific serotonergic antidepressant, was found in a small pilot study (40 breast cancer survivors) to be effective in reducing hot flashes, but compliance was an issue because of side effects (Biglia et al., 2007). Doses of these types of medications may need to be titrated to reach the maximal benefit with minimal side effects. Side effects can be problematic and decrease compliance. Some reported side effects include somnolence, weight gain, constipation, and sexual dysfunction. Importantly, certain selective serotonin reuptake inhibitors, particularly paroxetine and fluoxetine, have been postulated to decrease the effectiveness of tamoxifen and, as such, may be contraindicated. It has been suggested that alternative medicines be used, but such recommendations are controversial at this time. Gabapentin and citalopram are not considered potent CYP2D6 inhibitors. Bupropion also may affect tamoxifen metabolism but to a lesser degree (Desmarais & Looper, 2009). Because of the sexual side effects with some of the more commonly used antidepressants, it is important to ask whether patients note worsening sexual functioning while on these medications and to switch to a less problematic drug if so. However, given the number of side effects from many of these medications, women are increasingly seeking alternative ways to modify the severity of their vasomotor symptoms, even with minimal efficacy.

A newer but more invasive treatment for vasomotor symptoms is called stellate ganglion block. Lipov et al. (2008) found that the disease-free survivors on hormonal therapy who received this type of nerve block experienced a decrease in the number of hot flashes and night awakenings compared to controls in the first two weeks after the procedure and continued to have a decrease in symptoms over the remaining follow-up period (weeks 3–12). Of note, these women were experiencing severe symptoms that had not been controlled by conventional treatment measures over several months. They experienced temporary Horner syndrome (drooping of the eyelid, decreased pupil size, lack of sweating on affected side of face), indicating effectiveness of the block. Patients considered for this form of treatment should have explored other options first. Further study must be done before stellate ganglion block is deemed an acceptable first-line treatment strategy.

For women whose hot flashes continue to alter QOL or for those who are unable to tolerate the side effects of medications used to control symptoms, hormone replacement therapy can be considered. However, its concurrent use with antiestrogen therapies has not shown to be useful in ameliorating hot flashes (Osborne et al., 2009). It is essential that breast cancer survivors be provided with an adequate explanation of the possible risks and benefits of hormone replacement therapy, as there is a potential for increased risk of breast cancer recurrence (von Schoultz & Rutqvist, 2005). Hormonal medications that have been found to be useful include megestrol acetate and medroxyprogesterone acetate, but these are also associated with some unpleasant side effects (Bertelli et al., 2002; Pritchard, 2001). Switching to another form of antiestrogen therapy may also reduce the severity of symptoms in some patients, thereby enhancing compliance with therapy. Involving the patient in these decisions is critical. Fortunately, vasomotor symptoms have a tendency to decline in intensity over time in most women. Pharmacologic and nonpharmacologic self-care strategies for the management of hot flashes are described in Figure 9-9. The ONS PEP resource on hot flashes by Kaplan et al. (2011) deemed gabapentin and venlafaxine as treatments most likely to be effective. The authors ranked other medicinal agents and complementary therapies (clonidine, fluoxetine, mirtazapine, paroxetine, progestin therapy, sertraline, stellate ganglion block, tibolone, acupuncture, black cohosh, hypnosis, peer counseling, relaxation therapy, vitamin E, and yoga) as having unestablished efficacy.

## Osteoporosis

One of the most prevalent long-term sequelae of cancer therapy is osteoporosis, a disorder characterized by changes in bone density and quality. Patients with breast cancer are at in-

---

**Figure 9-9. Strategies for the Management of Hot Flash Symptoms in Breast Cancer Survivors**

| Environmental | Dietary | Complementary | Medication Therapy | Surgical Therapy |
|---|---|---|---|---|
| • Keep your room cool.<br>• Use fans; open windows.<br>• Dress in breathable fabrics.<br>• Dress in layers.<br>• Avoid high collars and clothing that fits tight at the neck.<br>• Wear hair shorter or off the neck.<br>• Identify and avoid personal triggers.<br>• Limit stressful situations.<br>• Control emotions. | • Have cool drinks available at all times.<br>• Avoid drinking alcohol.<br>• Avoid hot and spicy foods.<br>• Avoid eating late at night. | • Practice stress reduction techniques.<br>• Paced respirations<br>• Hypnosis<br>• Acupuncture<br>• Electroacupuncture<br>• Medication therapy<br>• Practice relaxation techniques. | • Switch to another type of hormone therapy.<br>• Take hormone replacement therapy.*<br>• Megestrol acetate<br>• Depot medroxyprogesterone acetate<br>• Vitamin E<br>• Gabapentin<br>• Venlafaxine<br>• Paroxetine +<br>• Fluoxetine +<br>• Citalopram<br>• Transdermal clonidine | • Stellate ganglion block |

* Relative contraindication in breast cancer survivors. Must be informed of inherent risks.

+ Have been found to reduce the effectiveness of tamoxifen

*Note.* Based on information from Bertelli et al., 2002; Biglia et al., 2009; Boekhout, 2006; Carpenter et al., 2002; Carson et al., 2009; Desmarais & Looper, 2009; Elkins et al., 2008; Hervik & Mjåland, 2009; Kaplan et al., 2010; Lipov et al., 2008; Nedstrand et al., 2005, 2006.

---

creased risk for cancer treatment–induced bone loss (CTIBL) as a result of hypogonadism from treatment and antiestrogen medication side effects (Pfeilschifter & Diel, 2000). The clinical consequences of osteoporosis, or decreased bone mass, are skeletal fractures, abdominal protrusion, height loss and kyphosis secondary to multiple vertebral fractures, chronic pain resulting from fractures, decreased respiratory capacity, and increased morbidity and mortality (Maxwell & Viale, 2005).

Bone undergoes a continual process of loss and formation throughout a woman's life. Women who go through natural menopause experience a sharp decrease in bone mass within five years after the end of menses, with gradual loss thereafter. Unless the bone formation rate increases, osteopenia, and eventually osteoporosis, will develop. Women undergoing chemotherapy-induced early menopause or receiving an aromatase inhibitor as part of their breast cancer therapy may experience accelerated bone density changes and increased fracture risk (Lønning, 2008). Many women with breast cancer who carry *BRCA1* and *BRCA2* mutations are opting for prophylactic oophorectomy, which further elevates their risk for premature bone loss.

Most breast cancers occur in women in the age group already at risk for osteoporosis—women older than 65. Premenopausal women with early-stage breast cancer who become amenorrheic experience accelerated bone loss of about 6%–8% in the first year compared to women undergoing natural menopause, and this loss persists for years after completion of chemotherapy in women who remain amenorrheic, primarily related to the loss of ovarian function (Saad et al., 2008). When postmenopausal women in the ATAC trial were evaluated for bone density after five years, women

on anastrozole who started therapy with a baseline T-score of less than –1.5 had a greater risk for developing osteoporosis compared to women taking tamoxifen (Eastell et al., 2008). Similar trials comparing the effectiveness of other aromatase inhibitors, namely letrozole and exemestane, to tamoxifen found similar results (Jones et al., 2008). Without treatment, the risk for bone fracture increases to 10% after five years of therapy with aromatase inhibitors based on the Breast International Group 1-98 and ATAC trials (ATAC Trialists' Group, 2008; Rabaglio et al., 2009). CTIBL can begin as soon as one year after chemotherapy. It can be accelerated with the use of all of the following aromatase inhibitors: anastrozole and letrozole in postmenopausal women and fulvestrant or tamoxifen in premenopausal women (Powles, Hickish, Kanis, Tidy, & Ashley, 1996). In a study by Sverrisdóttir, Fornander, Jacobsson, von Schoultz, and Rutqvist (2004), two years of ovarian ablation with goserelin therapy caused a significant reduction in bone mineral density, but a partial recovery occurred after cessation of treatment. Ovarian insufficiency generally develops within one year of therapy in 63%–96% of premenopausal women with breast cancer who receive cyclophosphamide, methotrexate, 5-fluorouracil, or doxorubicin. The risk of ovarian injury is related to the age of the patient at the time of treatment, the cumulative dose of the drug administered, and the duration of treatment (Pfeilschifter & Diel, 2000). The incidence of fractures caused by CTIBL has not been reported. However, the ATAC trial comparing anastrozole to tamoxifen indicated that the anastrozole group was more likely to experience bone loss. The incidence of fracture was 2.93% in the anastrozole group compared to 1.9% in the tamoxifen group during treatment, but the incidences were not significantly different following treatment (ATAC Trialists' Group, 2008).

The most important strategy that nurses can use to prevent bone loss in patients with breast cancer is to determine whether the patient is currently at high risk for osteoporosis development prior to the initiation of treatment and recommend appropriate screening and healthy lifestyle modifications. To assist in this assessment, the World Health Organization (WHO) has developed a Web-based tool called the Fracture Risk Assessment (FRAX®). The FRAX tool factors in height, weight, race, medication use, medical history, alcohol use, and bone mineral density T-scores at the femoral hip (WHO, n.d.). It can be accessed free of charge at www.shef.ac.uk/FRAX/index.jsp.

WHO has established criteria for categorizing bone density. Measurement of bone density by dual-energy x-ray absorptiometry (DEXA) scan is considered the gold standard. Results are reported as T-scores, which represent the number of standard deviations between an individual's bone mineral density and the mean value for a group of young adults of the same sex (National Osteoporosis Foundation [NOF], 2010). Women with T-scores above –1 are considered to have normal bone density with minimal risk of hip fracture. Women with T-scores of –1 to –2.5 have osteopenia and are at 2.6–7 times greater risk of hip fracture than normal controls. Women with T-scores less than –2.5 are considered to have osteoporosis and are at 7–11 times greater risk of having a hip fracture. Women with T-scores less than –2.5 who have already experienced one or more fractures are considered to have severe osteoporosis.

NOF recommends pharmacologic intervention when the bone mineral density T-score is between –1 and –2.5 and the 10-year probability of hip fracture is greater than or equal to 3% or the probability of major osteoporosis-related fracture is greater than 20% based on the U.S.-adapted FRAX tool. Unfortunately, the FRAX tool does not currently incorporate increased fracture risk associated with cancer-related hormone-ablative therapies. The rate of bone loss with aromatase inhibitors is greater than that seen with smoking but less than that associated with corticosteroid use. As such, the clinical fracture risk of about 10% after five years of aromatase inhibitor use places women at substantial fracture risk, thus supporting the need for pharmacologic intervention (Chlebowski & Tagawa, 2009).

Risk factors for the development of osteoporosis in healthy women are categorized as modifiable and nonmodifiable (see Figure 9-10). Nonmodifiable risks include female gender, increasing age, Caucasian or Asian ancestry, small body frame, family history of osteoporosis, certain medical conditions, and the need for certain types of medication therapy (glucocorticoids, heparin therapy, cyclosporine, gonadotropin-releasing hormone, proton pump inhibitors, aluminum-containing antacids, phenytoin, and phenobarbital). Modifiable risks include cigarette smoking, low calcium and vitamin D intake, sedentary lifestyle, alcohol intake, and low body weight. These risk factors should be taken into consideration to determine ad-

---

### Figure 9-10. Risk Factors for Developing Osteoporosis in Breast Cancer Survivors

**Modifiable**
- Lifestyle
- Smoking
- Excessive alcohol intake (more than three servings daily)
- Eating disorders
- Nutritional deficiencies (calcium, vitamin D)
- Low physical activity, especially lack of weight-bearing and resistance exercise
- High caffeine intake
- High salt intake
- High vitamin A intake
- Low sun exposure
- Intake of aluminum-containing antacids

**Nonmodifiable**
- Asian or Caucasian ethnicity
- Female gender
- Amenorrhea before age 45 or prolonged amenorrhea (longer than six months)
- Family history of osteoporosis
- Maternal or paternal history of hip fracture
- Postmenopausal status
- Increasing age (females older than 65, males older than 70)
- Personal history of low-impact fracture
- Small body frame
- Body mass index less than 20 kg/m²
- Medical conditions (hyperparathyroidism, hyperthyroidism, rheumatoid arthritis, prolonged corticosteroid use, diabetes mellitus, chronic liver or kidney disease)
- Cancer treatment with chemotherapy, fulvestrant, or hormonal therapy
- Prophylactic oophorectomy

*Note.* Based on information from Gass & Dawson-Hughes, 2006; National Osteoporosis Foundation, 2010.

---

ditive risks in women undergoing cancer treatment and provide appropriate counseling. It is important to note that the incidence of osteoporosis in women in the United States has increased in the past decade, placing more women at risk at the time of their breast cancer development (Gass & Dawson-Hughes, 2006; Kuehn, 2005; NOF, 2010).

The optimal timing of bone mineral density testing for CTIBL has not been established. Serum chemistries assessing for kidney or liver disease and parathyroid hormone, thyroid-stimulating hormone, vitamin D, serum calcium, phosphorus, and alkaline phosphatase levels may help in the evaluation (Pfeilschifter & Diel, 2000). Monitoring of serum vitamin D levels has become more common with the reports of deficiency seen in many patients with breast cancer at the time of diagnosis and increased risk for metastasis in these individuals compared to women with normal vitamin D levels (Holick & Chen, 2008; Moyad, 2008). However, recommending routine testing and treatment of vitamin D deficiencies requires further evaluation. A recent study by Khan et al. (2010) showed that treatment of vitamin D deficiency actually resulted in less joint pain in women who were taking letrozole, giving some credence to pretreatment testing of vitamin D levels. Treatment of deficiency may help promote patient comfort and compliance with aromatase inhibitor hormonal therapy.

According to the ASCO bone health guidelines for breast cancer survivors, women should be stratified into low- and high-risk groups depending on the presence of the aforementioned risk factors (Hillner et al., 2003). Breast cancer survivors considered high risk by ASCO are women age 65 and older, postmenopausal women receiving aromatase inhibitors, premenopausal women with premature menopause, and women ages 60–64 with general osteoporosis risk factors. These individuals should be advised to undergo a baseline hip and spine DEXA scan when initiating therapy and counseled about lifestyle and dietary changes (Hillner et al., 2003). It is recommended that patients with a T-score of –2.5 or lower be treated with bisphosphonates such as oral alendronate, oral or IV risedronate, IV zoledronic acid, IV pamidronate, or oral or IV ibandronate. Annual screening is recommended in the follow-up of women requiring treatment with these drugs to monitor response. ASCO recommends that low-risk patients not undergo bone density screening until age 65, but they should have an assessment of risk factors annually with ongoing counseling on diet and lifestyle changes (Hillner et al., 2003). Other clinicians have disagreed with this position and instead recommend baseline screening with repeat measurements performed every three to five years (Twiss et al., 2001).

Tamoxifen is modestly effective in preventing bone loss in postmenopausal women. Its protection of premenopausal women's bones has been questioned (Lønning, 2008; Ramaswamy & Sharpiro, 2003; Shapiro, Manola, & Leboff, 2001). However, the selective estrogen receptor modifier raloxifene was found to maintain bone mineral density and reduce spinal fractures in women at risk for osteoporosis with the same cardiac protective effects as tamoxifen (Jordan, 2007). In the Study of Tamoxifen and Raloxifene (or STAR) trial (Vogel et al., 2006), raloxifene also demonstrated chemoprotective effects in women at high risk for breast cancer development. As such, its use is now included in the NCCN guideline *Breast Cancer Risk Reduction* (NCCN, 2010b). Caution is advised because individuals who have taken tamoxifen or an aromatase inhibitor in the past should not take raloxifene concurrently or in the future.

A study by Reid et al. (2002) showed that a single yearly infusion of zoledronic acid significantly increased bone mineral density in healthy postmenopausal women with osteoporosis. On interim analysis, the Zometa®-Femara® (Novartis Pharmaceuticals Corp.) Adjuvant Synergy Trial in North America and a parallel study in Europe found that those patients given zoledronic acid at the initiation of therapy, rather than at the first sign of fracture or worsening bone density, had improvement in lumbar spine bone mineral density (Brufsky et al., 2008, 2009). Of specific interest, those patients who received up-front zoledronic acid had fewer disease recurrences and reduced mortality. In the Austrian Breast and Colorectal Cancer Study Group Trial 12, a four-arm trial of 1,800 premenopausal women with endocrine-responsive breast cancer randomized to ovarian suppression plus either tamoxifen or anastrozole, both either with or without zoledronic acid every

six months for three years, showed that the arms without zoledronic acid had significant bone loss (worse in the anastrozole arm), and although partial bone density recovery occurred, the women did not recover to baseline at five years of follow-up (Gnant et al., 2008). Further analysis at 48 months showed that the addition of zoledronic acid significantly improved disease-free survival (Gnant et al., 2009). A retrospective review of similar patients by Winter, Thorpe, Burkinshaw, Beevers, and Coleman (2008) showed both higher response rates following neoadjuvant chemotherapy with zoledronic acid and higher complete response rates, further increasing the interest in this mode of therapy. A recent update of the AZURE trial (Coleman et al., 2010) at the 2010 San Antonio Breast Cancer Symposium showed that zoledronic acid did not improve disease-free survival (DFS) in women who had undergone adjuvant chemotherapy with a median follow up of 5.9 months. However, in a subset analysis, they did find improved DFS and overall survival in those women treated with zoledronic acid five or more years after menopause. They hypothesized that the positive effects of zoledronic acid may require a low estrogen environment to be effective. The SABRE trial showed that risedronate was effective in preventing aromatase inhibitor–induced bone loss after 24 months of therapy (Van Poznak et al., 2010). The benefits of clodronate and risedronate have been demonstrated by the reduction of bone loss associated with chemotherapy-induced ovarian failure (Saarto, Vehmanen, Blomqvist, & Elomaa, 2008; Van Poznak et al., 2010). Ibandronate sodium has also been tested in breast cancer survivors and was found to be useful in the treatment of cancer-related bone loss (Body et al., 2004). Intranasal calcitonin has not been well studied in breast cancer survivors but can be a reasonable option for women who cannot tolerate the gastrointestinal side effects of oral medications. It has recently been shown to prevent vertebral fractures when compared with placebo in healthy women (MacLean et al., 2008).

Based on the increasing knowledge about the deleterious effects of aromatase inhibitors on bone health, Hadji et al. (2008) developed an algorithm that essentially recommends the use of IV zoledronic acid 4 mg every six months along with calcium and vitamin D for T-scores of less than –2 along with monitoring of bone mineral density every two years. They also recommended that if annual decrease in bone mineral density is more than 5%, secondary causes of bone loss should be considered.

For the most part, bisphosphonates are well tolerated. However, oral treatments have been associated with gastrointestinal upset. Of more concern have been reports of esophageal cancers with the use of oral therapy. IV therapy has been associated with renal toxicity, osteonecrosis of the jaw (ONJ), and atypical femur fractures in patients taking IV therapy for extended periods of time (more than three years) (Wysowski, 2009). ONJ occurred in up to 18.6% of patients with breast cancer taking bisphosphonates in IV form, with less risk for ONJ seen in patients taking ibandronate and pamidronate compared to zoledronic acid (Vahtsevanos et al., 2009). Special attention to dental health, with reporting of nonhealing oral sores and avoidance of tooth extractions after initiation of drug therapy, is imperative. Proper medication administration is also important. The patient should take the oral medication with a large glass of water and remain upright for 30 minutes. Generous hydration and monitoring of serum creatinine prior to each dose of IV medication are strongly advised. Patients also should be advised that flu-like symptoms are common after IV administration of bisphosphonates. See Table 9-7 for common pharmacologic treatments for osteoporosis in breast cancer survivors.

Although cancer therapies cause the biggest increase in osteoporosis risk in breast cancer survivors, patients also should be instructed about the importance of smoking cessation, moderation in alcohol consumption (three to four servings per week), and the importance of regular weight-bearing exercise (e.g., walking, running, weight training, stretching, resistance exercises, Tai Chi, yoga) prior to the initiation of therapy. A daily intake of 1,200–1,500 mg of calcium and 800–1,000 IU of vitamin D is recommended (Delaney, 2006; Hillner et al., 2003; Holick & Chen, 2008; NOF, 2010) above dietary intake.

Fall prevention is an important consideration for patients deemed to be at risk for fracture. Nurses should assess the patient's use of sedating drugs and assess environmental hazards (e.g., rugs, thresholds, poor lighting). Patients with a risk

| Table 9-7. Pharmacologic Interventions for Cancer Treatment–Induced Bone Loss | | |
|---|---|---|
| Drug | Dosage | Special Considerations and Side Effects |
| Calcium citrate | 1,200–1,500 mg daily in divided doses of 500 mg | Avoid taking with iron supplements and caffeine.<br>Drink with 8 oz of water.<br>Can cause constipation, bloating, and gas |
| Calcium carbonate | Same as above | Same as with calcium citrate<br>Concern with use in patients with renal insufficiency |
| Vitamin D | 800–1,000 IU | Can also be gained by 15 minutes of daily sun exposure |
| Calcitonin nasal spray | 200 units intranasally (one nostril per day)<br>Also available as a subcutaneous formulation | U.S. Food and Drug Administration approved for women who have been postmenopausal for at least five years.<br>Rhinitis and, rarely, epistaxis can occur. |
| Alendronate | 10 mg PO daily or 70 mg PO weekly (as treatment, not prevention) | Must be taken on an empty stomach<br>Take with 8 oz. of water.<br>Must stay upright for 30 minutes after taking medication<br>Can cause upper gastrointestinal irritation, myalgias, and arthralgias<br>Patients taking liquid formulation should take with at least 2 oz. plain water. |
| Risedronate | 5 mg PO daily or 35 mg PO weekly | Same as with alendronate |
| Raloxifene | 60 mg PO daily | Not recommended for use after tamoxifen therapy or with aromatase inhibitors<br>Can cause hot flashes, leg cramps, and, rarely, deep vein thrombosis |
| Tamoxifen | 10 mg PO BID or 20 mg PO daily | Should not be used with raloxifene or aromatase inhibitors<br>Can cause hot flashes, weight gain, cataract formation, deep vein thrombosis, and endometrial cancer<br>Has been found to promote bone loss in premenopausal women |
| Zoledronic acid | 5 mg IV once or twice annually, given over 15 minutes | Check creatinine clearance before each dose. Ensure adequate hydration. Avoid in people with history of aspirin-sensitive asthma.<br>Osteonecrosis of the jaw has occurred following dental procedures in people with prior or concurrent chemotherapy and dexamethasone therapy. Pretreatment dental examinations are advised. Good oral hygiene is important.<br>Patients should be advised to report oral sores or jaw pain.<br>Can cause flu-like symptoms, nausea, vomiting, fever, flushing, and loss of appetite |
| Ibandronate | 2.5 mg daily, 150 mg monthly, or 3 mg IV every 3 months given over 15–30 seconds | Must stay upright for 60 minutes after taking medication.<br>Take with 8 oz. of water.<br>Must be taken on empty stomach<br>Can cause upper gastrointestinal irritation, myalgias, and arthralgias<br>For IV formulation, checking of serum creatinine before each dose is advised. |

*Note.* Based on information from Brufsky et al., 2005; Hillner et al., 2003; Maxwell & Viale, 2005; National Osteoporosis Foundation, 2010.

for fainting, muscle weakness, dizziness, balance issues, foot neuropathy, and impaired vision also should be monitored closely. A cross-sectional prospective study of 72 breast cancer survivors found that those women with chemotherapy-induced amenorrhea and muscle weakness with poor balance had a heightened risk for falls and fractures (Winters-Stone, Nail, Bennett, & Schwartz, 2009).

The research on nonpharmacologic interventions for CTIBL has focused primarily on the use of exercise as an intervention. Waltman et al. (2003) tested a 12-month multicomponent intervention for preventing osteoporosis in 21 postmenopausal women who had completed breast cancer treatment (excluding tamoxifen). The intervention used a home-based strength and weight training exercise program combined with alendronate, vitamin D, and calcium, along with education about osteoporosis. Each of the participants had improvements in function, and 3 in 21 women who had measurable bone loss at baseline had normal bone mineral density after the intervention. A study by Schwartz, Winters-Stone, and Gallucci (2007) found that weight-bearing aerobic exercise over a six-month period of time, beginning with the onset of chemotherapy, attenuated declines in bone mineral density compared with patients who performed resistance exercise alone and controls. The average decline in the lumbar spine and whole body bone mineral density was –6.23% for the usual care controls, –4.92% for the resistance exercise group, and –0.76% for the aerobic exercise group. Just as with the exercise strategies recommended for women experiencing fatigue after breast cancer treatment, ways in which to overcome barriers and promote adherence to weight-bearing exercise and resistance exercise programs must be developed. Such interventions provide women with a proactive approach to health.

CTIBL is a significant health concern. Patients must be educated about the bone effects of treatment and should be encouraged to make lifestyle changes to promote bone health. The importance of the combined use of calcium and vitamin D and exercise along with recommended bisphosphonates for women with low bone mineral density must be emphasized. Healthcare professionals must be proactive in conducting follow-up studies to identify worsening bone health and take prompt corrective measures. For patients who are refractive to oral osteoporosis medications or are receiving aromatase inhibitors, serious consideration should be given to the use of IV bisphosphonate drug therapy sooner rather than later to prevent more costly sequelae.

## Conclusion

Symptom distress can adversely alter the experience of women diagnosed with breast cancer. Close review of the most commonly experienced side effects from treatment shows clear but complex interrelationships. Although most women with early-stage breast cancer do not experience se-

vere side effects, even minor symptoms can serve as a constant reminder of their cancer diagnosis. Promotion of self-care strategies in symptom management helps to empower women to take back control of their lives. Research into improved surgical techniques; kinder, gentler chemotherapy and hormonal therapy regimens; and more targeted symptom management strategies, taking into consideration genetic and gender differences, is needed to further improve women's QOL. The National Cancer Institute has a number of studies evaluating the effectiveness of complementary measures to address treatment-related side effects. A list of these trials can be accessed at http://clinicaltrials.gov.

Long-term follow-up of survivors is critical to enable prompt identification of post-treatment problems and to share medical updates. Education regarding cancer treatment side effects should be provided to all healthcare professionals involved in the care of these patients, including those in the primary care setting. Doing so will help to lessen patients' anxiety, avoid misconceptions, and reduce patients' fear of recurrence. As survivorship issues become a healthcare priority and the development of cancer treatment summaries becomes the norm, the emotional and physical well-being of millions of women who are breast cancer survivors will be enhanced.

## References

Ahlberg, K., Ekman, T., Gaston-Johansson, F., & Mock, V. (2003). Assessment and management of cancer-related fatigue in adults. *Lancet, 362,* 640–650. doi:10.1016/S0140-6736(03)14186-4

Ahles, T.A., Saykin, A.J., Furstenberg, C.T., Cole, B., Mott, L.A., Skalla, K., … Silberfarb, P.M. (2002). Neuropsychologic impact of standard-dose systemic chemotherapy in long-term survivors of breast cancer and lymphoma. *Journal of Clinical Oncology, 20,* 485–493. doi:10.1200/JCO.20.2.485

Ahles, T.A., Saykin, A.J., Noll, W.W., Furstenberg, C.T., Guerin, S., Cole, B., & Mott, L.A. (2003). The relationship of APOE genotype to neuropsychological performance in long-term cancer survivors treated with standard dose chemotherapy. *Psycho-Oncology, 12,* 612–619. doi:10.1002/pon.742

Alem, M., & Gurgel, M.S.C. (2008). Acupuncture in the rehabilitation of women after breast cancer surgery: A case series. *Acupuncture in Medicine, 26,* 87–93.

Alexander, S., Minton, O., Andrews, P., & Stone, P. (2009). A comparison of the characteristics of disease-free breast cancer survivors with or without cancer-related fatigue syndrome. *European Journal of Cancer, 45,* 384–392. doi:10.1016/j.ejca.2008.09.010

Allen, D.H., Von Ah, D., Jansen, C., Schiavone, R.M., Gagnon, P., Wulff, J., & Behrendt, R. (2011). ONS PEP resource: Cognitive impairment. In L.H. Eaton, J.M. Tipton, & M. Irwin (Eds.), *Putting evidence into practice: Improving oncology patient outcomes, volume 2* (pp. 23–30). Pittsburgh, PA: Oncology Nursing Society.

American Cancer Society. (2010). Exercises after breast surgery. Retrieved from http://www.cancer.org/Cancer/BreastCancer/MoreInformation/exercises-after-breast-surgery

Arimidex, Tamoxifen, Alone or in Combination Trialists' Group. (2008). Effect of anastrozole and tamoxifen as adjuvant treatment for early-stage breast cancer: 100-month analysis of the ATAC trial. *Lancet Oncology, 9,* 45–53. doi:10.1016/S1470-2045(07)70385-6

Armer, J.M., Radina, M.E., Porock, D., & Culbertson, S.D. (2003). Predicting breast cancer-related lymphedema using self-reported symptoms. *Nursing Research, 52,* 370–379.

Armer, J.M., Stewart, B.R., & Shook, R.P. (2009). 30-month post-breast cancer treatment lymphoedema. *Journal of Lymphoedema, 4,* 14–18.

Asmussen, P.D., & Strössenreuther, R.H.K. (2006). Compression therapy. In M. Földi & E. Földi (Eds.), *Földi's textbook of lymphology for physicians and lymphedema therapists* (2nd ed., pp. 563–629). Munich, Germany: Elsevier GmbH.

Avis, N.E., Stellato, R., Crawford, S., Bromberger, J., Ganz, P., Cain, V., & Kagawa-Singer, M. (2001). Is there a menopausal syndrome? Menopausal status and symptoms across racial/ethnic groups. *Social Science and Medicine, 52,* 345–356. doi:10.1016/S0277-9536(00)00147-7

Baglan, K.L., Sharpe, M.B., Jaffray, D., Frazier, R.C., Fayad, J., Kestin, L.L., … Vicini, F.A. (2003). Accelerated partial breast irradiation using 3D conformal radiation therapy (3D-CRT). *International Journal of Radiation Oncology, Biology, Physics, 55,* 302–311. doi:10.1016/S0360-3016(02)03811-7

Baney, T., McQuestion, M., Bell, K., Bruce, S., Feight, D., Weis-Smith, L., & Haas, M. (2011). ONS PEP resource: Radiodermatitis. In L.H. Eaton, J.M. Tipton, & M. Irwin (Eds.), *Putting evidence into practice: Improving oncology patient outcomes, volume 2* (pp. 57–75). Pittsburgh, PA: Oncology Nursing Society.

Baron, R.H., Fey, J.V., Borgen, P.I., Stempel, M.M., Hardick, K.R., & Van Zee, K.J. (2007). Eighteen sensations after breast cancer surgery: A 5-year comparison of sentinel lymph node biopsy and axillary lymph node dissection. *Annals of Surgical Oncology, 14,* 1653–1661. doi:10.1245/s10434-006-9334-z

Barsevick, A.M. (2007). The elusive concept of the symptom cluster. *Oncology Nursing Forum, 34,* 971–980. doi:10.1188/07.ONF.971-980

Barsevick, A.M., Whitmer, K., Sweeney, C., & Nail, L.M. (2002). A pilot study examining conservation for cancer treatment-related fatigue. *Cancer Nursing, 25,* 333–341.

Barton, D., & Loprinzi, C. (2002). Novel approaches to preventing chemotherapy-induced cognitive dysfunction in breast cancer: The art of the possible. *Clinical Breast Cancer, 3*(Suppl. 3), S121–S127.

Barton, D.L., Loprinzi, C.L., Quella, S.K., Sloan, J.A., Veeder, M.H., Egner, J.R., … Novotny, P. (1998). Prospective evaluation of vitamin E for hot flashes in breast cancer survivors. *Journal of Clinical Oncology, 16,* 495–500.

Beck, S.L., Dudley, W.N., & Barsevick, A. (2005). Pain, sleep disturbance, and fatigue in patients with cancer: Using a mediation model to test a symptom cluster [Online exclusive]. *Oncology Nursing Forum, 32,* E48–E55. doi:10.1188/04.ONF.E48-E55

Becker, C., Pham, D.N.M., Assoaud, J., Badia, A., Foucault, C., & Riquet, M. (2008). Postmastectomy neuropathic pain: Results of microsurgical lymph nodes transplantation. *Breast, 17,* 472–476. doi:10.1016/j.breast.2007.12.007

Bender, C.M., McDaniel, R.W., Murphy-Ende, K., Pickett, M., Rittenberg, C.N., Rogers, M.P., … Schwartz, R.N. (2002). Chemotherapy-induced nausea and vomiting. *Clinical Journal of Oncology Nursing, 6,* 94–102. doi:10.1188/02.CJON.94-102

Bender, C.M., Paraska, K.K., Sereika, S.M., Ryan, C.M., & Berga, S.L. (2001). Cognitive function and reproductive hormones in adjuvant therapy for breast cancer: A critical review. *Journal of Pain and Symptom Management, 21,* 407–424. doi:10.1016/S0885-3924(01)00268-8

Bendz, I., & Olsén, M.F. (2002). Evaluation of immediate versus delayed shoulder exercises after breast cancer surgery including lymph node dissection—A randomised controlled trial. *Breast, 11,* 241–248. doi:10.1054/brst.2001.0412

Benshushan, A., Rojansky, N., Chaviv, M., Arbel-Alon, S., Benmeir, A., Imbar, T., & Brzezinski, A. (2009). Climacteric symptoms in women undergoing risk-reducing bilateral salpingo-oophorectomy. *Climacteric, 12,* 404–409. doi:10.1080/13697130902780846

Berger, A.M. (2009). Update on the state of the science: Sleep-wake disturbances in adult patients with cancer [Online exclusive]. *Oncology Nursing Forum, 36,* E165–E177. doi:10.1188/09.ONF.E165-E177

Berger, A.M., Kuhn, B.R., Farr, L.A., Von Essen, S.G., Chamberlain, J., Lynch, J.C., & Agrawal, S. (2009). One year outcomes of a behavioral therapy intervention trial on sleep quality and cancer related fatigue. *Journal of Clinical Oncology, 27,* 6033–6040. doi:10.1200/JCO.2008.20.8306

Berger, A.M., Lockhart, K., & Agrawal, S. (2009). Variability of patterns of fatigue and quality of life over time based on different breast cancer adjuvant chemotherapy regimens. *Oncology Nursing Forum, 36,* 563–570. doi:10.1188/09.ONF.563-570

Berger, A.M., VonEssen, S., Kuhn, B.R., Piper, B.F., Farr, L., Agrawal, S., … Higginbotham, P. (2003). Adherence, sleep, and fatigue outcomes after adjuvant breast cancer chemotherapy: Results of a feasibility intervention study. *Oncology Nursing Forum, 30,* 513–522. doi:10.1188/03.ONF.513-522

Bertelli, G., Venturini, M., Del Mastro, L., Bergaglio, M., Sismondi, P., Biglia, N., … Rosso, R. (2002). Intramuscular depot medroxy-progesterone versus oral megestrol for the control of postmenopausal hot flashes in breast cancer patients: A randomized study. *Annals of Oncology, 13,* 883–888. doi:10.1093/annonc/mdf151

Beurskens, C.H., van Uden, C.J., Strobbe, L.J., Oostendorp, R.A., & Wobbes, T. (2007). The efficacy of physiotherapy upon shoulder function following axillary dissection in breast cancer, a randomized controlled study. *BMC Cancer, 7,* 166. doi:10.1186/1471-2407-7-166

Bieck, T., & Phillips, S. (2010). Appraising the evidence for avoiding lotions or topical agents prior to radiation therapy. *Clinical Journal of Oncology Nursing, 14,* 103–105. doi:10.1188/10.CJON.103-105

Biglia, N., Kubatzki, F., Sgandurra, P., Ponzone, R., Marenco, D., Peano, E., & Sismondi, P. (2007). Mirtazapine for the treatment of hot flushes in breast cancer survivors: A prospective pilot trial. *Breast Journal, 13,* 490–495. doi:10.1111/j.1524-4741.2007.00470.x

Biglia, N., Sgandurra, P., Peano, E., Marenco, D., Moggio, G., Bounous, V., … Sismondi, P. (2009). Non-hormonal treatment of hot flushes in breast cancer survivors: Gabapentin vs. vitamin E. *Climacteric, 12,* 310–318. doi:10.1080/13697130902736921

Boccia, R., Malik, I.A., Raja, V., Kahanic, L., Liu, R., Lillie, T., … Silberstein, P. (2006). Darbepoetin alfa administered every three weeks is effective for the treatment of chemotherapy-induced anemia. *Oncologist, 11,* 409–417. doi:10.1634/theoncologist.11-4-409

Body, J.J., Diel, I.J., Lichinitzer, M., Lazarev, A., Percherstorfer, M., Bell, R., … Bergstrom, B. (2004). Oral ibandronate reduces the risk of skeletal complications in breast cancer patients with metastatic bone disease: Results from two randomised, placebo-controlled phase III studies. *British Journal of Cancer, 90,* 1133–1137. doi:10.1038/sj.bjc.6601663

Boekhout, A.H., Beijnen, J.H., & Schellens, J.H.M. (2006). Symptoms and treatment in cancer therapy-induced early menopause. *Oncologist, 11,* 641–654. doi:10.1634/theoncologist.11-6-641

Booth, C.M., Clemons, M., Dranitsaris, G., Joy, A., Young, S., Callaghan, W., … Petrella, T. (2007). Chemotherapy-induced nausea and vomiting in breast cancer patients: A prospective observational study. *Journal of Supportive Oncology, 5,* 374–379.

Borger, J.H., Kemperman, H., Smitt, H.S., Hart, A., van Dongen, J., Lebesque, J., & Bartelink, H. (1994). Dose and volume effects on fibrosis after breast conservation. *International Journal of Radiation Oncology, Biology, Physics, 30,* 1073–1081.

Boris, M., Weindorf, S., & Lasinski, S. (1997). Persistence of lymphedema reduction after complex therapy. *Oncology, 11,* 99–109.

Bosompra, K., Ashikaga, T., O'Brien, P.J., Nelson, L., & Skelly, J. (2002). Swelling, numbness, pain, and their relationship to arm function among breast cancer survivors: A disablement process model perspective. *Breast Journal, 8,* 338–348. doi:10.1046/j.1524-4741.2002.08603.x

Boström, A., Lindman, H., Swartling, C., Berne, B., & Bergh, J. (2001). Potent corticosteroid cream (mometasone furoate) significantly reduces acute radiation dermatitis: Results from a double-blind, randomized study. *Radiotherapy and Oncology, 59,* 257–265. doi:10.1016/S0167-8140(01)00327-9

Boughey, J.C., Goravanchi, F., Parris, R.N., Kee, S.S., Frenzel, J.C., Hunt, K.K., ... Lucci, A. (2009). Improved postoperative pain control using thoracic paravertebral block for breast operations. *Breast Journal, 15,* 483–488. doi:10.1111/j.1524-4741.2009.00763.x

Bower, J.E., Ganz, P.A., Desmond, K.A., Bernaards, C., Rowland, J.H., Meyerowitz, B.E., & Belin, T.R. (2006). Fatigue in long-term breast carcinoma survivors: A longitudinal investigation. *Cancer, 106,* 751–758. doi:10.1002/cncr.21671

Box, R.C., Reul-Hirche, H.M., Bullock-Saxton, J.E., & Furnival, C.M. (2002). Shoulder movement after breast cancer surgery: Results of a randomised controlled study of postoperative physiotherapy. *Breast Cancer Research and Treatment, 75,* 35–50. doi:10.1023/A:1016571204924

Boykoff, N., Moieni, M., & Subramanian, S.K. (2009). Confronting chemobrain: An in depth look at survivors' reports of impact of work, social networks, and health care response. *Journal of Cancer Survivorship, 3,* 223–232. doi:10.1007/s11764-009-0098-x

Browse, N., Burnard, K.G., & Mortimer, P.S. (2003). *Diseases of the lymphatics.* London, England: Arnold.

Brufsky, A., Bundred, N., Coleman, R., Lambert-Falls, R., Mena, R., Hadji, P., ... Perez, E.A. (2008). Integrated analysis of zoledronic acid for prevention of aromatase inhibitor-associated bone loss in postmenopausal women with early breast cancer receiving adjuvant letrozole. *Oncologist, 13,* 503–514. doi:10.1634/theoncologist.2007-0206

Brufsky, A.M., Bosserman, L.D., Caradonna, R.R., Haley, B.B., Jones, C.M., Moore, H.C., ... Perez, E.A. (2009). Zoledronic acid effectively prevents aromatase inhibitor-associated bone loss in postmenopausal women with early breast cancer receiving adjuvant letrozole: Z-FAST study 36-month follow-up results. *Clinical Breast Cancer, 9,* 77–85. doi:10.3816/CBC.2009.n.015

Buijs, C., Mom, C.H., Willemse, P.H., Boezen, H.M., Maurer, J.M., Wymenga, A.N., ... Mourits, M.J. (2009). Venlafaxine versus clonidine for the treatment of hot flashes in breast cancer patients: A double-blind, randomized cross-over study. *Breast Cancer Research and Treatment, 115,* 573–580. doi:10.1007/s10549-008-0138-7

CancerCare. (2008a). Combating chemobrain: Keeping your memory sharp. Retrieved from http://www.cancercare.org/pdf/fact_sheets/fs_chemobrain_memory.pdf

CancerCare. (2008b). Improving your concentration: Three key steps. Retrieved from http://www.cancercare.org/pdf/fact_sheets/fs_chemobrain_concentration.pdf

Carpenter, J.S. (2005). State of the science: Hot flashes and cancer. Part 2: Management and future directions. *Oncology Nursing Forum, 32,* 969–978. doi:10.1188/04.ONF.969-978

Carpenter, J.S., Andrykowski, M.A., Cordova, M., Cunningham, L., Studts, J., McGrath, P., ... Munn, R. (1998). Hot flashes in postmenopausal women treated for breast carcinoma: Prevalence, severity, correlates, management, and relation to

quality of life. *Cancer, 82,* 1682–1691. doi:10.1002/(SICI)1097-0142(19980501)82:9<1682::AID-CNCR14>3.0.CO;2-0

Carpenter, J.S., Johnson, D.H, Wagner, L.J., & Andrykowski, M.A. (2002). Hot flashes and related outcomes in breast cancer survivors and matched comparison women [Online exclusive]. *Oncology Nursing Forum, 29,* E16–E25. doi:10.1188/02.ONF.E16-E25

Carson, J.W., Carson, K.M., Porter, L.S., Keefe, F.J., & Seewaldt, V.L. (2009). Yoga of Awareness program for menopausal symptoms in breast cancer survivors: Results from a randomized trial. *Supportive Care in Cancer, 17,* 1301–1309. doi:10.1007/s00520-009-0587-5

Casley-Smith, J.R., & Casley-Smith, J.R. (1997). *Modern treatment for lymphoedema* (5th ed.). Adelaide, Australia: Lymphoedema Association of Australia.

Casley-Smith, J.R., Casley-Smith, J.R., Lasinski, B.B., & Boris, M. (1996). The dangers of pumps in lymphoedema therapy. *Lymphology, 29,* 232–234.

Castellon, S.A., Ganz, P.A., Bower, J.E., Petersen, L., Abraham, L., & Greendale, G.A. (2004). Neurocognitive performance in breast cancer survivors exposed to adjuvant chemotherapy and tamoxifen. *Journal of Clinical and Experimental Neuropsychology, 26,* 955–969.

Cella, D., Dobrez, D., & Glaspy, J. (2003). Control of cancer-related anemia with erythropoietin agents: A review of evidence for improved clinical outcomes. *Annals of Oncology, 14,* 511–519. doi:10.1093/annonc/mdg167

Cella, D., & Fallowfield, L.J. (2008). Recognition and management of treatment-related side effects in breast cancer patients receiving adjuvant endocrine therapy. *Breast Cancer Research and Treatment, 107,* 167–180. doi:10.1007/s10549-007-9548-1

Cheville, A., & Gergich, N. (2004). Lymphedema: Implications for wound care. In P.J. Sheffield, A.P.S. Smith, & C. Fife (Eds.), *Wound care practice* (pp. 285–303). Flagstaff, AZ: Best Publishing Co.

Chikly, B. (2001). *Silent waves: The theory and practice of lymph drainage therapy: With applications for lymphedema, chronic pain, and inflammation.* Scottsdale, AZ: I.H.H. Publishing.

Chlebowski, R.T., & Tagawa, T. (2009). Early breast cancer and prostate cancer and clinical outcomes (fracture). *Oncology, 23*(Suppl. 14), 16–20.

Cinar, N., Seckin, U., Keskin, D., Bodur, H., Bozkurt, B., & Cengiz, O. (2008). The effectiveness of early rehabilitation in patients with modified radical mastectomy. *Cancer Nursing, 31,* 160–165. doi:10.1097/01.NCC.0000305696.12873.0e

Coleman, R.E., Thorpe, H., Cameron, D., Dodwell, D., Burkinshaw, R., Keane, M., ... Bell, R. (2010). Adjuvant treatment with zoledronic acid in stage II/III breast cancer: The AZURE trial: Big 1/04. San Antonio Breast Cancer Symposium, Abstract S4-5.

Collins, B., Mackenzie, J., Stewart, A., Bielajew, C., & Verma, S. (2009). Cognitive effects of chemotherapy in post-menopausal breast cancer patients 1 year after treatment. *Psycho-Oncology, 18,* 134–143. doi:10.1002/pon.1379

Couzi, R.J., Helzlsouer, K.J., & Fetting, J.H. (1995). Prevalence of menopausal symptoms among women with a history of breast cancer and attitudes toward estrogen replacement therapy. *Journal of Clinical Oncology, 13,* 2737–2744.

Curt, G.A., Breitbart, W., Cella, D., Groopman, J.E., Horning, S.J., Itri, L.M., ... Vogelzang, N.J. (2000). Impact of cancer-related fatigue on the lives of patients: New findings from the Fatigue Coalition. *Oncologist, 5,* 353–360.

Cuzick, J., Sestak, I., Cella, D., & Fallowfield, L. (2008). Treatment-emergent endocrine symptoms and the risk of breast cancer recurrence: A retrospective analysis of the ATAC trial. *Lancet Oncology, 9,* 1143–1148. doi:10.1016/S1470-2045(08)70259-6

Delaney, M.F. (2006). Strategies for the prevention and treatment of osteoporosis during early postmenopause. *American*

*Journal of Obstetrics and Gynecology, 194*(Suppl. 2), S12–S23. doi:10.1016/j.ajog.2005.08.049

Dell, D.D., Weaver, C., Kozempel, J., & Barsevick, A. (2008). Recovery after transverse rectus abdominis myocutaneous flap breast reconstruction surgery. *Oncology Nursing Forum, 35,* 189–196. doi:10.1188/08.ONF.189-196

Deng, G., Cassileth, B.R., & Yeung, K.S. (2004). Complementary therapies for cancer-related symptoms. *Journal of Supportive Oncology, 2,* 419–429.

Desmarais, J.E., & Looper, K.J. (2009). Interactions between tamoxifen and antidepressants via cytochrome P450 2D6. *Journal of Clinical Psychiatry, 70,* 1688–1697. doi:10.4088/JCP.08r04856blu

Deutsch, M., & Flickinger, J.C. (2001). Shoulder and arm problems after radiotherapy for primary breast cancer. *American Journal of Clinical Oncology, 24,* 172–176.

Deutsch, M., & Flickinger, J.C. (2003). Patient characteristics and treatment factors affecting cosmesis following lumpectomy and breast irradiation. *American Journal of Clinical Oncology, 26,* 350–353. doi:10.1097/01.COC.0000020589.75948.E7

Dibble, S.L., Casey, K., Nussey, B., Israel, J., & Luce, J. (2004). Chemotherapy-induced vomiting in women treated for breast cancer [Online exclusive]. *Oncology Nursing Forum, 31,* E1–E8. doi:10.1188/04.ONF.E1-E8

Dibble, S.L., Israel, J., Nussey, B., Casey, K., & Luce, J. (2003). Delayed chemotherapy-induced nausea in women treated for breast cancer [Online exclusive]. *Oncology Nursing Forum, 30,* E40–E47. doi:10.1188/03.ONF.E40-E47

Dibble, S.L., Luce, J., Cooper, B.A., Israel, J., Cohen, M., Nussey, B., & Rugo, H. (2007). Acupressure for chemotherapy-induced nausea and vomiting: A randomized clinical trial. *Oncology Nursing Forum, 34,* 813–820. doi:10.1188/07.ONF.813-820

Duff, M., Hill, A.D., McGreal, G., Walsh, S., McDermott, E.W., & O'Higgins, N.J. (2001). Prospective evaluation of the morbidity of axillary clearance for breast cancer. *British Journal of Surgery, 88,* 114–117. doi:10.1046/j.1365-2168.2001.01620.x

Dysesthesia. (n.d.). In *The free dictionary: Medical dictionary.* Retrieved from http://medical-dictionary.thefreedictionary.com/dysesthesia

Eastell, R., Adams, J.E., Coleman, R.E., Howell, A., Hannon, R.A., Cuzick, J., ... Clack, G. (2008). Effect of anastrozole on bone mineral density: 5-year results from the Anastrozole, Tamoxifen, Alone or in Combination Trial 18233230. *Journal of Clinical Oncology, 26,* 1051–1057. doi:10.1200/JCO.2007.11.0726

Eckert, R.M. (2001). Understanding anticipatory nausea. *Oncology Nursing Forum, 28,* 1553–1558.

Elkins, G., Marcus, J., Stearns, V., Perfect, M., Rajab, M.H., Ruud, C., ... Keith, T. (2008). Randomized trial of a hypnosis intervention for treatment of hot flashes among breast cancer survivors. *Journal of Clinical Oncology, 26,* 5022–5026. doi:10.1200/JCO.2008.16.6389

Enomoto, T.M., Johnson, T., Peterson, N., Homer, L., Walts, D., & Johnson, N. (2005). Combination glutathione and anthocyanins as an alternative for skin care during external-beam radiation. *American Journal of Surgery, 189,* 627–630. doi:10.1016/j.amjsurg.2005.02.001

Espie, C.A., Fleming, L., Cassidy, J., Samuel, L., Taylor, L.M., White, C.A., ... Paul, J. (2008). Randomized controlled clinical effectiveness trial of cognitive behavior therapy compared with treatment as usual for persistent insomnia in patients with cancer. *Journal of Clinical Oncology, 26,* 4651–4658. doi:10.1200/JCO.2007.13.9006

Eversley, R., Estrin, D., Dibble, S., Wardlaw, L., Pedrosa, M., & Favila-Penney, W. (2005). Post-treatment symptoms among ethnic minority breast cancer survivors. *Oncology Nursing Forum, 32,* 250–256. doi:10.1188/04.ONF.250-256

Fassoulaki, A., Sarantopoulos, C., Melemeni, A., & Hogan, Q. (2000). EMLA reduces acute and chronic pain after breast surgery for cancer. *Regional Anesthesia and Pain Medicine, 25,* 350–355. doi:10.1053/rapm.2000.7812

Fassoulaki, A., Triga, A., Melemeni, A., & Sarantopoulos, C. (2005). Multimodal analgesia with gabapentin and local anesthetics prevents acute and chronic pain after breast surgery for cancer. *Anesthesia and Analgesia, 101,* 1427–1432. doi:10.1213/01.ANE.0000180200.11626.8E

Feldman, J.L. (2005). The challenge of infection in lymphedema. *LymphLink, 17*(4), 1–2, 27.

Ferguson, R.J., & Ahles, T.A. (2003). Low neuropsychologic performance among adult cancer survivors treated with chemotherapy. *Current Neurology and Neuroscience Reports, 3,* 215–222.

Ferguson, R.J., Ahles, T.A., Saykin, A.J., McDonald, B.C., Furstenberg, C.T., Cole, B.F., & Mott, L.A. (2007). Cognitive-behavioral management of chemotherapy-related cognitive change. *Psycho-Oncology, 16,* 772–777. doi:10.1002/pon.1133

Fillion, L., Gagnon, P., Leblond, F., Gélinas, C., Savard, J., Dupuis, R., ... Larochelle, M. (2008). A brief intervention for fatigue management in breast cancer survivors. *Cancer Nursing, 31,* 145–159. doi:10.1097/01.NCC.0000305698.97625.95

Fisher, J., Scott, C., Stevens, R., Marconi, B., Champion, L., Freedman, G., ... Wong, G. (2000). Randomized phase III study comparing best supportive care to Biafine as a prophylactic agent for radiation-induced skin toxicity for women undergoing breast irradiation: Radiation Therapy Oncology Group (RTOG) 97-13. *International Journal of Radiation Oncology, Biology, Physics, 48,* 1307–1310. doi:10.1016/S0360-3016(00)00782-3

Földi, E., & Földi, M. (2006). Lymphostatic diseases. In M. Földi & E. Földi (Eds.), *Földi's textbook of lymphology for physicians and lymphedema therapists* (2nd ed., pp. 223–319). Munich, Germany: Elsevier GmbH.

Földi, M., & Földi, E. (2006). Physiology and pathology of the lymphatic system. In M. Földi & E. Földi (Eds.), *Földi's textbook of lymphology for physicians and lymphedema therapists* (2nd ed., pp. 179–222). Munich, Germany: Elsevier GmbH.

Friend, P.J., Johnston, M.P., Tipton, J.M., McDaniel, R.W., Barbour, L.A., Starr, P., ... Ripple, M.L. (2009). ONS PEP resource: Chemotherapy-induced nausea and vomiting. In L.H. Eaton & J.M. Tipton (Eds.), *Putting evidence into practice: Improving oncology patient outcomes* (pp. 71–83). Pittsburgh, PA: Oncology Nursing Society.

Ganz, P.A., Greendale, G.A., Petersen, L., Kahn, B., & Bower, J.E. (2003). Breast cancer in younger women: Reproductive and late health effects of treatment. *Journal of Clinical Oncology, 21,* 4184–4193. doi:10.1200/JCO.2003.04.196

Ganz, P.A., Greendale, G.A., Petersen, L., Zibecchi, L., Kahn, B., & Belin, T.R. (2000). Managing menopausal symptoms in breast cancer survivors: Result of a randomized controlled trial. *Journal of the National Cancer Institute, 92,* 1054–1065. doi:10.1093/jnci/92.13.1054

Gärtner, R., Jensen, M.B., Nielsen, J., Ewertz, M., Kroman, N., & Kehlet, H. (2009). Prevalence of and factors associated with persistent pain following breast cancer surgery. *JAMA, 302,* 1985–1992. doi:10.1001/jama.2009.1568

Gass, M., & Dawson-Hughes, B. (2006). Preventing osteoporosis-related fractures: An overview. *American Journal of Medicine, 119*(4, Suppl. 1), S3–S11. doi:10.1016/j.amjmed.2005.12.017

Gélinas, C., & Fillion, L. (2004). Factors related to persistent fatigue following completion of breast cancer treatment. *Oncology Nursing Forum, 31,* 269–278. doi:10.1188/04.ONF.269-278

Ghazinouri, R., Levy, C., Ben-Porat, L., & Stubblefield, M.D. (2005). Shoulder impairments in patients with breast cancer: A retrospective review. *Rehabilitation Oncology, 23*(2), 5–8.

Gnant, M., Mlineritsch, B., Luschin-Ebengreuth, G., Kainberger, F., Kässmann, H., Piswanger- Sölkner, J.C., ... Jakesz, R. (2008). Adjuvant endocrine therapy plus zoledronic acid in premenopausal women with early-stage breast cancer: 5-year follow-up of the ABCSG-12 bone-mineral density substudy. *Lancet Oncology, 9,* 840–849. doi:10.1016/S1470-2045(08)70204-3

Gnant, M., Mlineritsch, B., Schippinger, W., Luschin-Ebengreuth, G., Pöstlberger, S., Menzel, C., ... Greil, R. (2009). Endocrine therapy plus zoledronic acid in premenopausal breast cancer. *New England Journal of Medicine, 360,* 679–691. doi:10.1056/NEJMoa0806285

Goldberg, R.M., Loprinzi, C.L., O'Fallon, J.R., Veeder, M.H., Miser, A.W., Mailliard, J.A., ... Burnham, N.L. (1994). Transdermal clonidine for ameliorating tamoxifen-induced hot flashes. *Journal of Clinical Oncology, 12,* 155–158.

Graham, P., Browne, L., Capp, A., Fox, C., Graham, J., Hollis, J., & Nasser, E. (2004). Randomized, paired comparison of No-Sting Barrier Film versus sorbolene cream (10% glycerine) skin care during postmastectomy irradiation. *International Journal of Radiation Oncology, Biology, Physics, 58,* 241–246. doi:10.1016/S0360-3016(03)01431-7

Grunberg, S.M., Deuson, R.R., Mavros, P., Geling, O., Hansen, M., Cruciani, G., ... Daugaard, G. (2004). Incidence of chemotherapy-induced nausea and emesis after modern antiemetics. *Cancer, 100,* 2261–2268. doi:10.1002/cncr.20230

Guyton, A.C. (1997). The microcirculation and the lymphatic system: Capillary fluid exchange, interstitial fluid dynamics and lymph flow. In A.C. Guyton & J.E. Hall (Eds.), *Human physiology and mechanism of disease* (6th ed., pp. 162–174). Philadelphia, PA: Saunders.

Hadji, P., Body, J.J., Aapro, M.S., Brufsky, A., Coleman, R.E., Guise, T., ... Tubiana-Hulin, M. (2008). Practical guidance for the management of aromatase inhibitor-associated bone loss. *Annals of Oncology, 19,* 1407–1416. doi:10.1093/annonc/mdn164

Hanna, L.R., Avila, P.F., Meteer, J.D., Nicholas, D.R., & Kaminsky, L.A. (2008). The effects of a comprehensive exercise program on physical function, fatigue, and mood in patients with various types of cancer. *Oncology Nursing Forum, 35,* 461–469. doi:10.1188/08.ONF.461-469

Headley, J.A., Ownby, K.K., & John, L.D. (2004). The effect of seated exercise on fatigue and quality of life in women with advanced breast cancer. *Oncology Nursing Forum, 31,* 977–983. doi:10.1188/04.ONF.977-983

Heggie, S., Bryant, G.P., Tripcony, L., Keller, J., Rose, P., Glendenning, M., & Heath, J. (2002). A phase III study on the efficacy of topical aloe vera gel on irradiated breast tissue. *Cancer Nursing, 25,* 442–451.

Helms, G., Kühn, T., Moser, L., Remmel, E., & Kreienberg, R. (2009). Shoulder-arm morbidity in patients with sentinel node biopsy and complete axillary dissection—Data from a prospective randomised trial. *European Journal of Surgical Oncology, 35,* 696–701. doi:10.1016/j.ejso.2008.06.013

Henry, N.L., Rae, J.M., Li, L., Azzouz, F., Skaar, T.C., Desta, Z., ... Stearns, V. (2009). Association between CYP2D6 genotype and tamoxifen-induced hot flashes in a prospective cohort. *Breast Cancer Research and Treatment, 117,* 571–575. doi:10.1007/s10549-009-0309-1

Hermelink, K., Henschel, V., Untch, M., Bauerfeind, I., Lux, M.P., & Munzel, K. (2008). Short-term effects of treatment-induced hormonal changes on cognitive function in breast cancer patients. *Cancer, 113,* 2431–2439. doi:10.1002/cncr.23853

Herrstedt, J., Muss, H.B., Warr, D.G., Hesketh, P.J., Eisenberg, P.D., Raftopoulos, H., ... Skobieranda, F. (2005). Efficacy and tolerability of aprepitant for the prevention of chemotherapy-induced nausea and emesis over multiple cycles of moderately emetogenic chemotherapy. *Cancer, 104,* 1548–1555. doi:10.1002/cncr.21343

Hervik, J., & Mjåland, O. (2009). Acupuncture for the treatment of hot flashes in breast cancer patients, a randomized, controlled trial. *Breast Cancer Research and Treatment, 116,* 311–316. doi:10.1007/s10549-008-0210-3

Hillner, B.E., Ingle, J.N., Chlebowski, R.T., Gralow, J., Yee, G.C., Janjan, N.A., ... Brown, S. (2003). American Society of Clinical Oncology 2003 update on the role of bisphosphonates and bone health issues in women with breast cancer. *Journal of Clinical Oncology, 21,* 4042–4057. doi:10.1200/JCO.2003.08.017 [Erratum at doi:10.1200/JCO.2004.02.910]

Holick, M.F., & Chen, T.C. (2008). Vitamin D deficiency: A worldwide problem with health consequences. *American Journal of Clinical Nutrition, 87,* 1080S–1086S.

Howlader, N., Noone, A.M., Krapcho, M., Neyman, N., Aminou, R., Waldron, W., ... Edwards, B.K. (Eds.). (2011). SEER cancer statistics review, 1975–2008. Retrieved from http://seer.cancer.gov/csr/1975_2008

Hsieh, C.C., Sprod, L.K., Hydock, D.S., Carter, S.D., Hayward, R., & Schneider, C.M. (2008). Effects of supervised exercise intervention on recovery from treatment regimens in breast cancer survivors. *Oncology Nursing Forum, 35,* 909–915. doi:10.1188/08.ONF.909-915

Huberty, J.L., Vener, J., Waltman, N., Ott, C., Twiss, J., Gross, G., ... Dwyer, A. (2009). Development of an instrument to measure adherence to strength training in postmenopausal breast cancer survivors. *Oncology Nursing Forum, 36,* E266–E273. doi:10.1188/09.ONF.E266-E273

Hwang, J.H., Chang, H.J., Shim, Y.H., Park, W.H., Park, W., Huh, S.J., & Yang, J.H. (2008). Effects of supervised exercise therapy in patients receiving radiotherapy for breast cancer. *Yonsei Medical Journal, 49,* 443–450. doi:10.3349/ymj.2008.49.3.443

Inagaki, M., Yoshikawa, E., Matsuoka, Y., Sugawara, Y., Nakano, T., Akechi, T., ... Uchitomi, Y. (2006). Smaller regional volumes of brain gray and white matter demonstrated in breast cancer survivors exposed to adjuvant chemotherapy. *Cancer, 109,* 146–156. doi:10.1002/cncr.22368

Indelicato, D.J., Grobmyer, S.R., Newlin, H., Morris, C.G., Haigh, L.S., Copeland, E.M., III, & Mendenhall, N.P. (2006). Delayed breast cellulites: An evolving complication of breast conservation. *International Journal of Radiation Oncology, Biology, Physics, 66,* 1339–1346. doi:10.1016/j.ijrobp.2006.07.1388

Inomata, T., Narabayashi, I., Inada, Y., Shimbo, T., Takahashi, M., Tatsumi, T., ... Ogawa, Y. (2008). Patients' subjective evaluation of early and late sequelae in patients with breast cancer irradiated with short fractionation for breast conservation therapy: Comparison with conventional fractionation. *Breast Cancer, 15,* 93–100. doi:10.1007/s12282-007-0011-2

International Society of Lymphology. (2003). The diagnosis and treatment of peripheral lymphedema. Consensus document of the International Society of Lymphology. *Lymphology, 36,* 84–91.

Jacobsen, P.B., Donovan, K.A., Small, B.J., Jim, H.S., Munster, P.N., & Andrykowski, M.A. (2007). Fatigue after treatment for early stage breast cancer: A controlled comparison. *Cancer, 110,* 1851–1859. doi:10.1002/cncr.22993

Jansen, C., Miaskowski, C., Dodd, M., Dowling, G., & Kramer, J. (2005). Potential mechanisms for chemotherapy-induced impairments in cognitive function. *Oncology Nursing Forum, 32,* 1151–1163. doi:10.1188/04.ONF.1151-1163

Jansen, C.E., Miaskowski, C., Dodd, M., & Dowling, G. (2005). Chemotherapy-induced cognitive impairment in women with breast cancer: A critique of the literature. *Oncology Nursing Forum, 32,* 329–342. doi:10.1188/04.ONF.329-342

Jenkins, V., Shilling, V., Deutsch, G., Bloomfield, D., Morris, R., Allan, S., ... Winstanley, J. (2006). A 3-year prospective study of the effects of adjuvant treatment on cognition in women with early stage breast cancer. *British Journal of Cancer, 94,* 828–834. doi:10.1038/sj.bjc.6603029

Jim, H.S., Donovan, K.A., Small, B.J., Andrykowski, M.A., Munster, P.N., & Jacobsen, P.B. (2009). Cognitive functioning in breast cancer survivors: A controlled comparison. *Cancer, 115,* 1776–1783. doi:10.1002/cncr.24192

Jones, S., Stokoe, C., Sborov, M., Braun, M., Ethirajan, S., Kutteh, L., ... Asmar, L. (2008). The effect of tamoxifen or exemestane on bone mineral density during the first 2 years of adjuvant treatment of postmenopausal women with early breast cancer. *Clinical Breast Cancer, 8,* 527–532. doi:10.3816/CBC.2008.n.065

Jordan, V.C. (2007). SERMs: Meeting the promise of multifunctional medicines. *Journal of the National Cancer Institute, 99,* 350–356. doi:10.1093/jnci/djk062

Jud, S.M., Fasching, P.A., Maihöfner, C., Heusinger, K., Loehberg, C.R., Hatko, R., ... Bani, M.R. (2010). Pain perception and detailed visual pain mapping in breast cancer survivors. *Breast Cancer Research and Treatment, 119,* 105–110. doi:10.1007/s10549-009-0485-z

Kairaluoma, P.M., Bachmann, M.S., Rosenberg, P.H., & Pere, P.J. (2006). Preincisional paravertebral block reduces the prevalence of chronic pain after breast surgery. *Anesthesia and Analgesia, 103,* 703–708. doi:10.1213/01.ane.0000230603.92574.4e

Kalso, E., Tasmuth, T., & Neuvonen, P.J. (1996). Amitriptyline effectively relieves neuropathic pain following treatment of breast cancer. *Pain, 64,* 293–302. doi:10.1016/0304-3959(95)00138-7

Kaplan, M., Mahon, S., Cope, D., Hill, S., Keating, E., & Jacobson, M. (2011). ONS PEP resource: Hot flashes. In L.H. Eaton, J.M. Tipton, & M. Irwin (Eds.), *Putting evidence into practice: Improving oncology patient outcomes, volume 2* (pp. 39–48). Pittsburgh, PA: Oncology Nursing Society.

Kärki, A., Simonen, R., Mälkiä, E., & Selfe, J. (2005). Impairments, activity limitations and participation restrictions 6 and 12 months after breast cancer operation. *Journal of Rehabilitation Medicine, 37,* 180–188. doi:10.1080/16501970410024181

Katz, J., Poleshuck, E.L., Andrus, C.H., Hogan, L.A., Jung, B.F., Kulick, D.I., & Dworkin, R.H. (2005). Risk factors for acute pain and its persistence following breast cancer surgery. *Pain, 119,* 16–25. doi:10.1016/j.pain.2005.09.008

Kaufman, S.A., DiPetrillo, T.A., Price, L.L., Midle, J.B., & Wazer, D.E. (2007). Long-term outcome and toxicity in a phase I/II trial using high-dose-rate multicatheter interstitial brachytherapy for T1/T2 breast cancer. *Brachytherapy, 6,* 286–293. doi:10.1016/j.brachy.2007.09.001

Kelly, D.G. (2002). *A primer on lymphedema.* Upper Saddle River, NJ: Prentice Hall.

Khan, Q.J., Reddy, P.S., Kimler, B.F., Sharma, P., Baxa, S.E., O'Dea, A.P., ... Fabian, C.J. (2010). Effect of vitamin D supplementation on serum 25-hydroxy vitamin D levels, joint pain, and fatigue in women starting adjuvant letrozole treatment for breast cancer. *Breast Cancer Research and Treatment, 119,* 111–118. doi:10.1007/s10549-009-0495-x

Kim, S.C., Kim, D.W., Moadel, R.M., Kim, C.K., Chatterjee, S., Shafir, M.K., ... Krynyckyi, B.R. (2005). Using the intraoperative hand held probe without lymphoscintigraphy or using only dye correlates with higher sensory morbidity following sentinel lymph node biopsy in breast cancer: A review of the literature [Electronic version]. *World Journal of Surgical Oncology, 3,* 64. doi:10.1186/1477-7819-3-64

King, C.R. (1997). Nonpharmacologic management of chemotherapy-induced nausea and vomiting. *Oncology Nursing Forum, 24*(Suppl. 7), 41–48.

Knobf, M.T. (2002). Carrying on: The experience of premature menopause in women with early stage breast cancer. *Nursing Research, 51,* 9–17.

Knobf, M.T., & Sun, Y. (2005). A longitudinal study of symptoms and self-care activities in women treated with primary radiotherapy for breast cancer. *Cancer Nursing, 28,* 210–218.

Ko, D.S.C., Lerner, R., Klose, G., & Cosimi, A.B. (1998). Effective treatment of lymphedema of the extremities. *Archives of Surgery, 133,* 452–458.

Kohli, S., Fisher, S.G., Tra, Y., Adams, M.J., Mapstone, M.E., Wesnes, K.A., ... Morrow, G.R. (2009). The effect of modafinil on cognitive function in breast cancer survivors. *Cancer, 115,* 2605–2616. doi:10.1002/cncr.24287

Koul, R., Dufan, T., Russell, C., Guenther, W., Nugent, Z., Sun, X., & Cooke, A.L. (2007). Efficacy of complete decongestive therapy and manual lymphatic drainage on treatment-related lymphedema in breast cancer. *International Journal of Radiation Oncology, Biology, Physics, 67,* 841–846. doi:10.1016/j.ijrobp.2006.09.024

Kronenberg, F. (1990). Hot flashes: Epidemiology and physiology. *Annals of the New York Academy of Sciences, 592,* 52–86. doi:10.1111/j.1749-6632.1990.tb30316.x

Kronenberg, F., & Fugh-Berman, A. (2002). Complementary and alternative medicine for menopausal symptoms: A review of randomized, controlled trials. *Annals of Internal Medicine, 137,* 805–813.

Kudel, I., Edwards, R.R., Kozachik, S., Block, B.M., Agarwal, S., Heinberg, L.J., ... Raja, S.N. (2007). Predictors and consequences of multiple persistent postmastectomy pains. *Journal of Pain and Symptom Management, 34,* 619–627. doi:10.1016/j.jpainsymman.2007.01.013

Kuehn, B.M. (2005). Better osteoporosis management a priority: Impact predicted to soar with aging population. *JAMA, 293,* 2453–2458. doi:10.1001/jama.293.20.2453

Lacomba, M.T., Del Moral, O.M., Zazo, J.L.C., Sánchez, M.J.Y., Ferrandez, J.C., & Goñi, A.Z. (2009). Axillary web syndrome after axillary dissection in breast cancer: A prospective study. *Breast Cancer Research and Treatment, 117,* 625–630. doi:10.1007/s10549-009-0371-8

Langer, I., Guller, U., Berclaz, G., Koechli, O.R., Schaer, G., Fehr, M.K., ... Zuber, M. (2007). Morbidity of sentinel lymph node biopsy (SLN) alone versus SLN and completion axillary lymph node dissection after breast cancer surgery: A prospective Swiss multicenter study on 659 patients. *Annals of Surgery, 245,* 452–461. doi:10.1097/01.sla.0000245472.47748.ec

Layeeque, R., Hochberg, J., Siegel, E., Kunkel, K., Kepple, J., Henry-Tillman, R.S., ... Klimberg, V.S. (2004). Botulinum toxin infiltration for pain control after mastectomy and expander reconstruction. *Annals of Surgery, 240,* 608–614.

Lee, J., Dodd, M.J., Dibble, S.L., & Abrams, D.I. (2008). Nausea at the end of adjuvant cancer treatment in relation to exercise during treatment in patients with breast cancer. *Oncology Nursing Forum, 35,* 830–835. doi:10.1188/08.ONF.830-835

Lee, T.S., Kilbreath, S.L., Sullivan, G., Refshauge, K.M., & Beith, J.M. (2010). Patient perceptions of arm care and exercise advice after breast cancer surgery. *Oncology Nursing Forum, 37,* 85–91. doi:10.1188/10.ONF.85-91

Lerner, R. (2000). Chronic lymphedema. In J.B. Chang, E. Olsen, P. Kailash, & B. Sumpio (Eds.), *Textbook of angiology* (pp. 1227–1236). New York, NY: Springer.

Liguori, V., Guillemin, C., Pesce, G.F., Mirimanoff, R.O., & Bernier, J. (1997). Double-blind, randomized clinical study comparing hyaluronic acid cream to placebo in patients treated with radiotherapy. *Radiotherapy and Oncology, 42,* 155–161. doi:10.1016/S0167-8140(96)01882-8

Lipov, E.G., Joshi, J.R., Sanders, S., Wilcox, K., Lipov, S., Xie, H., ... Slavin, K. (2008). Effects of stellate-ganglion block on hot flushes and night awakenings in survivors of breast cancer: A pilot study. *Lancet Oncology, 9,* 523–532. doi:10.1016/S1470-2045(08)70131-1

Lønning, P.E. (2008). Endocrine therapy and bone loss in breast cancer: Time to close in the RANK(L)? *Journal of Clinical Oncology, 26,* 4859–4861. doi:10.1200/JCO.2008.18.0851

Loprinzi, C.L., Barton, D.L., Sloan, J.A., Zahasky, K.M., Smith, D.A., Pruthi, S., … Christensen, B.J. (2002). Pilot evaluation of gabapentin for treating hot flashes. *Mayo Clinic Proceedings, 77,* 1159–1163. doi:10.4065/77.11.1159

Loprinzi, C.L., Kugler, J.W., Sloan, J.A., Mailliard, J.A., La Vasseur, B.I., Barton, D.L., … Christensen, B.J. (2000). Venlafaxine in management of hot flashes in survivors of breast cancer: A randomised controlled trial. *Lancet, 356,* 2059–2063. doi:10.1016/S0140-6736(00)03403-6

Loprinzi, C.L., Sloan, J.A., Perez, E.A., Quella, S.K., Stella, P.J., Mailliard, J.A., … Rummans, T.A. (2002). Phase III evaluation of fluoxetine for treatment of hot flashes. *Journal of Clinical Oncology, 20,* 1578–1583. doi:10.1200/JCO.20.6.1578

Lower, E.E., Fleishman, S., Cooper, A., Zeldis, J., Faleck, H., Yu, Z., & Manning, D. (2009). Efficacy of dexmethylphenidate for the treatment of fatigue after cancer chemotherapy: A randomized clinical trial. *Journal of Pain and Symptom Management, 38,* 650–662. doi:10.1016/j.jpainsymman.2009.03.011

Lymphology Association of North America. (2005). *Certification makes a difference.* Wilmette, IL: Author.

Macdonald, L., Bruce, J., Scott, N.W., Smith, W.C., & Chambers, W.A. (2005). Long-term follow up of breast cancer survivors with post-mastectomy pain syndrome. *British Journal of Cancer, 92,* 225–230. doi:10.1038/sj.bjc.6602304

MacLean, C., Newberry, S., Maglione, M., McMahon, M., Ranganath, V., Suttorp, M., … Grossman, J. (2008). Systematic review: Comparative effectiveness of treatments to prevent fractures in men and women with low bone density or osteoporosis. *Annals of Internal Medicine, 148,* 197–213.

Magnan, M.A., & Mood, D.W. (2003). The effects of health state, hemoglobin, global symptom distress, mood disturbance, and treatment site on fatigue onset, duration, and distress in patients receiving radiation therapy [Online exclusive]. *Oncology Nursing Forum, 30,* E33–E39. doi:10.1188/03.ONF.E33-E39

Maiche, A., Isokangas, O., & Gröhn, P. (1994). Skin protection by sucralfate cream during electron beam therapy. *Acta Oncologica, 33,* 201–203.

Mar Fan, H.G., Clemons, M., Xu, W., Chemerynsky, I., Breunis, H., Braganza, S., & Tannock, I.F. (2008). A randomised, placebo-controlled, double-blind trial of the effects of d-methylphenidate on fatigue and cognitive dysfunction in women undergoing adjuvant chemotherapy for breast cancer. *Supportive Care in Cancer, 16,* 577–583. doi:10.1007/s00520-007-0341-9

Mar Fan, H.G., Houédé-Tchen, N., Chemerynsky, I., Yi, Q.L., Xu, W., Harvey, B., & Tannock, I.F. (2009). Menopausal symptoms in women undergoing chemotherapy-induced and natural menopause: A prospective controlled study. *Annals in Oncology, 21,* 983–987. doi:10.1093/annonc/mdp394

Marrs, J. (2007). Lymphedema and implications for oncology nursing practice. *Clinical Journal of Oncology Nursing, 11,* 19–21. doi:10.1188/07.CJON.19-21

Masferrer, J.P., Mejía, M.M., Fernández, M.V., Astudillo, A.A., Armenteros, M.L.H., Hernández, V.M., … Ferre, A.M. (2010). Prophylaxis with a cream containing urea reduces the incidence and severity of radio-induced dermatitis. *Clinical and Translational Oncology, 12,* 43–48.

Maxwell, C., & Viale, P.H. (2005). Cancer treatment-induced bone loss in patients with breast or prostate cancer. *Oncology Nursing Forum, 32,* 589–601. doi:10.1188/04.ONF.589-603

McAnaw, M.B., & Harris, K.W. (2002). The role of physical therapy in the rehabilitation of patients with mastectomy and breast reconstruction. *Breast Disease, 16,* 163–174.

McCredie, M.R.E., Dite, G.S., Porter, L., Maskiell, J., Giles, G.G., Phillips, K.-A., … Hopper, J.L. (2001). Prevalence of self-reported arm morbidity following treatment for breast cancer in the Australian Breast Cancer Family Study. *Breast, 10,* 515–522. doi:10.1054/brst.2000.0291

McQuestion, M. (2006). Evidence-based skin care management in radiation therapy. *Seminars in Oncology Nursing, 22,* 163–173. doi:10.1016/j.soncn.2006.04.004

McQuestion, M. (2010). Radiation-induced skin reactions. In M.L. Haas & G.J. Moore-Higgs (Eds.), *Principles of skin care and the oncology patient* (pp. 115–139). Pittsburgh, PA: Oncology Nursing Society.

Mitchell, S.A. (2009). Cancer-related fatigue. In C.G. Brown (Ed.), *A guide to oncology symptom management* (pp. 271–297). Pittsburgh, PA: Oncology Nursing Society.

Mitchell, S.A., Beck, S.L., Hood, L.E., Moore, K., & Tanner, E.R. (2009). ONS PEP resource: Fatigue. In L.H. Eaton & J.M. Tipton (Eds.), *Putting evidence into practice: Improving oncology patient outcomes* (pp. 155–174). Pittsburgh, PA: Oncology Nursing Society.

Mock, V., & Olsen, M. (2003). Current management of fatigue and anemia in patients with cancer. *Seminars in Oncology Nursing, 19*(4, Suppl. 2), 36–41.

Mock, V., Pickett, M., Ropka, M.E., Lin, E.M., Stewart, K.J., Rhodes, V.A., … McCorkle, R. (2001). Fatigue and quality of life outcomes of exercise during cancer treatment. *Cancer Practice, 9,* 119–127. doi:10.1046/j.1523-5394.2001.009003119.x

Moller, J.F., Nikolajsen, L., Rodt, S.A., Ronning, H., & Carlsson, P.S. (2007). Thoracic paravertebral block for breast cancer surgery: A randomized double-blind study. *Anesthesia and Analgesia, 105,* 1848–1851. doi:10.1213/01.ane.0000286135.21333.fd

Morimoto, T., Tamura, A., Ichihara, T., Minakawa, T., Kuwamura, Y., Miki, Y., & Sasa, M. (2003). Evaluation of a new rehabilitation program for postoperative patients with breast cancer. *Nursing and Health Sciences, 5,* 275–282. doi:10.1046/j.1442-2018.2003.00163.x

Morrison, J.E., Jr., & Jacobs, V.R. (2003). Reduction or elimination of postoperative pain medication after mastectomy through use of temporarily placed local anesthetic pump vs. control group. *Zentralblatt für Gynäkologie, 125,* 17–22.

Morrow, G.R., Ryan, J.L., & Kohli, S. (2006). Modafinil (Provigil®) for persistent post-treatment fatigue: An open label study of 82 women with breast cancer. *MASCC International Symposia,* Abstract No. 11-070.

Mota, D.D., & Pimenta, C.A. (2006). Self-report instruments for fatigue assessment: A systematic review. *Research and Theory for Nursing Practice, 20,* 49–78.

Moyad, M.A. (2008). Vitamin D: A rapid review. *Urologic Nursing, 28,* 343–349.

Mulrooney, T. (2008). Cognitive impairment after breast cancer. *Clinical Journal of Oncology Nursing, 12,* 678–680. doi:10.1188/08.CJON.678-680

Muscari, E. (2004). Lymphedema: Responding to our patients' needs. *Oncology Nursing Forum, 31,* 905–912. doi:10.1188/04.ONF.905-912

Mustian, K.M., Sprod, L.K., Palesh, O.G., Peppone, L.J., Janelsins, M.C., Mohile, S.G., & Carroll, J. (2009). Exercise for the management of side effects and quality of life among cancer survivors. *Current Sports Medicine Reports, 8,* 325–330. doi:10.1249/JSR.0b013e3181c22324

Nail, L. (2002). Fatigue in patients with cancer. *Oncology Nursing Forum, 29,* 537–545. doi:10.1188/ONF.537-546

National Cancer Institute. (2007). Radiation therapy and you: A guide to self-help during cancer treatment. Retrieved from http://www.cancer.gov/cancertopics/radiation-therapy-and-you

National Comprehensive Cancer Network. (2010a). *NCCN Clinical Practice Guidelines in Oncology™: Adult cancer pain* [v.1.2010]. Retrieved from http://www.nccn.org/professionals/physician_gls/pdf/pain.pdf

National Comprehensive Cancer Network. (2010b). *NCCN Clinical Practice Guidelines in Oncology™: Breast cancer risk reduction* [v.2.2010]. Retrieved from http://www.nccn.org/professionals/physician_gls/PDF/breast_risk.pdf

National Comprehensive Cancer Network. (2010c). *NCCN Clinical Practice Guidelines in Oncology™: Cancer- and chemotherapy-induced anemia* [v.2.2011]. Retrieved from http://www.nccn.org/professionals/physician_gls/PDF/anemia.pdf

National Comprehensive Cancer Network. (2010d). *NCCN Clinical Practice Guidelines in Oncology™: Cancer-related fatigue* [v.1.2011]. Retrieved from http://www.nccn.org/professionals/physician_gls/PDF/fatigue.pdf

National Comprehensive Cancer Network. (2011). *NCCN Clinical Practice Guidelines in Oncology™: Antiemesis* [v.1.2011]. Retrieved from http://www.nccn.org/professionals/physician_gls/PDF/antiemesis.pdf

National Lymphedema Network Medical Advisory Committee. (2005). Position statement of the National Lymphedema Network. Topic: Training of lymphedema therapists. Retrieved from http://www.lymphnet.org/pdfDocs/nlntraining.pdf

National Lymphedema Network Medical Advisory Committee. (2008a). Position statement of the National Lymphedema Network. Topic: Air travel. Retrieved from http://www.lymphnet.org/pdfDocs/nlnairtravel.pdf

National Lymphedema Network Medical Advisory Committee. (2008b). Position statement of the National Lymphedema Network. Topic: Exercise. Retrieved from http://www.lymphnet.org/pdfDocs/nlnexercise.pdf

National Lymphedema Network Medical Advisory Committee. (2008c). Position statement of the National Lymphedema Network. Topic: Lymphedema risk reduction practices. Retrieved from http://www.lymphnet.org/pdfDocs/nlnriskreduction.pdf

National Osteoporosis Foundation. (2010). *Clinician's guide to prevention and treatment of osteoporosis.* Retrieved from http://www.nof.org/sites/default/files/pdfs/NOF_ClinicianGuide2009_v7.pdf

Nedstrand, E., Wijman, K., Wyon, Y., & Hammar, M. (2005). Vasomotor symptoms decrease in women with breast cancer randomized to treatment with applied relaxation or electroacupuncture: A preliminary study. *Climacteric, 8,* 243–250. doi:10.1080/13697130500118050

Nedstrand, E., Wyon, Y., Hammar, M., & Wijman, K. (2006). Psychological well-being improves in women with breast cancer after treatment with applied relaxation or electroacupuncture for vasomotor symptoms. *Journal of Psychosomatic Obstetrics and Gynaecology, 27,* 193–199.

Nieboer, P., Buijs, C., Rodenhuis, S., Seynaeve, C., Beex, L.V., van der Wall, E., ... de Vries, E.G. (2005). Fatigue and relating factors in high-risk breast cancer patients treated with adjuvant standard or high-dose chemotherapy: A longitudinal study. *Journal of Clinical Oncology, 23,* 8296–8304. doi:10.1200/JCO.2005.10.167

Nystedt, K.E., Hill, J.E., Mitchell, A.M., Goodwin, F., Rowe, L.A., Wong, F.L., & Kind, A.L. (2005). The standardization of radiation skin care in British Columbia: A collaborative approach. *Oncology Nursing Forum, 32,* 1199–1205. doi:10.1188/04.ONF. 1199-1205

Okhuma, M. (1990). Cellulitis seen in lymphoedema. In M. Mishi, S. Uchino, & S. Yabukis (Eds.), *Progress in lymphology XII. Excerpto medica, International Congress Series 887* (pp. 401–402). Amsterdam, Netherlands: Elsevier.

Okumura, S., Mitsumori, M., Kokubo, M., Yamauchi, C., Kawamura, S., Oya, N., ... Hiraoka, M. (2003). Late skin and subcutaneous soft tissue changes after 10-Gy boost for breast conserving therapy. *Breast Cancer, 10,* 129–133.

Olsen, D.L., Raub, W., Jr., Bradley, C., Johnson, M., Macias, J.L., Love, V., & Markoe, A. (2001). The effect of aloe vera gel/mild soap versus mild soap alone in preventing skin reactions in patients undergoing radiation therapy. *Oncology Nursing Forum, 28,* 543–547.

Osborne, C.R., Duncan, A., Sedlacek, S., Paul, D., Holmes, F., Vukelja, S., ... O'Shaughnessy, J.A. (2009). The addition of hormone therapy to tamoxifen does not prevent hot flashes in women at high risk for developing breast cancer. *Breast Cancer Research and Treatment, 116,* 521–527. doi:10.1007/s10549-008-0284-y

O'Shaughnessy, J.A., Vukelja, S.J., Holmes, F.A., Savin, M., Jones, M., Royall, D., ... Von Hoff, D. (2005). Feasibility of quantifying the effects of epoetin alfa therapy on cognitive function in women with breast cancer undergoing adjuvant or neoadjuvant chemotherapy. *Clinical Breast Cancer, 5,* 439–446.

Palesh, O.G., Roscoe, J.A., Mustian, K.M., Roth, T., Savard, J., Ancoli-Israel, S., ... Morrow, G.R. (2010). Prevalence, demographics, and psychological associations of sleep disruption in patients with cancer: University of Rochester Cancer Center–Community Clinical Oncology Program. *Journal of Clinical Oncology, 28,* 292–298. doi:10.1200/JCO.2009.22.5011

Payne, J.K., Held, J., Thorpe, J., & Shaw, H. (2008). Effect of exercise on biomarkers, fatigue, sleep disturbances, and depressive symptoms in older women with breast cancer receiving hormonal therapy. *Oncology Nursing Forum, 35,* 635–642. doi:10.1188/08.ONF.635-642

Perera, F., Chisela, F., Stitt, L., Engel, J., & Venkatesan, V. (2005). TLD skin dose measurements and acute and late effects after lumpectomy and high-dose rate brachytherapy only for early breast cancer. *International Journal of Radiation Oncology, Biology, Physics, 62,* 1283–1290. doi:10.1016/j.ijrobp.2005.01.007

Petrek, J.A., Peters, M.M., Nori, S., Knauer, C., Kinne, D.W., & Rogatko, A. (1990). Axillary lymphadenectomy. A prospective, randomized trial of 13 factors influencing drainage, including early or delayed arm mobilization. *Archives of Surgery, 125,* 378–382.

Pfeilschifter, J., & Diel, I.J. (2000). Osteoporosis due to cancer treatment: Pathogenesis and management. *Journal of Clinical Oncology, 18,* 1570–1593.

Phillips, K.A., & Bernhard, J. (2003). Adjuvant breast cancer treatment and cognitive function: Current knowledge and research directions. *Journal of the National Cancer Institute, 95,* 190–197. doi:10.1093/jnci/95.3.190

Pignol, J.P., Olivotto, I., Rakovitch, E., Gardner, S., Sixel, K., Beckham, W., ... Paszat, L. (2008). A multicenter randomized trial of breast intensity modulated radiation therapy to reduce acute radiation dermatitis. *Journal of Clinical Oncology, 26,* 2085–2092. doi:10.1200/JCO.2007.15.2488

Polovich, M., White, J.M., & Olsen, M. (Eds.). (2009). *Chemotherapy and biotherapy guidelines and recommendations for practice* (3rd ed.). Pittsburgh, PA: Oncology Nursing Society.

Pommier, P., Gomez, F., Sunyach, M.P., D'Hombres, A., Carrie, C., & Montbarbon, X. (2004). Phase III randomized trial of Calendula officinalis compared with trolamine for the prevention of acute dermatitis during irradiation for breast cancer. *Journal of Clinical Oncology, 22,* 1447–1453. doi:10.1200/JCO.2004.07.063

Póti, Z., Nemeskéri, C., Fekésházy, A., Sáfrány, G., Bajzik, G., Nagy, Z.P., ... Esik, O. (2004). Partial breast irradiation with interstitial 60 CO brachytherapy results in frequent grade 3 or 4 toxicity. Evidence based on a 12-year follow-up of 70 patients. *International Journal of Radiation Oncology, Biology, Physics, 58,* 1022–1033. doi:10.1016/j.ijrobp.2003.08.013

Powles, T.J., Hickish, T., Kanis, J.A., Tidy, A., & Ashley, S. (1996). Effect of tamoxifen on bone mineral density measured by dual-energy x-ray absorptiometry in healthy premenopausal and post-menopausal women. *Journal of Clinical Oncology, 14*, 78–84.

Pritchard, K.I. (2001). Hormone replacement in women with a history of breast cancer. *Oncologist, 6*, 353–362.

Quesnel, C., Savard, J., & Ivers, H. (2009). Cognitive impairments associated with breast cancer treatments: Results from a longitudinal study. *Breast Cancer Research and Treatment, 116*, 113–123. doi:10.1007/s10549-008-0114-2

Rabaglio, M., Sun, Z., Price, K.N., Castiglione-Gertsch, M., Hawle, H., Thürlimann, B., … Coates, A.S. (2009). Bone fractures among postmenopausal patients with endocrine-responsive early breast cancer treated with 5 years of letrozole or tamoxifen in the BIG 1-98 trial. *Annals of Oncology, 20*, 1489–1498. doi:10.1093/annonc/mdp033

Ramaswamy, B., & Shapiro, C.L. (2003). Osteopenia and osteoporosis in women with breast cancer. *Seminars in Oncology, 30*, 763–775. doi:10.1053/j.seminoncol.2003.08.028

Reeder, R., Carter, D.L., Howell, K., Henkenberns, P., Tallhamer, M., Johnson, T., … Leonard, C.E. (2009). Predictors for clinical outcomes after accelerated partial breast intensity-modulated radiotherapy. *International Journal of Radiation Oncology, Biology, Physics, 74*, 92–97. doi:10.1016/j.ijrobp.2008.06.1917

Reid, I.R., Brown, J.P., Burckhardt, P., Horowitz, Z., Richardson, P., Trechsel, U., … Meunier, P.J. (2002). Intravenous zoledronic acid in postmenopausal women with low bone mineral density. *New England Journal of Medicine, 346*, 653–661. doi:10.1056/NEJMoa011807

Reuben, S.S., Makari-Judson, G., & Lurie, S.D. (2004). Evaluation of efficacy of the perioperative administration of venlafaxine XR in the prevention of postmastectomy pain syndrome. *Journal of Pain and Symptom Management, 27*, 133–139. doi:10.1016/j.jpainsymman.2003.06.004

Rietman, J.S., Dijkstra, P.U., Hoekstra, H.J., Eisma, W.H., Szabo, B.G., Groothoff, J.W., & Geertzen, J.H. (2003). Late morbidity after treatment of breast cancer in relation to daily activities and quality of life: A systematic review. *European Journal of Surgical Oncology, 29*, 229–238. doi:10.1053/ejso.2002.1403

Rogers, L.Q., Shah, P., Dunnington, G., Greive, A., Shanmugham, A., Dawson, B., & Courneya, K.S. (2005). Social cognitive theory and physical activity during breast cancer treatment. *Oncology Nursing Forum, 32*, 807–815. doi:10.1188/04.ONF.807-815

Roscoe, J.A., Bushunow, P., Morrow, G.R., Hickok, J.T., Kuebler, P.J., Jacobs, A., & Banerjee, T.K. (2004). Patient expectation is strong predictor of severe nausea after chemotherapy. *Cancer, 101*, 2701–2708. doi:10.1002/cncr.20718

Rowland, J.H., Desmond, K.A., Meyerowitz, B.E., Belin, T.R., Wyatt, G.E., & Ganz, P.A. (2000). Role of breast reconstructive surgery in physical and emotional outcomes among breast cancer survivors. *Journal of the National Cancer Institute, 92*, 1422–1429. doi:10.1093/jnci/92.17.1422

Royer, H.R., Phelan, C.H., & Heidrich, S.M. (2009). Older breast cancer survivors' symptom beliefs. *Oncology Nursing Forum, 36*, 463–470. doi:10.1188/09.ONF.463-470

Rugo, H.S., & Ahles, T. (2003). The impact of adjuvant therapy for breast cancer on cognitive function: Current evidence and directions for research. *Seminars in Oncology, 30*, 749–762. doi:10.1053/j.seminoncol.2003.09.008

Ryan, J.L., Heckler, C., Dakhil, S.R., Kirshner, J., Flynn, P.J., Hickok, J.T., & Morrow, G.R. (2009). Ginger for chemotherapy-related nausea in cancer patients: A URCC CCOP randomized, double-blind, placebo-controlled clinical trial of 644 cancer patients. *Journal of Clinical Oncology, 27*(Suppl. 15), Abstract No. 9511.

Saad, F., Adachi, J.D., Brown, J.P., Canning, L.A., Gelmon, K.A., Josse, R.G., & Pritchard, K.I. (2008). Cancer treatment-induced bone loss in breast and prostate cancer. *Journal of Clinical Oncology, 26*, 5465–5476. doi:10.1200/JCO.2008.18.4184

Saarto, T., Vehmanen, L., Blomqvist, C., & Elomaa, I. (2008). Ten-year follow-up of 3 years of oral adjuvant clodronate therapy shows significant prevention of osteoporosis in early-stage breast cancer. *Journal of Clinical Oncology, 26*, 4289–4295. doi:10.1200/JCO.2007.15.4997

Sagen, A., Kåresen, R., Sandvik, L., & Risberg, M.A. (2009). Changes in arm morbidities and health-related quality of life after breast cancer surgery—A five-year follow-up study. *Acta Oncologica, 48*, 1111–1118. doi:10.3109/02841860903061691

Savard, M.H., Savard, J., Quesnel, C., & Ivers, H. (2009). The influence of breast cancer treatment on the occurrence of hot flashes. *Journal of Pain and Symptom Management, 37*, 687–697. doi:10.1016/j.jpainsymman.2008.04.010

Saykin, A.J., Ahles, T.A., & McDonald, B.C. (2003). Mechanisms of chemotherapy-induced cognitive disorders: Neuropsychological, pathophysiological, and neuroimaging perspectives. *Seminars in Clinical Neuropsychiatry, 8*, 201–216.

Schagen, S.B., Muller, M.J., Boogerd, W., Rosenbrand, R.M., van Rhijn, D., Rodenhuis, S., & van Dam, F.S. (2002). Late effects of adjuvant chemotherapy on cognitive function: A follow-up study in breast cancer patients. *Annals of Oncology, 13*, 1387–1397. doi:10.1093/annonc/mdf241

Schilder, C.M., Seynaeve, C., Beex, L.V., Boogerd, W., Linn, S.C., Gundy, C.M., … Schagen, S.B. (2010). Effects of tamoxifen and exemestane on cognitive functioning of postmenopausal patients with breast cancer: Results from the neuropsychological side study of tamoxifen and exemestane adjuvant multinational trial. *Journal of Clinical Oncology, 28*, 1294–1300. doi:10.1200/JCO.2008.21.3553

Schmitz, K. (2010). Weight lifting and LE: Clearing up misconceptions. Retrieved from http://www.lymphnet.org/lymphedemaFAQs/weightliftingLE.htm

Schmitz, K.H., Ahmed, R.L., Troxel, A., Cheville, A., Smith, R., Lewis-Grant, L., … Greene, Q.P. (2009). Weight lifting in women with breast-cancer–related lymphedema. *New England Journal of Medicine, 361*, 664–673. doi:10.1056/NEJMoa0810118

Schneider, C.M., Hsieh, C.C., Sprod, L.K., Carter, S.D., & Hayward, R. (2007). Effects of supervised exercise training on cardiopulmonary function and fatigue in breast cancer survivors during and after treatment. *Cancer, 110*, 918–925. doi:10.1002/cncr.22862

Schnell, F.M. (2003). Chemotherapy-induced nausea and vomiting: The importance of acute antiemetic control. *Oncologist, 8*, 187–198.

Schwartz, A.L., Winters-Stone, K., & Gallucci, B. (2007). Exercise effects on bone mineral density in women with breast cancer receiving adjuvant chemotherapy. *Oncology Nursing Forum, 34*, 627–633. doi:10.1188/07.ONF.627-633

Sekine, H., Kobayashi, M., Honda, C., Aoki, M., Nakagawa, M., & Kanehira, C. (2000). Skin reactions after breast-conserving therapy and prediction of late complications using physiological functions. *Breast Cancer, 7*, 142–148.

Sener, S.F., Winchester, D.J., Martz, C.H., Feldman, J.L., Cavanaugh, J.A., Winchester, D.P., … Morehead, C. (2001). Lymphedema after sentinel lymphadenectomy for breast carcinoma. *Cancer, 92*, 748–752. doi:10.1002/1097-0142(20010815)92:4<748::AID-CNCR1378>3.0.CO;2-V

Shamley, D.R., Barker, K., Simonite, V., & Beardshaw, A. (2005). Delayed versus immediate exercises following surgery for breast cancer: A systematic review. *Breast Cancer Research and Treatment, 90*, 263–271. doi:10.1007/s10549-004-4727-9

Shapiro, C.L., Manola, J., & Leboff, M. (2001). Ovarian failure after adjuvant chemotherapy is associated with rapid bone loss in women with early-stage breast cancer. *Journal of Clinical Oncology, 19*, 3306–3311.

Shilling, V., Jenkins, V., Morris, R., Deutsch, D., & Bloomfield, D. (2005). The effects of adjuvant chemotherapy on cognition in women with breast cancer—Preliminary results of an observational longitudinal study. *Breast, 14,* 142–150. doi:10.1016/j.breast.2004.10.004

Sidiropoulou, T., Buonomo, O., Fabbi, E., Silvi, M.B., Kostopanagiotou, G., Sabato, A.F., & Dauri, M. (2008). A prospective comparison of continuous wound infiltration with ropivacaine versus single-injection paravertebral block after modified radical mastectomy. *Anesthesia and Analgesia, 106,* 997–1001. doi:10.1213/ane.0b013e31816152da

Simon, M.S., & Cody, R.L. (1992). Cellulitis after axillary node dissection for carcinoma of the breast. *American Journal of Medicine, 93,* 543–548. doi:10.1016/0002-9343(92)90583-W

Smoot, B., Wampler, M., & Topp, K.S. (2009). Breast cancer treatments and complications: Implications for rehabilitation. *Rehabilitation Oncology, 27,* 16–26.

So, W.K.W., Marsh, G., Ling, W.M., Leung, F.Y., Lo, J.C.K., Yeung, M., & Li, G.K.H. (2009). The symptom cluster of fatigue, pain, anxiety and depression and the effect on the quality of life of women receiving treatment for breast cancer: A multicenter study [Online exclusive]. *Oncology Nursing Forum, 36,* E205–E214. doi:10.1188/09.ONF.E205-E214

Stanton, A.W., Levick, J.R., & Mortimer, P.S. (1996). Current puzzles presented by postmastectomy oedema (breast cancer related lymphoedema). *Vascular Medicine, 1,* 213–225.

Stearns, V., & Hayes, D.F. (2002). Cooling off hot flashes. *Journal of Clinical Oncology, 20,* 1436–1438.

Stearns, V., & Loprinzi, C.L. (2003). New therapeutic approaches for hot flashes in women. *Journal of Supportive Oncology, 1,* 11–21.

Stearns, V., Slack, R., Greep, N., Henry-Tilman, R., Osborne, M., Bunnell, C., ... Isaacs, C. (2005). Paroxetine is an effective treatment for hot flashes: Results from a prospective randomized clinical trial. *Journal of Clinical Oncology, 23,* 6919–6930. doi:10.1200/JCO.2005.10.081

Stricker, C.T., Drake, D., Hoyer, K.A., & Mock, V. (2004). Evidence-based practice for fatigue management in adults with cancer: Exercise as an intervention. *Oncology Nursing Forum, 31,* 963–976. doi:10.1188/04.ONF.963-976

Strössenreuther, R.H.K. (2006). Decongestive kinesiotherapy, respiratory therapy, physiotherapy and other physical therapy techniques. In M. Földi & E. Földi (Eds.), *Földi's textbook of lymphology for physicians and lymphedema therapists* (2nd ed., pp. 547–562). Munich, Germany: Elsevier GmbH.

Strunk, B., & Maher, K. (1993). Collaborative nurse management of multifactorial moist desquamation in a patient undergoing radiotherapy. *Journal of ET Nursing, 20,* 152–157.

Su, H.I., Sammel, M.D., Springer, E., Freeman, E.W., DeMichele, A., & Mao, J.J. (2010). Weight gain is associated with increased risk of hot flashes in breast cancer survivors on aromatase inhibitors. *Breast Cancer Research and Treatment, 124,* 205–211. doi:10.1007/s10549-010-0802-6

Sverrisdóttir, A., Fornander, T., Jacobsson, H., von Schoultz, E., & Rutqvist, L.E. (2004). Bone mineral density among premenopausal women with early breast cancer in a randomized trial of adjuvant endocrine therapy. *Journal of Clinical Oncology, 22,* 3694–3699. doi:10.1200/JCO.2004.08.148

Swenson, K.K., Nissen, M.J., Ceronsky, C., Swenson, L., Lee, M.W., & Tuttle, T.M. (2002). Comparison of side effects between sentinel lymph node and axillary lymph node dissection for breast cancer. *Annals of Surgical Oncology, 9,* 745–753.

Tannock, I.F., Ahles, T.A., Ganz, P.A., & van Dam, F.S. (2004). Cognitive impairment associated with chemotherapy for cancer: Report of a workshop. *Journal of Clinical Oncology, 22,* 2233–2239. doi:10.1200/JCO.2004.08.094

Taylor, M.E., Perez, C.A., Halverson, K.J., Kuske, R.R., Philpott, G.W., Garcia, D.M., ... Rush, C. (1995). Factors influencing cosmetic results after conservation therapy for breast cancer. *International Journal of Radiation Oncology, Biology, Physics, 31,* 753–764. doi:10.1016/0360-3016(94)00480-3

Théberge, V., Harel, F., & Dagnault, A. (2009). Use of axillary deodorant and effect on acute skin toxicity during radiotherapy for breast cancer: A prospective randomized noninferiority trial. *International Journal of Radiation Oncology, Biology, Physics, 75,* 1048–1052. doi:10.1016/j.ijrobp.2008.12.046

Thomas, R., Williams, M., Marshall, C., & Walker, L. (2008). Switching to letrozole or exemestane improves hot flushes, mood and quality of life in tamoxifen intolerant women. *British Journal of Cancer, 98,* 1494–1499. doi:10.1038/sj.bjc.6604323

Thomas-MacLean, R.L., Hack, T., Kwan, W., Towers, A., Miedema, B., & Tilley, A. (2008). Arm morbidity and disability after breast cancer: New directions for care. *Oncology Nursing Forum, 35,* 65–71. doi:10.1188/08.ONF.65-71

Twiss, J.J., Waltman, N., Ott, C.D., Gross, G.J., Lindsey, A.M., & Moore, T.E. (2001). Bone mineral density in postmenopausal breast cancer survivors. *Journal of the American Academy of Nurse Practitioners, 13,* 276–284.

Vahtsevanos, K., Kyrgidis, A., Verrou, E., Katodritou, E., Triaridis, S., Andreadis, C.G., ... Antoniades, K. (2009). Longitudinal cohort study of risk factors in cancer patients of bisphosphonate-related osteonecrosis of the jaw. *Journal of Clinical Oncology, 27,* 5356–5362. doi:10.1200/JCO.2009.21.9584

van Dam, F.S., Schagen, S.B., Muller, M.J., Boogerd, W., Wall, E., Fortuyn, M.E.D., & Rodenhuis, S. (1998). Impairment of cognitive function in women receiving adjuvant treatment for high-risk breast cancer: High-dose versus standard-dose chemotherapy. *Journal of the National Cancer Institute, 90,* 210–218.

Van Poznak, C., Hannon, R.A., Mackey, J.R., Campone, M., Apffelstaedt, J.P., Clack, G., ... Eastell, R. (2010). Prevention of aromatase inhibitor–induced bone loss using risedronate: The SABRE trial. *Journal of Clinical Oncology, 28,* 967–975. doi:10.1200/JCO.2009.24.5902

Vicini, F.A., Chen, P., Wallace, M., Mitchell, C., Hasan, Y., Grills, I., ... Martinez, A. (2007). Interim cosmetic results and toxicity using 3D conformal external beam radiotherapy to deliver accelerated partial breast irradiation in patients with early-stage breast cancer treated with breast-conserving therapy. *International Journal of Radiation Oncology, Biology, Physics, 69,* 1124–1130. doi:10.1016/j.ijrobp.2007.04.033

Vogel, V.G., Costantino, J.P., Wickerham, D.L., Cronin, W.M., Cecchini, R.S., Atkins, J.N., ... Wolmark, N. (2006). Effects of tamoxifen vs. raloxifene on the risk of developing invasive breast cancer and other disease outcomes: The NSABP Study of Tamoxifen and Raloxifene (STAR) P-2 trial. *JAMA, 295,* 2727–2741. doi:10.1001/jama.295.23.joc60074

Von Ah, D., Russell, K.M., Storniolo, A.M., & Carpenter, J.S. (2009). Cognitive dysfunction and its relationship to quality of life in breast cancer survivors. *Oncology Nursing Forum, 36,* 326–334. doi:10.1188/09.ONF.326-334

Von Ah, D.M., Kang, D.H., & Carpenter, J.S. (2008). Predictors of cancer-related fatigue in women with breast cancer before, during and after adjuvant therapy. *Cancer Nursing, 31,* 134–144. doi:10.1097/01.NCC.0000305704.84164.54

von Schoultz, E., & Rutqvist, L.E. (2005). Menopausal hormone therapy after breast cancer: The Stockholm randomized trial. *Journal of the National Cancer Institute, 97,* 533–535. doi:10.1093/jnci/dji071

Wagner, L.I. (2010). Coping with "chemobrain": Brief cognitive behavioral therapy to manage chemotherapy-related cognitive impairments. *Oncology Nurse Edition, 24,* 50–54.

Wallace, M.S., Wallace, A.M., Lee, J., & Dobke, M.K. (1996). Pain after breast surgery: A survey of 282 women. *Pain, 66,* 195–205. doi:10.1016/0304-3959(96)03064-3

Waltman, N.L., Twiss, J.J., Ott, C.D., Gross, G.J., Lindsey, A.M., Moore, T.E., & Berg, K. (2003). Testing an intervention for preventing osteoporosis in postmenopausal breast cancer survivors. *Journal of Nursing Scholarship, 35,* 333–338. doi:10.1111/j.1547-5069.2003.00333.x

Waltzman, R., Croot, C., Justice, G.R., Fesen, M.R., Charu, V., & Williams, D. (2005). Randomized comparison of epoetin alfa (40,000 U weekly) and darbepoetin alfa (200 μg every 2 weeks) in anemic patients with cancer receiving chemotherapy. *Oncologist, 10,* 642–650. doi:10.1634/theoncologist.10-8-642

Warr, D.G., Hesketh, P.J., Gralla, R.J., Muss, H.B., Herrstedt, J., Eisenberg, P.D., ... Skobieranda, F. (2005). Efficacy and tolerability of aprepitant for the prevention of chemotherapy-induced nausea and vomiting in patients with breast cancer after emetogenic chemotherapy. *Journal of Clinical Oncology, 23,* 2822–2830. doi:10.1200/JCO.2005.09.050

Wefel, J., Lenzi, R., Theriault, R.L., Davis, R.N., & Meyers, C.A. (2004). The cognitive sequelae of standard-dose adjuvant chemotherapy in women with breast carcinoma. *Cancer, 100,* 2292–2299. doi:10.1002/cncr.20393

Wefel, J.S., Lenzi, R., Theriault, R., Buzdar, A.U., Cruickshank, S., & Meyers, C.A. (2004). "Chemobrain" in breast carcinoma. *Cancer, 101,* 466–475. doi:10.1002/cncr.20393

Weinfurt, K.P., Wait, S.L., Boyko, W., & Schulman, K.A. (1998). Psychosocial quality of life in a phase III trial of letrozole [Abstract]. *Proceedings of the American Society of Clinical Oncology,* Abstract No. 417. Retrieved from http://www.asco.org

Weissleder, H., & Schuchhardt, C. (2001). *Lymphedema: Diagnosis and therapy* (3rd ed.). Cologne, Germany: Viavital Verlag.

Wells, M., Macmillan, M., Raab, G., MacBride, S., Bell, N., MacKinnon, K., ... Munro, A. (2004). Does aqueous or sucralfate cream affect the severity of erythematous radiation skin reactions? A randomised controlled trial. *Radiotherapy and Oncology, 73,* 153–162. doi:10.1016/j.radonc.2004.07.032

Wengström, Y., Häggmark, C., Strander, H., & Forsberg, C. (2000). Perceived symptoms and quality of life in women with breast cancer receiving radiation therapy. *European Journal of Oncology Nursing, 4,* 78–90. doi:10.1054/ejon.1999.0052

Whelan, T.J., Pignol, J., Levine, M.N., Julian, J.A., MacKenzie, R., Parpia, S., ... Freeman, C. (2010). Long-term results of hypofractionated radiation therapy for breast cancer. *New England Journal of Medicine, 362,* 513–520. doi:10.1056/NEJMoa0906260

Whiteman, M.K., Staropoli, C.A., Langenberg, P.W., McCarter, R.J., Kjerulff, K.H., & Flaws, J.A. (2003). Smoking, body mass, and hot flashes in midlife women. *Obstetrics and Gynecology, 101,* 264–272.

Wickham, R. (2004). Nausea and vomiting. In C.H. Yarbro, M.H. Frogge, & M. Goodman (Eds.), *Cancer symptom management* (3rd ed., pp. 187–207). Sudbury, MA: Jones and Bartlett.

Wielgus, K.K., Berger, A.M., & Hertzog, M. (2009). Predictors of fatigue 30 days after completing anthracycline plus taxane adjuvant chemotherapy for breast cancer. *Oncology Nursing Forum, 36,* 38–48. doi:10.1188/09.ONF.38-48

Williams, M.S., Burk, M., Loprinzi, C.L., Hiel, M., Schomberg, P.J., Nearhood, K., ... Eggleston, W.D. (1996). Phase III double-blind evaluation of an aloe vera gel as a prophylactic agent for radiation-induced skin toxicity. *International Journal of Radiation Oncology, Biology, Physics, 36,* 345–349. doi:10.1016/S0360-3016(96)00320-3

Winter, M.C., Thorpe, H.C., Burkinshaw, R., Beevers, S.J., & Coleman, R.E. (2008). The addition of zoledronic acid to neoadjuvant chemotherapy may influence pathological response-exploratory evidence for direct anti-tumor activity in breast cancer. *Cancer Research, 69*(2, Suppl. 1), Abstract No. 5101. doi:10.1158/0008-5472.SABCS-5101

Winters-Stone, K.M., Bennett, J.A., Nail, L., & Schwartz, A. (2008). Strength, physical activity, and age predict fatigue in older breast cancer survivors. *Oncology Nursing Forum, 35,* 815–821. doi:10.1188/08.ONF.815-821

Winters-Stone, K.M., Nail, L., Bennett, J.A., & Schwartz, A. (2009). Bone health and falls: Fracture risk in breast cancer survivors with chemotherapy-induced amenorrhea. *Oncology Nursing Forum, 36,* 315–325. doi:10.1188/09.ONF.315-325

Woo, B., Dibble, S.L., Piper, B.F., Keating, S.B., & Weiss, M.C. (1998). Differences in fatigue by treatment methods in women with breast cancer. *Oncology Nursing Forum, 25,* 915–920.

World Health Organization. (n.d.). FRAX®. WHO Fracture Risk Assessment Tool. Retrieved from http://www.shef.ac.uk/FRAX/tool.jsp?locationValue=1

Wu, H.-S., Dodd, M.J., & Cho, M.H. (2008). Patterns of fatigue and effect of exercise in patients receiving chemotherapy for breast cancer [Online exclusive]. *Oncology Nursing Forum, 35,* E90–E99. doi:10.1188/08.ONF.E90-E99

Wyon, Y., Wijma, K., Nedstrand, E., & Hammar, M. (2004). A comparison of acupuncture and oral estradiol treatment of vasomotor symptoms in postmenopausal women. *Climacteric, 7,* 153–164.

Wysowski, D.K. (2009). Reports of esophageal cancer with oral bisphosphonate use [Letter to the editor]. *New England Journal of Medicine, 360,* 89–90. doi:10.1056/NEJMc0808738

Yaffe, K., Krueger, K., Sarkar, S., Grady, D., Barrett-Connor, E., Cox, D.A., & Nickelsen, T. (2001). Cognitive function in postmenopausal women treated with raloxifene. *New England Journal of Medicine, 344,* 1207–1213. doi:10.1056/NEJM200104193441604

Yamada, T.H., Denburg, N.L., Beglinger, L.J., & Schultz, S.K. (2010). Neuropsychological outcomes of older breast cancer survivors: Cognitive features ten or more years after chemotherapy. *Journal of Neuropsychiatry and Clinical Neuroscience, 22,* 48–54. doi:10.1176/appi.neuropsych.22.1.48

Yang, E.J., Park, W.B., Seo, K.S., Kim, S.W., Heo, C.Y., & Lim, J.Y. (2010). Longitudinal change of treatment related upper limb dysfunction and its impact on late dysfunction in breast cancer survivors: A prospective study. *Journal of Surgical Oncology, 101,* 84–91. doi:10.1002/jso.21435

# CHAPTER 10

# Psychosocial Issues

## Suzanne M. Mahon, RN, DNSc, AOCN®, APNG

## Introduction

Although adjusting to the many physical changes associated with breast cancer and its treatment is a complex process, the changes in emotional state, body image, and family roles and adjustment to the psychosocial difficulties that also accompany a diagnosis of breast cancer can be equally challenging. Psychosocial care is no longer considered an optional component of oncology care. Psychosocial care, with its goals of relieving emotional distress and promoting well-being, is central to efforts to improve the quality of patients' lives.

Many patients who could benefit from psychosocial care do not receive the help they need. Psychosocial care that is ineffective may be worse than no care at all (Jacobsen & Jim, 2008). Improving patients' access to psychosocial care is important; however, ensuring that the care made available has been shown to be effective is just as important. Oncology nurses play an enormous role in ensuring both access to and delivery of appropriate, quality psychosocial care. This chapter will identify areas of concern and explore ways in which healthcare professionals can support women with breast cancer, their families, and significant others.

## Psychosocial Distress Associated With Breast Cancer

The literature on the psychosocial aspects of breast cancer suggests that the vast majority of women eventually adjust well to the diagnosis of breast cancer and manage to endure the complex and sometimes toxic treatments associated with primary therapy (Coughlin, 2008). Fortunately, most women manage their psychosocial distress relatively well using personally available support systems (spouse, family, friends, clergy), as well as some professional resources that are ac-

cessible within many clinical settings (nurses, social workers, community resources, support groups). However, women uniformly report that they appreciate the attention and support from their healthcare team and referral to appropriate resources as necessary (Ganz, 2008). Many women will underestimate and not fully anticipate all of the side effects and complications of breast cancer treatment, so professional guidance and more intensive support as appropriate is appreciated and ultimately results in improved quality of life (QOL).

The diagnosis of breast cancer undoubtedly brings immediate and significant change and associated distress to both patients and their loved ones. Everyone reacts to the diagnosis differently. A diagnosis of breast cancer is a stressful event and often is accompanied with an increase in anxiety and depression (Jacobsen & Jim, 2008). Women diagnosed with breast cancer consistently score lower than the general female population on QOL measures during their cancer diagnosis and treatment and for as long as one year following treatment (Schou, Ekeberg, Sandvik, Hjermstad, & Ruland, 2005). Not only is the diagnostic period stressful, but the treatment and follow-up periods also can have potentially negative psychological consequences. Nurses need to be aware of the salient psychosocial aspects of diagnosis, treatment, and survival and implement appropriate strategies to assist patients and family members in coping. Figure 10-1 provides an overview of common psychosocial concerns in women diagnosed with breast cancer.

Some patients are at increased risk for psychosocial distress. These include people with a history of prior psychosocial or psychiatric diagnoses, communication problems, cognitive problems, or inadequate social support; those living alone; those with a history of abuse; and those experiencing financial problems (National Comprehensive Cancer Network [NCCN], 2010). Oncology nurses need to be especially aware of these at-risk groups and continually assess for psychosocial distress to promote early intervention.

*The author would like to acknowledge Gail Osterman, PhD, for her contribution to this chapter that remains unchanged from the first edition of this book.*

## Definition of Distress

Individuals may experience psychosocial distress as a result of cancer or its treatment. Psychosocial distress often is manifested as fears of recurrence or death, more generalized symptoms of worry, trouble sleeping, fatigue, and difficulty concentrating. According to NCCN (2010),

> Distress is a multifactorial unpleasant emotional experience of a psychological (cognitive, behavioral, emotional), social, and/or spiritual nature that may interfere with the ability to cope effectively with cancer, its physical symptoms, and its treatment. Distress extends along a continuum, ranging from common normal feelings of vulnerability, sadness, and fears to problems that can become disabling, such as depression, anxiety, panic, social isolation, and existential and spiritual crisis. (p. DIS-2)

The NCCN (2010) guideline that addresses psychosocial issues is titled *Distress Management*. Oncology nurses should be familiar with this guideline, which is continually updated. The term *distress* was chosen because (a) it carries fewer stigmas than psychiatric, psychosocial, or emotional problems, (b) it seems more "normal," and (c) it can be measured by simple self-report tools. For similar reasons, nurses may want to consider this strategy when addressing patients and their significant others.

Estimates suggest that approximately 35%–45% of women with a diagnosis of breast cancer show significant distress at some point during the illness and its treatment (NCCN, 2010). A significant proportion of women will experience at least some degree of depression and anxiety (Institute of Medicine, 2004). These symptoms may be brief adjustment reactions that decrease as patients receive more information about the diagnosis and treatment, or they may be present intermittently or long term throughout the cancer continuum. Unfortunately, although up to 45% of women who have breast cancer experience significant psychological distress, at most only 30% of those who experience this distress receive a psychosocial intervention (Azzone, Frank, Pakes, Earle, & Hassett, 2009).

## Impact of Psychosocial Distress

The diagnosis of breast cancer is almost always a threat to patients' sense of security and order in life. The source and magnitude of the distress can be variable. Possible sources are varied and include problems predating the cancer diagnosis and reactions to the diagnosis of a severe and possibly life-threatening illness, as well as the presence of unpleasant symptoms (such as pain, nausea, or fatigue). Concerns about disruptions in life plans, diminished QOL, and disease recurrence or progression also can produce anxiety and depression. In addition, the physiologic side effects of certain treatments on the central nervous system may directly produce anxiety or depression. Studies indicate that heightened anxiety and depression are not limited to the active treatment period and may persist for months or even years following successful treatment (Jacobsen & Jim, 2008).

The psychological functioning of patients should be addressed throughout all phases of the cancer trajectory. Psychosocial health affects patients' QOL as well as treatment outcomes. Potentially better disease status and longer survival have been documented in patients with fewer psychosocial disturbances (Aukst-Margetić, Jakovljević, Margetić, Biscán, & Samija, 2005; NCCN, 2010).

## Psychosocial Service Providers

Oncology caregivers should provide psychosocial services as part of total medical care. This responsibility initially falls to oncologists (medical, surgical, and radiation) and oncology nurses (inpatient, outpatient, and hospice). Often, referrals to specialists in psycho-oncology are indicated. This may include psychologists, psychiatrists, social workers, pastoral counselors, plastic and reconstructive surgeons, pharmacists, dietitians, prosthesis fitters, patient educators and navigators, genetics professionals, occupational therapists, physical therapists, and other professionals. Although the availability of such specialists may be limited in some practice settings, all women diagnosed with breast cancer should have a psychosocial assessment and often it is rendered by a variety of professionals.

Several barriers exist that prevent women from receiving adequate psychosocial care (Institute of Medicine, 2004). Care has gradually shifted from the inpatient to outpatient setting. Many outpatient clinics lack a full complement of specialists in psychosocial care. Furthermore, insurance coverage for

---

**Figure 10-1. Psychosocial Concerns of Women Diagnosed With Breast Cancer**

- Fear of recurrence
- Physical symptoms, including fatigue, sleep disturbances, nausea, and pain
- Body image changes, including those related to surgery, weight, skin, and hair
- Sexual dysfunction (e.g., painful intercourse, vaginal dryness, early menopause, decreased libido)
- Treatment-related anxieties (e.g., concerns about chemotherapy side effects, nausea, vomiting, alopecia, fatigue, undergoing venipuncture)
- Emotional distress (e.g., cognitive dysfunction, anxiety, depression, grief, helplessness, anger, low self-esteem)
- Persistent anxiety or intrusive distressing thoughts about body and illness
- Marital or partner communication issues
- Social isolation or difficulty communicating with friends
- Fears of vulnerability
- Difficulties completing duties associated with career or other roles
- Financial concerns
- Existential concerns and related fears of death

mental health services often is limited, and many women lack the financial means to afford such specialty care. Busy clinical settings also may discourage women from discussing psychosocial concerns, as they may have a stigma or be perceived as unnecessary extras. Figure 10-2 provides an overview of the barriers to assessing and promoting psychosocial care.

---

### Figure 10-2. Barriers to Appropriate Use of Psychosocial Services

- Poor access to services because of a lack of readily available providers in some settings
- Under-recognition of the importance of psychosocial care
- Healthcare providers' lack of awareness of community services
- Lack of communication between healthcare providers and patients about psychosocial concerns
- Poor health insurance coverage for psychosocial services
- Lack of financial resources at institutions for additional services such as psychosocial care
- Fragmentation among care providers
- Lack of a systematic method to routinely assess patients for psychosocial distress
- Lack of widespread adoption of clinical practice guidelines to promote psychosocial functioning
- General misconceptions about mental health care and psychological functioning
- Inadequate quality assurance and accountability for psychosocial care

---

## Psychosocial Functioning in Specific Groups and Phases of the Breast Cancer Trajectory

The assessment of psychosocial distress is important because distress is so prevalent. Predictors of increased stress include younger age at diagnosis, fewer social supports, and lower socioeconomic status. Figure 10-3 provides an overview of areas in which to facilitate psychosocial adaptation. Some populations and situations have specific issues that need to be addressed.

Distress affects one's family life, employment, and psychosocial functioning. Asking an objective question such as, "How is your pain today on a scale of 0 to 10?" makes it easier and more comfortable for caregivers to learn about patients' pain. Similarly, asking patients, "How is your distress today on a scale of 0 to 10?" opens a dialogue for a discussion of emotions that is more acceptable. This assessment also serves as an indicator of the magnitude of distress that a patient or family is experiencing and the potential impact on QOL.

Effective communication is important in both the assessment and management of psychosocial distress. Nurses need to be aware of their communication styles and develop a style that promotes psychosocial adjustment (Sivesind & Pairé, 2009). Table 10-1 provides some suggested communication approaches that oncology nurses might want to incorporate into their care.

---

### Figure 10-3. Suggested Measures to Facilitate Psychosocial Adaptation

- Clarify the diagnosis, treatment options, and side effects. Take time to ensure that patients understand each issue.
- Instruct patients that cancer has a trajectory and that needs will change over time. Assure patients and families that they will receive support during each phase as needed.
- Teach patients and families about social and community resources early in the trajectory and encourage them to mobilize the resources early.
- Remind patients that psychosocial health is just as important as physical health. Instruct them that this is why psychosocial assessment is conducted regularly.
- Acknowledge that distress is common. Inform patients of expected points for when distress might increase, and tell patients that they need to communicate about distress just as healthcare providers need to assess for distress.
- Suggest concrete recommendations for coping with distress, including journaling, speaking with a trained counselor (such as a psychologist, nurse, chaplain, or social worker), or joining a support group.
- Coordinate resources, and make referrals as indicated.
- Manage symptoms promptly, and assess the effectiveness of interventions.

---

Often, information related to a diagnosis of cancer is bad news. The manner and delivery of bad news can affect the patient's comprehension of information, satisfaction with medical care, sense of hope, and subsequent psychological adjustment (Jacobsen & Jackson, 2009). The SPIKES protocol (see Figure 10-4) is one method that is often effective in delivering distressing or bad news (Baile et al., 2000). Phases in the trajectory when communication is especially likely to be challenging include at the initial diagnosis, when treatment is unsuccessful, when recurrence or metastasis occurs, when treatment options become limited, or when hospice should be considered (Hughes, 2009).

### Younger Women

A diagnosis of breast cancer in women younger than age 40 can be particularly challenging and puts these women at increased risk for psychosocial distress. Studies repeatedly suggest that younger women with breast cancer are at greater risk for psychological distress (Shaha & Bauer-Wu, 2009). Patients with breast cancer who are premenopausal face a potential shorter life span along with the potential long-term consequences of treatment, including premature menopause and infertility. Evidence exists that young women with breast cancer experience lower QOL than their older counterparts do, not only during the treatment period but also during the years after the diagnosis and treatment. Being diagnosed with a life-threatening disease such as breast cancer during a period that is usually marked by establishing roots, developing meaningful relationships and careers, and giving birth can be shattering to young women and can interfere with their ability to adjust to important life events. Younger women diagnosed with breast cancer often report feeling different from their peers (Katz, 2007). Breast cancer not only affects the woman but also influences her family and work life (Shaha & Bauer-Wu, 2009). If the diagnosis is made during a pregnancy or shortly after a delivery, the woman must confront the diagnosis while managing the demands of a family and infant. The threat of early menopause or infertility also is associated with increased

## Table 10-1. Communication Skills That Enhance the Psychosocial Care of Patients With Cancer

| Skill | Application |
|---|---|
| Listening with interest and empathy | Use thoughtful silence to encourage the patient to talk. Make and maintain eye contact. |
| Exploring the patient's feelings (helping the patient to put feelings into words) | "Tell me more about feeling out of control." |
| Validating the patient's feelings | "It must be very difficult to manage all of this—your anger is a normal feeling." |
| Clarifying misconceptions that may exaggerate fear or isolation | "I'm not sure I understand what is troubling you. Could you explain that further?" |
| Inquiring about the patient's response to the diagnosis, treatment, and prognosis | "Tell me what you understand about the seriousness of your cancer." |
| Using questions and comments that encourage open communication | "That sounds interesting; tell me more." |
| Respecting the patient's views and efforts | "Help me understand what you mean. Your views are important. We will work together on these problems." |
| Reassuring the patient with realistic hope | "We can help manage your pain and distress" instead of "Don't worry. Everything will be all right." |
| Summarizing your interactions with the patient and validating mutual understanding | "Let me summarize what we just discussed." (This reinforces your attentiveness to the patient and provides structure for closure to your interaction.) |

*Note.* From "Coping With Cancer: Patient and Family Issues," by D.M. Sivesind and S. Pairé in C.C. Burke (Ed.), *Psychosocial Dimensions of Oncology Nursing Care* (2nd ed., pp. 3–4), 2009, Pittsburgh, PA: Oncology Nursing Society. Copyright 2009 by the Oncology Nursing Society. Reprinted with permission.

## Figure 10-4. SPIKES Approach to Communication

S—**S**etting up the interview
- The provider should devise a plan for telling the patients and how to respond to their emotional reactions or difficult questions.
- Arrange for some privacy with tissues readily available.
- Sit down at a comfortable distance.
- Ask permission, and if desired, involve significant others.
- Allow adequate time and minimize interruptions.

P—Patient's **p**erception of the situation
- Use open-ended questions to reasonably understand and have an accurate picture of how patients perceive the medical situation.
  - "What have you been told about your diagnosis so far?"
  - "What is your understanding of the reasons we did the scan?"

I—**I**nvitation from the patient to give information
- Ask patients directly how they would like to receive information.
  - "How would you like me to give the information about the test results?"

K—Giving **k**nowledge and information to the patient
- Warning patients that bad news is coming may lessen the shock that can follow the disclosure of bad news.
  - "Unfortunately I've got some bad news to tell you" or "I'm sorry to tell you that . . . ."
  - "As you know, we did this test to determine . . . ."

E—**E**xplore emotions and empathize with the patient's response
- Until an emotion is acknowledged, it is difficult to go on to discuss other issues.
- Clinicians can also use empathetic responses to acknowledge their own sadness or other emotions.
  - "I can see how upsetting this information is to you."
  - "Tell me more about this."
  - "Could you explain what you feel?"

S—**S**trategize and summarize
- Making the plan for the future as clear as possible decreases anxiety.
- Checking patients' understanding of the information allows for the correction of misconceptions.
  - "What can we do now?"

*Note.* Based on information from Baile et al., 2000; Finlay & Casarett, 2009; Jacobsen & Jackson, 2009.

psychological distress. Furthermore, trying to juggle work and career development can be challenging for younger women (Thewes, Butow, Girgis, & Pendlebury, 2004). Often, the families of younger women are unprepared for and have difficulty in managing the changes that occur with a diagnosis of breast cancer and could benefit from psychosocial intervention.

Breast cancer has the potential to be devastating to the sexual function and self-esteem of premenopausal women (Shaha & Bauer-Wu, 2009). This may be related to ovarian failure, premature menopause, and significant hormonal disruption. They also may have more concerns about feminine self-image and intimacy. Protection of fertility is a significant concern that cannot be underestimated.

## Older Women

Women 65 years and older comprise approximately 50% of the population newly diagnosed with breast cancer, and the five-year survival rate after a breast cancer diagnosis in women older than 50 years is as high as 84% (American Cancer Society [ACS], 2010). Despite the high survival rate, experiencing and managing cancer in old age can be stressful because of age-related health declines, including multiple and often chronic symptoms, late effects of cancer treatments, and comorbidities. Cancer often leaves numerous physical health sequelae that persist for decades despite successful treatments.

Women are living longer, and thus, over a lifetime, are more likely to develop breast cancer. They are staying in the workforce longer, and a diagnosis of breast cancer can cause difficulty in maintaining financial and social independence. Some older women may be at increased risk for other physical function problems and chronic illnesses. They may or may not have a social support system, especially if they are widowed or divorced. Although they may experience less disruption in routines than younger women, they are at risk for psychosocial distress.

Older women may perceive breast cancer as less threatening to their lives in the future, but they may be more vulnerable in terms of their physical health and functioning. Psychological effects reported by older women include concerns with emotional function, fear of recurrence, lack of social support, body image concerns, and cognitive changes. All of these effects may have an impact on QOL outcomes in older women. Cognitive changes and deficits in concentration may be more prominent in older women (Loerzel, McNees, Powel, Su, & Meneses, 2008). Benefits related to religion and spirituality have been reported in older women with breast cancer. Older women have felt that religion and faith gave them support, comfort, and a feeling of connectedness. Faith also has helped older women to cope and make meaning of their illness (Loerzel et al., 2008).

Older breast cancer survivors may have difficulties in interpreting symptoms, identifying their causes, and deciding whether they should report them to their healthcare providers (Yeom & Heidrich, 2009). Older cancer survivors may think that their healthcare providers should focus on high-priority topics and that talking about symptoms that older adults may view as age-related may distract the providers from providing more important care, or that reporting symptoms may cause them to be labeled a "difficult" patient. Taken together, these beliefs may keep older cancer survivors from communicating with their healthcare providers about symptoms or psychosocial concerns, even if they worry that symptoms may be signs of a cancer recurrence.

## Men With Breast Cancer

Male breast cancer makes up only 1% of all breast cancers reported in the United States; unfortunately, it is frequent-ly diagnosed at a later stage (ACS, 2010). Public awareness of male breast cancer is relatively low because of the overwhelming association of breast cancer with women. One reason that men often present with advanced breast cancer is possibly because of a general lack of awareness about the disease, as the vast majority of men with breast cancer were unaware that the disease could affect men (Donovan & Flynn, 2007). Breast cancer usually occurs, initially, as a painless breast mass. Because these cancers are rarely symptomatic or tender, men are unlikely to notice them during normal activity and are more likely to dismiss them once found, often later resulting in guilt for ignoring the symptoms (Robinson, Metoyer, & Bhayani, 2008). When men disclose their diagnosis to friends and family, they often find their potential social supports equally unaware, especially other men (Pant & Dutta, 2008). Very few celebrity spokespeople and few screening guidelines exist for male breast cancer.

Male breast cancer and associated interventions, such as mastectomy, may lead to a distorted self-image. Breasts most often are associated with femininity and sexuality, with many men discounting male breasts as simple anatomy. Conversely, male breasts (or more commonly called "pecs") are viewed by most men in today's society as a symbol of masculinity and strength. Consequently, men often experience significant stress after total or modified radical mastectomy, as evidenced by several studies showing their reluctance to go shirtless in public postoperatively (Pant & Dutta, 2008).

Because of the significantly higher incidence of breast cancer in women, male-specific or even gender-neutral information is lacking. Everything from marathons to logos, including the pink ribbon, and brochures are geared to women with breast cancer. The psychosocial implications of this disease are myriad and made more complex by the pink branding of breast cancer. Breast cancer literature often includes tips on menstruation, breast reconstruction, and bra fittings, specific to women, which can discourage a male patient. In fact, most men report receiving most of their information verbally rather than as patient information literature and find it distressing that no literature is really available that is appropriate to their situation (Donovan & Flynn, 2007).

## Breast Cancer During Pregnancy

An estimated 1.3 diagnoses of breast cancer occur during pregnancy per 10,000 live births (Molckovsky & Madarnas, 2008). The average age of patients with breast cancer diagnosed during pregnancy ranges from 32 to 38 years. Because increasing age is a risk factor for breast cancer, the frequency of concurrent breast cancer and pregnancy has the potential to increase as women in the United States delay childbearing to a later age.

For any woman diagnosed with breast cancer, many decisions arise, and typically many emotions, including fear, anger, and distress. For women diagnosed with breast cancer during pregnancy, the medical decisions become even more complicated and emotionally loaded (Theriault & Hahn, 2007). This is tempered by whether the pregnancy was planned or unplanned, whether the partner is involved or not, whether it is the first pregnancy, and other conception issues.

The hardest part of treatment planning is balancing when a conflict exists between the best known treatment for the mother and the well-being of the fetus (Theriault & Hahn, 2007). A woman who is found to have breast cancer during a pregnancy may have hard choices to make and requires expert help. Her obstetrician will need to work with her surgeon, oncologist, radiation oncologist, and others. Through all this, the woman with breast cancer will need emotional support, and often a counselor or psychologist should be part of her care team (Molckovsky & Madarnas, 2008).

## Breast Cancer in Middle Adulthood

When breast cancer occurs during middle adulthood, life plans are immediately altered. Often, this diagnosis occurs when women are achieving career goals and adjusting to children transitioning through their academic careers and leaving the home. Women may be adjusting to menopausal changes that are exacerbated by treatment.

The woman may have already noticed changes in body image, such as graying of hair, changes in skin texture, possibly weight gain, or decreases in muscle mass. Treatment for breast cancer that results in surgical scars, skin changes from radiation, alopecia, or further weight changes compounds psychosocial distress.

Middle-aged women may have a stable support system with a partner, may have never partnered, or may be recently widowed, separated, or divorced. Children may be physically separated from the woman because of their own career or academic paths. The availability or lack of availability of a support system contributes to how women manage the distress associated with the diagnosis.

## Breast Cancer in Lesbians

Little information is available about the needs of lesbians diagnosed with breast cancer. An estimated 2%–3% of the population identifies themselves as lesbian, so oncology professionals need to be sensitive to the needs of this population (Katz, 2007). The estimated relative risk of invasive breast cancer among lesbians is 1.74, which is likely due to reproductive-related differences; lesbians typically have fewer pregnancies and live births (Brown & Tracy, 2008). Moreover, lesbians who are estranged from family members may not have access to family or genetic history or be able to share the history of their diagnosis with the family. This estrangement often makes it difficult to accurately assess breast cancer risk.

Many lesbians do not tell their healthcare providers about their sexual orientation because they do not want discrimina-

tion to affect the quality of the health care they receive. This can make it harder for them to establish a strong connection with a provider. Fear of encountering a negative experience with a healthcare provider can lead some women to delay or avoid medical care, especially routine care such as early detection tests. Missing routine cancer screenings can lead to cancer being diagnosed at a later stage, when it is more difficult to treat (Brandenburg, Matthews, Johnson, & Hughes, 2007). When compared with heterosexual women, lesbians report more stress associated with the diagnosis, lower satisfaction with care, and lower satisfaction with the available emotional support (Brandenburg et al., 2007).

Furthermore, lesbian women must deal with the legal and financial barriers regarding end-of-life care, which can complicate an already difficult time. Many health insurance policies do not cover unmarried partners. This makes it harder for many lesbians and bisexual women to get quality health care (Arena et al., 2006).

The education of service providers is a key variable in bringing the health needs of lesbians to the forefront, and educating lesbians via health promotion campaigns and programs that specifically address risk reduction can be instrumental in ensuring that their health needs are met (Katz, 2007). Many find it difficult to attend support programs that target the needs of heterosexual women. Partners also need support and need to be included in care (Katz, 2007).

## Women in the Diagnostic Phase

The diagnostic period can be an extremely anxiety-provoking time. An estimated 10%–20% of breast biopsies are positive, which means that more than two million women annually will undergo some procedure to evaluate a breast change (Chappy, 2004). The psychosocial needs of women in this phase of the cancer trajectory should not be overlooked. Finding a lump can be a frightening experience, as can an undefined or suspicious finding on a routine mammogram. This leads to additional appointments for more radiologic studies and often a biopsy. A period of days to a week or more can separate each phase of the diagnostic process. This can be a period of great anxiety and fear. Women undergoing any type of biopsy may have escalated feelings of uncertainty and anxiety because of the potential diagnosis and its implications for their relationships, mortality, and sexuality. Some evidence suggests that women awaiting breast biopsy may be more distressed than women awaiting curative breast cancer surgery (Schnur et al., 2008). The experience of uncertainty prior to a biopsy may be more anxiety provoking than the actual cancer diagnosis. This often is the first significant experience a woman has with the healthcare system or surgical procedures. Care during this time can be very fragmented, as a woman may need to see radiologists, technicians, or surgeons. Specific psychosocial care services are very limited during this phase.

Waiting for the results of a pathologic diagnosis can be extremely difficult. It often takes nearly a week for a final report to become available, during which time women sometimes feel as though their lives are "on hold." Although many women eventually receive the good news that their biopsy was benign, a portion of women will receive a diagnosis of malignancy. Assisting women in finding a supportive environment and individuals during this phase is critical, especially when the diagnosis is a malignancy. Women who are inadequately informed as to what to expect during a biopsy usually have much higher levels of anxiety (Chappy, 2004). Scheduling problems and long waits for appointments and test results can increase stress. All efforts should be made to reduce the time between the initial identification of the problem and the biopsy and to provide continuity of care with an identified provider who can answer questions and provide guidance each step of the way. Comprehensive breast centers often have nurses who work in this capacity.

## Reactions to the Diagnosis

Receiving a diagnosis of breast cancer, contemplating the uncertainty of the future, and anticipating the daunting process of choosing and undergoing treatments can induce distress. For a significant percentage of new patients, this initial distress can be extreme and persistent, often presaging a psychiatric disorder, such as major depression. About one-third of patients with breast cancer experience significant emotional distress and functional impairment (Hegel et al., 2008).

Although women fear a diagnosis of breast cancer, the initial response when the diagnosis is confirmed and disclosed is often one of shock and disbelief (Institute of Medicine, 2004). Even though it is well publicized that a woman's lifetime risk of breast cancer is 1 in 8 (ACS, 2010), a breast cancer diagnosis at any point in a woman's life can be very stressful, very sudden, and unexpected. Without warning or choice, a woman is forced to abandon her current identified life to attend doctors' appointments and undergo tests that are unfamiliar and uncomfortable. Women frequently feel as though they have lost control of their life during the days surrounding the initial diagnosis. Common reactions include denial, anger, fear, stress, anxiety, depression, sadness, guilt, and loneliness. Informing women that these are common reactions is the first step in facilitating their adjustment to the diagnosis and its treatment.

Denial is frequently experienced. The disbelief that the diagnosis has been made is actually psychologically protective, unless it persists for extended periods of time or impairs decision making regarding appropriate treatment. Short-term denial can be helpful because it gives patients time to enable their families and themselves to adjust to the diagnosis. Most patients work through the denial quickly and have some acceptance of the disease by the time treatment begins.

Anger is another reaction that must be acknowledged and dealt with. Patients and families can be angry about the diagnosis and specifically with healthcare providers, family, friends, and sometimes an existential power. Encouraging individuals to discuss their feelings of anger can be an effective tool.

A wide range of fears and concerns can accompany the diagnosis of breast cancer. Patients and families most often are initially fearful of existential concerns and mortality. As the reality of the diagnosis surfaces, fears may shift toward experiencing pain, alopecia, nausea and vomiting, surgery, unknown healthcare procedures, and fatigue; managing the day-to-day activities of the family; paying for the costs of treatment; and keeping a job. Patients with cancer also may have many fears and concerns about how to discuss the diagnosis with friends and others. Identification of specific fears and developing concrete strategies to manage each specific problem can be very effective in reducing stress.

Reactive depression commonly occurs when the diagnosis is initially made. Signs of depression include feelings of helplessness, hopelessness, and loss of interest in family, friends, and activities. Physical manifestations of depression might include loss of appetite, changes in energy level, or sleep disturbances. Depending on the seriousness of the depression and the length of obvious symptoms, short- or long-term intervention may be indicated. Women and their families need to be counseled that these interventions are not being delivered because the person is "weak" but rather to improve QOL and facilitate tolerance of the treatment. Any suicidal thoughts require immediate intervention, and patients and families should be instructed on this point.

Guilt is another common reaction to the diagnosis of breast cancer. Some women feel guilt related to prior use of hormone replacement therapy or birth control pills. Others feel guilt if they believe they have a hereditary predisposition for developing breast cancer and fear they have passed the susceptibility gene on to a child. Others feel guilty because they perceive themselves to be a burden to others. Acknowledging that these feelings are common, as well as encouraging patients to discuss them, may be helpful.

## Information Seeking and Treatment Decision Making

Once the diagnosis of breast cancer has been made, the patient, family, and physicians will begin to discuss treatment. Most women are unprepared for the diagnosis and even less prepared for the array of medical consultants they will be scheduled to see in a relatively short period of time, as well as the number of treatment decisions they will have to make. Lives and work schedules usually are abruptly interrupted for not only the patients but also those supporting them during the decision-making and treatment process.

The first few days and weeks after the biopsy involve more diagnostic workups, which can be a frightening and unfamiliar experience for patients. This is necessary to determine the stage of disease and other prognostic factors. This information can be technically complex. Many times, healthcare providers have difficulty explaining the details of the pathology reports, and patients can have significant difficulty understanding the findings. This can lead to more anxiety and distress for women with cancer and those supporting them.

Following the discussion of the pathologic findings come the decisions regarding treatment. This can be a very overwhelming experience. Often, more than one treatment is discussed or suggested, which may require the patient to make choices about the best treatment or treatments for her. Women frequently are asked to decide about the type of treatment (mastectomy with or without reconstruction or lumpectomy with radiation) and subsequent treatment (standard or investigational). Essentially, patients must make important treatment decisions about which they usually have little knowledge and background and to choose a medical care team with which they are comfortable. Some patients find that this decision-making process restores a sense of control, whereas others find these choices very stressful. Patients' ability to make informed decisions may be influenced by their educational level, stress level, family and social support systems, and previous experiences with the healthcare system. Women need to be reminded that although they must make a decision, they should not be too hasty, which can result in decisions that are later regretted (Institute of Medicine, 2004). Patients can be encouraged to seek a second opinion with another group of specialists to help ensure that treatment decisions are appropriate.

Information and education about cancer are the support services most frequently requested by patients (Institute of Medicine, 2008). Patients similarly rate information needs pertaining to their illness and treatments as very important. Information should be tailored to each patient's expectations and preferences, as well as to the patient's individual diagnosis and clinical situation. Most patients have a wide range of information needs (such as information specific to their type and stage of cancer, treatment, prognosis, rehabilitation, achievement and maintenance of maximal health, coping, and financial and legal concerns) that change over time.

Communication and patient education can be challenging because of the shock of the diagnosis. Shock and anxiety can limit one's ability to comprehend and register information (Kerr, Engel, Schlesinger-Raab, Sauer, & Hölzel, 2003). Acceptance of the disease and its treatment comes at different rates for different individuals. Lack of information increases anxiety, and adequate information can provide individuals with some sense of control. Striking a balance is important.

Psychosocial distress also can be increased during this time because women may have to deal with multiple specialists. Although these providers ideally are seen as a team, wom-

en often must go from office to office or to different departments. Fragmentation of care can be an additional psychosocial burden (Institute of Medicine, 2004).

Decisions regarding treatment lie with the patient but must be made based on information from the physician, the nurse, and other resources. Some treatment alternatives are based on the size or location of the tumor, whereas other treatments may be suggested because of preexisting or comorbid conditions. With the decision to have surgery, patients then face the additional choice of lumpectomy versus mastectomy. This is a personal choice for women and may be based on fear, preconceived ideas about the surgery and body image changes, or financial concerns. Some women may fear recurrence of the breast cancer and feel they will have a better chance for survival if their entire breast or even both breasts are removed.

Nurses should assess women's preferences for the amount, timing, and sources of information desired and not make assumptions based on age or education level alone. It also is important for nurses to recognize that women receive information from a variety of sources, and they should support them in finding accurate information. Finally, women should be supported in decision making and allowed sufficient time during the pretreatment period to continue gathering and reviewing information, even if they appear to have already made a treatment choice. All of these nursing interventions facilitate patients' adjustment to the diagnosis and confidence in the treatment decision (Lally, 2009).

Body image plays a major role in treatment decisions. Some patients may choose a lumpectomy because they feel unable to handle the changes made by a mastectomy. Other women believe they will no longer "feel like a woman" without breasts. Some patients may agree to a mastectomy if immediate reconstruction can be done. This may be possible for some patients, but for others, a medical reason may necessitate a delay in reconstruction, especially if postoperative chemotherapy or radiation therapy is needed. The treatment team, including the medical oncologist, radiation oncologist, surgeon, nurse, and patient, should discuss the reasons behind the delay. For other women, the possibility of cancer remaining in the breast makes mastectomy a logical choice. Supporting women in whatever choice they make, as long as they are informed, is an important nursing responsibility.

A subset of women have a germ-line genetic predisposition for developing breast cancer, and these women may choose to undergo prophylactic surgery on the unaffected breast. A prophylactic mastectomy will reduce the chances of a second primary cancer occurring in the other breast and may improve cosmesis (see Chapter 2). The treatment team must discuss these issues and should explore the psychological consequences of patients' choices throughout the decision-making process.

Financial concerns also may play a role in the choice of treatment. Financial assistance programs are available to help defray the costs of some treatments. Patients should be encouraged to discuss their financial concerns with the medical team to minimize anxiety about payment; a consult to the institution's social worker should be initiated at that point to manage potential problems proactively. Other support agencies, such as ACS (see www.cancer.org), are available to help patients in dealing with financial problems throughout treatment. In some geographic locations, the local affiliate of Susan G. Komen for the Cure may be able to assist with treatment-related costs.

Women with breast cancer who have been actively involved in deciding about their treatment tend to be more satisfied with the care they receive, have higher overall QOL, experience higher physical and social functioning, and report fewer side effects. Patients with breast cancer who participated in consultation planning were more satisfied and reported fewer barriers to communicating with their oncologist (Stacey, Samant, & Bennett, 2008).

## Active Treatment

Once the treatment plan is determined, patients may feel some sense of relief, but then new fears and concerns related to the treatment usually surface. The shift toward outpatient and short-stay surgical procedures adds to the psychosocial distress for some families. Distress may be related to the presence of drains and dressings or to limited mobility because someone must be available to help with the management of the incision and household tasks. Careful assessment of the support system available to patients is necessary for successful care. Often, those who assist patients will have psychosocial concerns that also need to be addressed.

As active treatment begins, women must make decisions about when, how, and to whom they will disclose the diagnosis. Although the emotional expression about a diagnosis of breast cancer has been shown to reap psychological benefits, decisions to disclose can be hampered by stigma and fear around breast cancer (Yoo, Aviv, Levine, Ewing, & Au, 2010). Emotional work and disclosure about illness inherently involves risk and vulnerability; it requires thinking about how individuals will react emotionally to the communication and often results in the patient feeling a need to anticipate and find ways to manage the emotions of others (Katz, 2009). Telling others about one's illness takes emotional resources and opens the individual up to vulnerability, scrutiny, and possibly rejection. Paradoxically, disclosure is also required in order to enlist and secure support. This task can be emotionally taxing. Disclosure can have emotional consequences, such as strained relationships, inability to handle the responses of others, and loss of control and autonomy. When women disclose a new diagnosis of breast cancer to others, they also need to be willing and open to receive support, sometimes in surprising ways and from unexpected people. Often, women are surprised by how others, such as family members, friends, and coworkers, can react with strength, compassion, and support.

Some women find it helpful to share the diagnosis with one or two close, supportive friends and then have their friends help share the information with others (Katz, 2009). Nurses need to prepare and guide women in disclosing the diagnosis to others.

Communicating with friends can be challenging. Friends want to be updated and share their support. CaringBridge is a nonprofit group that provides free Web sites that families of a seriously ill person can construct to keep family and friends updated on the health and condition of the loved one. Families can add photos, and visitors can leave messages. Families can choose to restrict access if they want. Although it is not a substitute for real visits, it keeps people informed with consistent and accurate information, especially when family members may need a rest. It also helps visitors to have a more realistic picture of what is occurring. More information can be found at www.caringbridge.org.

Following the initial adjustment to the diagnosis of cancer, patients begin the journey of treatment. Treatment may include any combination of surgery, chemotherapy, radiation therapy, hormonal therapy, or close follow-up. Treatment results in a change in physical health, which also affects patients' psychosocial health. These include side effects from therapy, role changes, and body image alterations. Teaching often is less effective in patients who experience high anxiety levels secondary to a cancer diagnosis (Williams & Schreier, 2005). If a patient is experiencing significant anxiety or pain, it must be addressed prior to the delivery of an educational message. Pain or anxiety can greatly limit a patient's ability to participate in and understand educational messages and materials. However, patient safety may depend on adequate understanding of the side effects of treatment and managing them at home. Optimal teaching plans ensure that the extent, content, and timing of information given to patients are tailored to meet their needs (Balmer, 2005). Patients who have difficulty using standard written materials or those who learn best from auditory or visual information may require innovative and nontraditional teaching methods.

For most women, active treatment begins with a surgical procedure. The early phase of surgical recovery often is referred to in the literature as the *subacute* phase and consists of the first four to six weeks after surgery (Wyatt, Beckrow, Gardiner, & Pathak, 2008). The ability to identify predictors of postsurgical physical and psychological well-being during the subacute phase and before adjuvant therapy begins will allow healthcare providers to better assess which patients may need additional physical and psychological supportive services.

Depression and anxiety can increase as side effects worsen, which can intensify the physical symptoms. Depression can increase anxiety and pain, cause difficulty with concentration, and result in insomnia (Sharp, 2010). This cycle (depression causing physical symptoms, and physical symptoms causing more depression) is difficult to identify and even harder to break. Psychosocial support can help to control some side effects, ultimately affecting patients' tolerance to treatment.

Managing work commitments can be a major challenge for patients and family members. Maintaining employment can be important to ensure continued income and benefits, including health care. The Family and Medical Leave Act of 1993 (FMLA) is a labor law requiring larger employers to provide employees with up to 12 weeks of job-protected unpaid leave if they are unable to perform their job because of a serious health condition or to care for a sick family member. The FMLA is administered by the Wage and Hour Division within the U.S. Department of Labor. An "eligible" employee allowed leave under the FMLA is an employee who has been employed with the company for at least 1,250 hours during a 12-month period prior to the start of the leave. The 12 months do not need to be consecutive months. FMLA leave can be taken on an intermittent basis, allowing the employee to work on a less than full-time schedule. FMLA leave can help relieve stress for some patients, and nurses may advise patients and family members to explore this option.

## Long-Term Survivors

The end of treatment can be a time of mixed emotions. The stress associated with the transition often is underestimated. Separation from frequent contact with the medical team may heighten overall psychological distress as well as uncertainty about the future and may reflect reduction of an important kind of social support (Garofalo, Choppala, Hamann, & Gjerde, 2009). Patients may feel a sense of joy in completing treatment but may also have a fear of leaving the close monitoring of the healthcare team. A sense of comfort comes from having chemotherapy or radiation therapy that will fight the cancer. When treatment is over, the sense of control over the cancer also is taken away for some patients. Talking with others who have completed treatment may help to normalize these feelings.

Patients also may have feelings of anxiety and depression about taking hormonal therapy after completion of surgery, chemotherapy, or radiation. The risk of future serious side effects frightens some women, ultimately affecting their adjustment to the end of treatment. Psychosocial support can help patients to identify their fears and find ways of discussing them with family, friends, and the healthcare team.

Many survivors are unprepared for the lingering effects of therapy, including fatigue, cognitive dysfunction, and menstrual symptoms (Ganz, 2008). Researchers have found that general oncology clinicians spend much time preparing patients for the acute toxicities of treatment (e.g., nausea, vomiting, fatigue, alopecia) and much less time on what to expect in the pattern of recovery and adjustment following active treatment. Although clinicians may tell patients that it takes as much time to recover as it did to complete the therapy, little is specifically known about how this recovery takes place and how long it takes.

Throughout the diagnosis and treatment period, it is common for a woman to identify herself as a patient with cancer. Other roles, such as wife, mother, or career woman, are put on hold, and cancer becomes the main focus. Although often difficult, it is important for patients with cancer to learn to integrate the cancer and related treatments into their lives. Some patients may find strength in groups where other women discuss how they returned to normal lives (i.e., their lives without cancer), whereas others may prefer individual counseling to help them to understand the meaning of the illness and return to a normal life. The ultimate goal is to understand the effects of the cancer on the individual and the best way to move forward with life. For some, this may mean a change in career, whereas others may find they have a different perspective on life after having experienced a serious illness. They may be less bothered by everyday nuisances, or they may find themselves searching for new meaning in their lives.

Following the end of treatment, some women find the possibility of a recurrence frightening and almost paralyzing. The transition from active treatment and from patient to survivor may be a particularly important point in recovery, and the quality of psychosocial adjustment at this point appears to affect the future well-being of cancer survivors. Where focused efforts to treat the disease and deal with the adverse effects of treatment had been primary stressors, survivors must now cope with more diffuse threats, such as recurrence, social stigmatization, and the long-term consequences of medical treatment. Premorbid disposition, coping styles, and stress burden also can affect one's susceptibility to poor long-term adjustment.

For some, this fear manifests as an increased dependence on the healthcare team. Although the concerns may seem excessive to everyone other than the patient, a cancer survivor may consider every ache and pain to be related to a recurrence of the cancer. This can create unnecessary stress on both the patient and the healthcare team. Women may need to be reassured that late effects, such as aches and pains or fatigue, caused by past anticancer treatments are not a sign of recurrence (Ganz, 2008).

The fear of recurrence can affect a survivor's willingness to continue medical follow-up. These fears can be addressed in a support group setting or with individual psychosocial support. Many women find strength in having faced breast cancer. Peer support programs in which people communicate and share experiences with others having a common personal experience often are an effective mechanism for building self-efficacy, which is the belief that one is capable of carrying out a course of action to reach a desired goal (Institute of Medicine, 2008). Self-efficacy is a critical determinant of how well knowledge and skills are obtained and is an excellent predictor of behavior.

Healthy living habits after the diagnosis of and treatment for breast cancer can influence long-term survivorship. Exercise has been associated with higher QOL at least

10 years after cancer diagnosis (Kendall, Mahue-Giangre-co, Carpenter, Ganz, & Bernstein, 2005; Vallance, Courneya, Jones, & Reiman, 2005; van Weert et al., 2005), as well as with a decrease in long-term fatigue, which often is felt following treatment for cancer (Bower, 2005). Exercise can have a positive effect on body image of breast cancer survivors and should be encouraged in patients throughout the cancer continuum.

Healthcare professionals should not underestimate the stressors and fears that often are present in long-term survivors. Although follow-up visits for these patients are not as complicated, these women and their families still require and benefit from careful psychosocial assessment and intervention. Figure 10-5 shows some helpful strategies to suggest to patients.

## Recurrent and Advanced Disease

Although the overall prognosis for breast cancer is good (75% are alive at 15 years after diagnosis), especially for those who have early-stage disease, some women will experience a recurrence of breast cancer (ACS, 2010). Some

will be diagnosed with advanced or metastatic disease. Recurrence is defined as the return of the disease after an initial course of treatment with a disease-free period. Although recurrence does not necessarily lead to terminal illness, patients with recurrent disease usually are much more aware of the reality of and potential mortality of their diagnosis. Often this event occurs years after the initial diagnosis. For many, it is considered a failure for both the patient and the treatment team. Because recurrence frequently is associated with clinical symptoms from the cancer, including increased pain, cough, headaches, or other changes, patients have a tangible, constant reminder that their condition is serious and perhaps life limiting. This can lead to enormous stress for both patients and families.

Recurrent disease may involve the same treatment as the initial cancer, a similar treatment, or something completely different. Women may feel overwhelmed by the treatment and their potential mortality. Recurrent disease is a distinctly different emotional event than the initial diagnosis (Ganz, 2008). Women with recurrent breast cancer may have more anxiety about treatment because of their previous experiences, as well as more symptom distress, including

### Figure 10-5. Strategies and Interventions to Prepare Individuals and Families for Long-Term Survivorship

- Give patients and families a range of what to expect that could potentially happen in terms of prognosis, physical symptoms, emotional concerns, and sexual function.
- Remind patients and significant others that they may never return to "normal" and that they may need to establish a new normalcy.
- Specifically define what symptoms should promptly be reported for further evaluation.
- Describe the anticipated follow-up schedule for office visits, scans, and laboratory work with the rationale for the proposed schedule.
- Teach patients what tertiary prevention is and what specific tertiary screening measures will be recommended (i.e., colon screening, bone densitometry, gynecologic screening).
- Develop a wellness plan, including a specific strategy for exercise, diet, skin cancer prevention, and smoking cessation when indicated.
- Remind patients and significant others that it is common to have "trigger" events that are upsetting, such as the anniversary of the diagnosis, the diagnosis of a loved one with a similar disease, or feelings of anxiety surrounding things that remind patients of unpleasant aspects of treatment.
- Discuss that recovery from treatment is a gradual process and that it may take a year or more before full energy returns.
- Assess for mental health problems. Manage depression and anxiety early. Remind patients and family members that it is common to have some feelings of depression, anxiety, or being overwhelmed even though treatment is completed. Discuss with them that treatments are available to manage these symptoms, and advise patients to bring these concerns to the attention of healthcare providers to explore the best means to improve this quality-of-life aspect.
- Acknowledge that patients may need to adopt a new self-image in terms of energy, physical appearance, and sexuality. For many, staying active and exploring new hobbies and activities helps them to develop a new self-image.
- Assess for financial problems. Survivors may be paying for the costs of care long after treatment is complete. If appropriate, remind patients that social services may be able to assist them.
- Discuss the importance of maintaining continuous healthcare coverage. If the patient or family member carrying the insurance wants to change jobs or something else occurs that would lead to a lapse in coverage, he or she should consider a referral to social services.
- Patients and significant others may want to consider becoming an advocate for others with cancer or volunteering in some other way. Some individuals find benefit from continued participation in a support group.
- Instruct patients to inform their healthcare provider if they are experiencing problems or changes with memory or concentration after chemotherapy, as some strategies can decrease the impact of these problems.
- Advise patients and their family members to consider learning more about genetic risk if the family history suggests hereditary susceptibility for developing the cancer and they have not yet received counseling about genetic testing.
- Instruct survivors that they may need to plan what they want to disclose, how to disclose it, and how much to disclose. When meeting new people or dating, it can be awkward to know when to disclose that one has completed cancer treatment. Talking with other survivors can help patients to feel more comfortable with how and when to disclose.
- Advise patients that they may still face challenges in the workplace related to follow-up care, energy levels, or other health-related concerns. Encourage them to discuss these needs with their employer. If problems cannot be resolved, a referral to social services, local cancer advocacy services, or perhaps legal resources may be indicated.

fatigue and pain. Patients also may have anger, self-blame, and regret about prior treatment choices. Women may be less hopeful because the first treatment did not completely eradicate the disease.

As the disease progresses, attention to symptom and pain relief becomes paramount. This phase of the illness also may be accompanied by spiritual and existential concerns. Patients encounter many fears in the advanced phases of disease, including fear of the unknown, pain, suffering, abandonment, loss of control, loss of identity, loss of body image, loss of loved ones, and loss of hope (Gorman, 2006). Acknowledgment of these fears and the fact that they are common reactions is the first step in helping patients to cope with these overwhelming feelings. Open communication with family members and significant others may decrease some distress and offer an opportunity for closure, not only for patients but also for those involved in their care.

## End of Life

As women approach the terminal phases of the disease, they may express a fear of death (Hughes, 2009). A helpful nursing intervention is to identify the woman's specific fears and then take concrete steps to address the concerns. If the woman is afraid of pain, information about and a plan for pain control can be implemented. If the woman is afraid of dying alone, a plan for continual care can be implemented. Without proper assessment, it is impossible to develop an effective plan of care to promote QOL and decrease psychosocial distress.

Many women are angry that therapy is no longer effective and that their life may end prematurely. Acknowledging that this is a common reaction is important. Assisting the patient to find ways to direct the energy expended in anger can be helpful.

Some women feel regret over the choices they have made in the past or things they have not or will not have the opportunity to accomplish. Once again, acknowledging that this is a common reaction can be helpful. Some patients benefit from leaving some small legacy, such as a letter, photo album, or other item (Hughes, 2009). Quality conversations with loved ones can be beneficial for both the patient and family members.

A discussion of advance directives helps to ensure that the woman's wishes are carried out in the event she is unable to direct her care (Wasserman, 2008). Signing a living will, durable power of attorney, and do-not-resuscitate orders can be difficult steps but often bring a sense of peace when completed. Nurses need to encourage patients to complete these forms.

Many women could benefit from hospice services. Often this referral comes late; earlier referral actually promotes QOL (Hill & Hacker, 2010). Some women want to stay at home, whereas others choose to go to an assisted living center, a nursing home, or an inpatient hospice program. The goal of hospice care is to help patients to live their last days as alert and pain free as possible (Hughes, 2009). Hospice care aims to manage symptoms so that a person's last days may be spent with dignity and quality, surrounded by loved ones. Hospice affirms life and neither hastens nor postpones death. Hospice focuses on quality rather than quantity of life. It provides family-centered care, involving the patient and family in all decisions. Bereavement care is typically available for family members after death.

## Assessment Strategies

A knowledge of the specific needs of various groups of women and phases of the cancer trajectory forms the base for assessment of psychosocial distress. Better assessment of distress results in better and more appropriate supportive care. Supporting the patient also means supporting the family. Clinicians should assess the needs of the family at the time of diagnosis. Issues such as intimacy and sexuality, femininity, role changes, childcare needs, and ways to talk to partners or children about the diagnosis require assessment and often intervention.

### Prior Psychosocial Functioning

Assessment of patients' past psychosocial history is beneficial. The diagnosis and treatment of breast cancer is stressful and potentially could exacerbate preexisting conditions that have been under control. For instance, a patient with a long-standing history of clinical depression may find that the diagnosis of breast cancer increases the depression, and she may require more intensive intervention. Assessment and understanding of past effective coping strategies may provide insight into how to manage the multiple stressors that accompany a diagnosis of breast cancer.

### Assessment of Support Systems

Family and friends also play a critical role in patients' decisions regarding treatment. A patient may have a family member or friend who was diagnosed with and treated for breast cancer, which could cause the newly diagnosed patient to assume she will have the same reactions. As part of the initial assessment, the healthcare team needs to determine whether the patient has any preconceived ideas based on reports from other patients, family members, or friends. This will provide an opportunity to dispel any misconceptions regarding the patient's diagnosis and provides an estimate of the baseline information that the woman and her family have about the diagnosis and its treatment.

Research suggests that the first year following the diagnosis is a critical time for women and their partners (Ganz, 2008). During this time, they need to adjust to the ramifications of having a potentially life-threatening diagnosis, recover and adjust to surgery and adjuvant treatment, cope with the side effects of therapy, and begin to establish a new normalcy and routine. When families have additional outside stressors, the disease is more likely to be perceived as threatening, and QOL is decreased (Ganz, 2008). Higher levels of support from a partner, family members, or friends are associated with the use of more positive coping strategies and indirectly contribute to improved mood. Adjustment shortly after the diagnosis is related to later levels of adjustment. For this reason, early assessment and intervention of potential problems are important.

The diagnosis of breast cancer in mothers with children living at home is disruptive to the routines in the home and especially to the accessibility and availability of the mothers to the children. Ultimately, this often results in negative effects on the overall tension in the home and marriage (Herbenick, Reece, Hollub, Satinsky, & Dodge, 2008). Cancer brings change to any family, whether it is a young couple, a couple with children, an older couple, single people, widowed people, or individuals living in nontraditional relationships. Healthcare providers need to assess the impact of the diagnosis and its subsequent changes in each specific situation. This includes an assessment of finances (including whether the patient can work during treatment), living arrangements (so that someone is available to assist the patient), and management of daily activities, which can be especially important in families with children. A clear and thorough assessment helps to identify potential problems to enable early intervention.

## Assessment Instruments

Many instruments are available for the assessment of psychosocial distress for patients with breast cancer. Most instruments address issues of psychological functioning, physical functioning, social functioning, and symptoms and side effects. Many cancer-specific assessment tools are available to identify women who need more support throughout their treatment. Figure 10-6 provides some examples of commonly used instruments.

One of the biggest challenges that health professionals face is finding an assessment tool that is brief and easy to administer that also rapidly identifies individuals and families who are at significant risk for psychosocial problems. A 1–10 scale is an easy way to assess patients' symptoms and can easily be communicated to the rest of the healthcare team. This scale can be used at each appointment to track changes and allows for additional consultation as needed. A score of four or higher may alert the assessor of the need for specific referrals to mental health professionals (NCCN, 2010). If the distress responds to a combination of psychotherapy or cognitive-behavioral therapy with or without pharmacologic intervention, the patient's follow-up can be

### Figure 10-6. Selected Tools Used in the Psychosocial Assessment of People With Breast Cancer

- **The Beck Depression Inventory (BDI-II)** is a 21-question self-report, multiple-choice format for measuring the severity of depression. The BDI-II is designed for individuals aged 13 and older and is composed of items related to symptoms of depression, such as hopelessness and irritability, and cognitions, such as guilt or feelings of being punished, as well as physical symptoms, such as fatigue, weight loss, and lack of interest in sex.
- **Brief Symptom Inventory (BSI):** The BSI is a 53-item measure of psychological distress written at a sixth-grade reading level and requiring five to seven minutes to complete. Each item is referenced to the past seven days.
- **Cancer Rehabilitation Evaluation System (CARES):** CARES generates a report for both patients and healthcare professionals. There is a format for clinical use and one for research. The clinical format allows patients to check a box if they desire help with a certain problem. It focuses on quality of life and related cancer-specific needs. Patients complete the instrument by rating problem statements on a scale of 0–4 as it applies to the previous month. It can include up to 193 items that focus on physical and psychosocial concerns, medical interactions with the care team, marital issues, and sexual issues.
- **Distress thermometer and problem list from the National Comprehensive Cancer Network (NCCN):** This tool is based on the NCCN guidelines for distress management in clinical practice. It uses a 0–10 scale to measure a variety of psychosocial problems.
- **European Organisation for Research and Treatment of Cancer (EORTC) Quality of Life Questionnaire:** The EORTC questionnaire is used to assess quality of life in individuals with cancer who are participating in clinical trials. It considers physical symptoms, cognitive issues, fatigue, pain, nausea and vomiting, global health, and quality of life.
- **Functional Assessment of Cancer Therapy–Breast (FACT-B):** The FACT-B is a 46-item self-report scale that measures quality of life in the physical, social/family, emotional, and functional realms on a five-point rating scale.
- **Quality of Life Breast Cancer Instrument from City of Hope National Medical Center:** Nineteen of the items are specific to breast cancer.
- **Hospital Anxiety and Depression Scale (HADS):** The HADS is a brief tool that provides separate scores for anxiety and depression with suggested cutoff points to identify a possible mood disorder.
- **The Medical Outcomes Study Short Form (SF-36):** The SF-36 was designed for use in clinical practice, research health policy evaluations, and general surveys. It measures eight areas of functional status, well-being, and self-perceived health: limitations in physical activities because of health problems, limitations in usual role activities because of physical health problems, bodily pain, general health perceptions, vitality (energy and fatigue), limitations in social activities because of physical or emotional problems, limitations in usual role activities because of emotional problems, and mental health (psychological distress and well-being).

*Note.* Based on information from Institute of Medicine, 2004; National Comprehensive Cancer Network, 2010; Sharp, 2010; Sheldon, 2010.

delegated to the oncology team. If the response is not adequate, continued intervention with a mental health professional is indicated.

The 1–10 scale is also effective because it can be used repeatedly to assess improvements and new problems with distress. NCCN (2010) provides a detailed schema including the distress thermometer for managing distress. This tool can and should be used throughout the cancer trajectory. The accompanying problem list may be very helpful in identifying specific problems that merit further evaluation and intervention.

## Specific Interventions to Promote Psychosocial Health

### Bibliotherapy

Bibliotherapy is a form of therapy in which selected reading materials are used to help to identify and solve problems. The amount of information available regarding a diagnosis of breast cancer can be very overwhelming. Web sites, books, pamphlets, and help lines are available to provide information about the diagnosis and treatment options and the use or misuse of complementary and alternative treatments. Although many of these resources provide quality information, a wide range of medical misinformation and misrepresentation can be found in both the academic and popular press.

Helping patients to identify appropriate sources of information regarding breast cancer should be a priority for healthcare professionals throughout the cancer trajectory. During the initial assessment, healthcare professionals should determine whether the patient wants a large amount of information or if only the essential information should be provided over time. Reliable resources are available through many Web sites to help patients understand breast cancer and its treatment modalities.

Traditional oncology teaching tools include written booklets and teaching sheets, which can be expensive to print, require significant storage space, and need periodic updates. Because of these constraints, educational materials housed in healthcare facilities may be limited, and information about rare cancers or unusual procedures may be difficult to find. Despite these limitations, printed literature still has a place in patient education. Most importantly, it can serve as a reinforcement of information after the patient leaves the medical setting and can be easily shared with other family members and friends (Karten, 2007).

The premise behind both complex and easy-to-read booklets is that they are intended to help patients and caregivers communicate with healthcare providers about their treatment and support needs. The easy-to-read booklets often are developed for newly diagnosed patients and individuals with lower reading levels. Sometimes as patients become more knowl-edgeable about the disease and its treatment, they desire and request more complex information. This information is available from many agencies, including the National Institutes of Health, ACS, and NCCN. Many of these more detailed guides can be accessed or downloaded from the agency's Web site.

For such publications to be a useful adjunct to education, patients must be able to comprehend the material, which requires varying degrees of health literacy. Nurses need to assess for health literacy and choose appropriate materials. Approximately one in five Americans is functionally illiterate, and an estimated one in five Americans reads at a fifth-grade level or lower (Balmer, 2005). This is not necessarily due to learning disorders or low IQ. It is often linked to poverty, unemployment, being part of a minority group, or advancing age. People who are illiterate may be very functional, as they have learned to compensate in other ways for their lack of reading skills. These statistics need to be considered in the development and selection of patient education materials.

Another often overlooked issue with literacy in patients with cancer is the increased risk of cognitive dysfunction compared with those who have never had cancer or cancer treatment (Evens & Eschiti, 2009). Cognitive dysfunction is a frequent finding in people with cancer, but it may go unnoticed. Cognitive problems result from many causes, including the direct effects of cancer on the central nervous system, indirect effects of certain cancers, and effects of cancer treatment on the brain. Cognitive dysfunction is often compounded by the mental and emotional aspects of dealing with a cancer diagnosis, including information overload, the stress of living with uncertainty and making treatment decisions, changes in schedule, anxiety, fear, and financial pressures. Ultimately, cognitive dysfunction also influences literacy and can make some information difficult to process and comprehend.

### Internet

The Internet has influenced the ways in which patients learn about and cope with their disease. Advantages associated with the use of the Internet include access 24 hours a day, seven days a week to current information in a variety of patient-friendly formats. Although the Internet may be a source of empowerment for patients, it can overwhelm users because of the sheer amount of information that is available. Others may be unable to access Internet resources because of barriers associated with income, education, physical limitations, or ethnic background. Issues of trustworthiness and security are concerns in all cases where online sources are used for health-related information. Nurses are uniquely suited to use online resources to aid in patient education and support.

For many patients, the Internet has become one of the first places to go for important information, including health information that ultimately guides treatment decisions. An enormous amount of cancer information exists on the Internet. This information can help people facing cancer to make decisions about their illness and treatment. Patients and families need to understand that just because a wealth of information is available, it does not provide any guarantee that the information is current or accurate. Web sites can provide basic facts about certain types of cancer, assist in locating the most current clinical trials, and provide information and support in dealing with cancer. It is possible to access information on research articles, doctors and hospitals, cancer treatment guidelines, drug information, and information on complementary and alternative therapies.

Finding sites that are responsible, accurate, and applicable to an individual's specific concern or question can be more challenging than it appears. One approach to help women access safe information is to provide them with a list of addresses to reputable Web sites. Considerations when selecting sites include who runs the site (professional or commercial), peer review policies, how often it is updated, whether it includes current and appropriate references, and the purpose of the site. Working from a list of sites that have been reviewed by a health professional, patients can type in the exact Web address and visit the sites. This approach ensures patients' access to safe information; however, problems can occur if the user follows links from the site that eventually lead to unreliable sources. If the site does not have the information the patient is searching for, this method can be a source of frustration. Nurses can integrate Internet resources into practice by first reviewing reputable sites and then incorporating the information into teaching sessions with patients.

## Treatment Setting Orientation

A simple intervention to promote psychosocial adaptation and decrease distress is a brief (15–20 minutes) clinic tour for new patients in a medical oncology clinic. Tours can include an opportunity to see the phlebotomy, nursing, and chemotherapy areas. This information can be reinforced by the distribution of written materials about clinic hours, telephone numbers, and procedures. The potential effectiveness of this intervention should not be underestimated. In one study, 150 consecutively referred patients with a variety of cancers were randomly assigned to either the clinic orientation or to standard care (Coughlin, 2008). Patients who received an orientation showed less anxiety, less mood disturbance, and fewer depressive symptoms at a one-week follow-up. In addition, these patients reported more knowledge of clinic procedures, more confidence in their physicians, and higher levels of satisfaction and hope.

## Journaling

Journaling is often an effective technique to decrease distress. It can help to identify symptoms that can be managed, as well as the positive things occurring in one's life. For some patients, it serves as a way to leave a legacy of what they experienced. It also is a means to organize thoughts and ideas.

Women are expected to take part in their treatment decision making, but this can be very stressful. Specific strategies to help decrease stress include encouraging patients and family members to write down questions as they occur. One way to encourage this is to provide patients with a small notebook or journal specifically for this purpose. This notebook also can be used to write down notes during visits. Encouraging patients to keep all written materials, reports, telephone numbers, medication lists, and family history information in one place can provide them with a sense of control over the situation.

## Cancer Information Centers

A cancer information or resource center can provide education and information. A nurse who provides the education and support usually staffs an information center. Resource centers often distribute brochures, videos, educational models, wigs, head coverings, and temporary prostheses, which help to facilitate psychosocial adjustment. The nurses in these centers can provide guidance on Internet searches and answer specific questions. Many institutions now offer these services, and healthcare providers should encourage and refer patients.

Nurse navigators can assist patients throughout the cancer trajectory. They can provide psychosocial support and make appropriate referrals. See Chapter 11 for more information about nurse navigators.

## Complementary and Alternative Medicine

No discussion of supportive and psychological care in breast cancer is complete without addressing the attraction and use of complementary and alternative medicine (CAM) for the treatment of side effects associated with cancer and its treatment. This is a rapidly emerging field, and CAM use can have a direct effect, either positive or negative, on cancer treatment. For this reason, nurses need to be aware of CAM and take direct steps to accurately assess whether women are incorporating these strategies into their cancer care, especially to manage side effects and associated psychosocial distress.

*Complementary medicine* is used along with standard medical treatments. One example is the use of acupuncture to help with the side effects of cancer treatment. *Alternative medicine* is used in place of standard medical treatments. An example is using a special diet to treat cancer instead of a method that an oncologist suggests. *Integrative medicine* is a total approach to care that involves the patient's mind, body, and spirit. It combines standard medicine with the CAM practices that have shown the most promise. For example, some women use relaxation as a way to reduce stress during chemotherapy. To date, no CAM practice has been proved to be universally effective in the treatment of cancer, but promising research has shown that they may be a valuable adjunct to treatment (Chong, 2006). CAM therapies can be categorized into five areas (see Figure 10-7).

**Figure 10-7. Categories of Complementary and Alternative Medicine (CAM) Therapies**

**Mind-body medicines:** CAM practices based on the belief that one's mind is able to affect one's body. Some examples include
- Meditation
- Biofeedback
- Hypnosis
- Yoga
- Imagery
- Art, music, or dance therapy.

**Biologically based practices:** CAM that uses natural products, such as dietary supplements and herbal products. Some examples are
- Vitamins
- Herbs
- Foods
- Special diets.

**Manipulative and body-based practices:** CAM practices based on working or moving one or more body parts. Some examples include
- Massage
- Chiropractic care
- Reflexology.

**Energy medicine:** CAM practices based on the belief that the body has energy fields that can be used for healing and wellness. Some examples are
- Tai Chi
- Reiki
- Therapeutic touch.

**Whole medical systems:** CAM practices that consider the mind, body, and spirit. Some examples are
- Ayurvedic medicine
- Chinese medicine
- Acupuncture
- Homeopathy
- Naturopathic medicine.

*Note.* Based on information from Astin et al., 2003; Smith, 2005.

The challenge of nurses and other healthcare providers is to be supportive of patients who use CAM while also being appropriate advocates. CAM can be promoted by imposters and con artists who seek out the vulnerable (Smith, 2005). The obligation of healthcare providers is to help patients sort through massive amounts of information; focus on those options that are promising, effective, and safe; and support studies that generate documented effectiveness data.

Some women with breast cancer are concerned that their healthcare providers will not approve of the use of CAM. Communication with a healthcare provider is important to avoid dangerous interactions between traditional cancer therapies and CAM. For this reason, nurses need to directly and continually assess whether patients are using CAM. An environment of open communication will help prevent complications.

The prevalence of CAM use in the general population has increased substantially during the past 30 years and especially in the past decade. In December 2008, the National Center for Complementary and Alternative Medicine (NCCAM) released new findings on Americans' use of CAM. In the United States, approximately 38% of adults with cancer use some form of CAM (NCCAM, 2008). People of all backgrounds use CAM; however, its use among adults is greater among women and those with higher levels of education and higher incomes (NCCAM, 2008).

CAM users are likely to use more than one CAM therapy in conjunction with conventional medicine. Commonly cited reasons for use include the beliefs that these therapies can boost immune function, prevent cancer recurrence, improve QOL, increase the feelings of being in control, and palliate the symptoms of cancer treatment (Chong, 2006).

Preferences for CAM therapies vary. Several studies report a high prevalence of the use of prayer, dietary supplements, massage, and relaxation techniques. The use of dietary supplements is estimated to be particularly popular in patients with breast cancer (Smith, 2005).

Nondisclosure of CAM use by patients with cancer has been well documented, with studies reporting rates from 40% to 70% (Chong, 2006). Patients' reasons for nondisclosure were that they felt it was not important for the doctor to know and because the doctor never asked. It is also speculated that patients do not see CAM's potential to affect their standard cancer treatment and that patients did not perceive the therapy they were using as CAM (especially if it is marketed as a natural supplement, vitamin, or food product). Other possible reasons are feared disinterest or negative response by the provider or the view that the discussion of CAM is a poor use of time or inappropriate (Smith, 2005). The reality that patients do not reveal CAM use to the healthcare team is of particular concern because the safety and efficacy of some CAM therapies are not yet fully known.

In 1998, the National Institutes of Health established NCCAM, the purpose of which was to conduct basic and clinical research, train researchers, and educate and communicate findings concerning therapeutic and preventive CAM therapies. NCCAM is the lead agency in the United States for scientific research on CAM. Nurses should learn to access the many resources available at the NCCAM Web site (http://nccam.nih.gov) if they have specific questions about a treatment. The site contains a comprehensive list of CAM therapies that includes a description of the therapy, pictures when available, the scientific basis of the therapy, and safety considerations. Patients also can be referred to this Web site if they have additional questions. The usefulness of this resource for both healthcare professionals and patients should not be underestimated.

## Acupuncture

Acupuncture is a technique in which very thin needles of varying lengths are inserted through the skin to treat a variety of conditions. It may help treat nausea caused by chemotherapy drugs and surgical anesthesia (Sherman et al., 2005). A recent analysis of 11 studies looked at the effect of acupuncture in reducing nausea and vomiting related to chemotherapy (Ezzo et al., 2006). The report suggested that acupuncture may reduce the vomiting that occurs shortly after chemotherapy is given, even though it had little effect on nausea. It does not seem to help with delayed vomiting (Mayo Clinic, 2007).

When performed by a trained professional, acupuncture is generally considered safe. The reported complications are relatively few, but there is a risk that a patient may be harmed if the acupuncturist is not well trained (Ernst, Strzyz, & Hagmeister, 2003). Although the needles used in traditional needle acupuncture are very fine, they can cause dizziness, fainting, local internal bleeding, nerve damage, and increased pain. The risk of infection is low because acupuncturists in the United States use sterile needles that are discarded after a single use.

## Aromatherapy

Aromatherapy is the use of fragrant substances, called essential oils, distilled from plants to alter mood or improve health. These highly concentrated aromatic substances are either inhaled or applied during massage. Approximately 40 essential oils are commonly used in aromatherapy; among the most commonly used are lavender, rosemary, eucalyptus, chamomile, marjoram, jasmine, peppermint, lemon, and geranium (Mayo Clinic, 2007).

The underlying mechanism of action of aromatherapy is not fully understood. Scent receptors in the nose are known to send chemical messages through the olfactory nerve to the brain's limbic region, which influences emotional responses, heart rate, blood pressure, and respiration (Smith, 2005). These connections explain the effects of essential oils' pleasant smells. The effects may depend partly on previous associations of the person with a particular scent. Laboratory studies suggest that the oils can affect organ function, but whether this can be useful is not yet clear (Campenni, Crawley, & Meier, 2004). Many aromatherapists are trained as massage therapists, psychologists, social workers, or chiropractors and use the oils as part of their practices. The essential oils can be used one at a time or in combination and may be inhaled or applied to the skin.

Early clinical trials suggest that aromatherapy may have some benefit in reducing stress, pain, nausea, and depression. However, some studies show no difference in outcome between massage with aromatherapy oils and massage without them (Soden, Vincent, Craske, Lucas, & Ashley, 2004). There are also reports that inhaled peppermint, ginger, and cardamom oil seem to relieve the nausea caused by chemotherapy and radiation (Smith, 2005).

Aromatherapy is generally safe (Lee, 2003). Essential oils should not be taken internally, as many of them are poisonous. Some oils can cause sensitization or allergies, and others may cause irritation if applied undiluted to the skin.

## Art Therapy

Art therapy is the use of creative activities to express emotions to help people manage physical and emotional problems. It provides a way for people to come to terms with emotional conflicts, increase self-awareness, and express unspoken and often unconscious concerns about their illness and their lives. It may include dance and movement, drama, poetry, and photography, as well as the more traditional art methods.

In art therapy, patients are given the tools they need to produce paintings, drawings, sculptures, and many other types of artwork. Art therapists work with patients individually or in groups. The role of the art therapist is to help patients express themselves through their creations and to talk to patients about their emotions and concerns as they relate to their art.

Case studies have reported that art therapy benefits patients with both emotional and physical illnesses (Walsh, Martin, & Schmidt, 2004). Some of the potential uses of art therapy include reducing anxiety levels, improving recovery times, decreasing hospital stays, improving communication and social function, and controlling pain.

Art therapy is considered safe when conducted by a skilled therapist. It may be useful as a complementary therapy to help people with cancer to deal with their emotions. Although uncomfortable feelings may be stirred up at times, this is considered part of the healing process. More information about art therapy, including how to locate a licensed art therapist, is available through the American Art Therapy Association at www.arttherapy.org.

## Biofeedback

Biofeedback is a treatment method that uses monitoring devices to help people consciously control physical processes, such as heart rate, blood pressure, temperature, sweating, and muscle tension, that are usually controlled automatically. By helping the patient to change the heart rate, skin temperature, breathing rate, muscle control, and other such activities in the body, biofeedback can reduce stress and muscle tension and promote relaxation. Through a greater awareness of bodily functions, the person can regulate or alter other physical functions. Biofeedback often is a matter of trial and error as patients learn to adjust their thinking and connect changes in thought, breathing, posture, and muscle tension with changes in physical functions that are usually controlled unconsciously.

Biofeedback has no direct effect on the development or progression of cancer, but it can improve the QOL for some people with cancer (Astin, Shapiro, Eisenberg, & Forys, 2003). Biofeedback often is used with relaxation for the best results.

Biofeedback is thought to be a safe technique. It is noninvasive. Biofeedback requires a trained and certified professional to manage equipment, interpret changes, and monitor the patient. Physical therapists often provide this therapy. A typical session takes 30–60 minutes (Mayo Clinic, 2007).

## Cognitive-Behavioral Therapy, Psychotherapy, and Family and Couples Therapy

Cognitive-behavioral therapy works by identifying and correcting inaccurate thoughts associated with depression or anxiety. This often is accomplished through developing and practicing problem-solving skills (NCCN, 2010).

Psychotherapy covers a wide range of approaches designed to help people change their ways of thinking, feeling, or behaving. Psychotherapy can help people, including those with cancer, find the inner strength they need to improve their coping skills, thereby allowing them to more fully enjoy their lives. Psychotherapy can be used to help people deal with the diagnosis and treatment of cancer. It also can be useful in overcoming depression and anxiety, which are common in people with cancer (NCCN, 2010).

Psychotherapy is available in many forms. People may seek individual therapy, which is a one-on-one relationship with a therapist. Therapists also can work with couples or entire families to help them deal with the impact of the cancer and its diagnosis on those most closely affected. Psychotherapy may be practiced with groups, in which a number of people meet together to discuss common experiences and issues and to learn specific coping techniques.

Psychotherapists vary in the amount of their training and experience in dealing with the issues that are important for people with cancer. Psychotherapy may be performed by practitioners with a number of different qualifications, including psychologists, marriage and family therapists, licensed clinical social workers, counselors, psychiatric nurses, and psychiatrists (Smith, 2005). Healthcare providers should be familiar with reputable providers for referrals. Some institutions have a psychotherapist on staff, which increases access.

## Guided Imagery

Guided imagery involves the use of the imagination to create sights, sounds, smells, tastes, or other sensations to develop a type of purposeful daydream. The techniques can help to reduce stress, anxiety, and depression; manage pain; lower blood pressure; ease some of the side effects of chemotherapy; and create feelings of being in control (Astin et al., 2003).

For people with cancer, guided imagery can relieve nausea and vomiting from chemotherapy, relieve stress that is associated with having cancer, enhance the immune system, combat depression, and lessen pain (Astin et al., 2003). Imagery techniques are considered safe, especially under the guidance of a trained health professional. Guided imagery may be provided by counselors, music therapists, or psychiatric nurses with specialized training.

## Massage

Massage involves manipulation, rubbing, and kneading of the body's muscle and soft tissue to enhance function of those tissues and promote relaxation (Mayo Clinic, 2007). In all forms of massage, therapists use their hands (and some-times forearms, elbows, and massage tools) to manipulate the body's soft tissue. Massage strokes can vary from light and shallow to firm and deep and from slow, steady pressure to quick tapping. The choice will depend on the health and needs of the individual and the training and style of the massage therapist. Massage therapy has been shown to reduce pain, stress, depression, fatigue, and anxiety in randomized controlled trials (Deng & Cassileth, 2005).

Massage or manipulation of a bone in an area of cancer metastasis could result in a bone fracture (Mayo Clinic, 2007). Also, people who have had radiation may find even light touch on or near the treatment area to be uncomfortable. Women with cancer should consult with their physicians before undergoing any type of therapy that involves the manipulation of joints and muscles. It is contraindicated in people with significant risk for a deep vein thrombosis (Mayo Clinic, 2007).

## Meditation

Meditation is a mind-body process that uses concentration or reflection to relax the body and calm the mind. Meditation may be done by choosing a quiet place free from distraction, sitting or resting quietly with eyes closed, noticing breathing and physical sensations, and noticing and then letting go of all intruding thoughts. The person also may achieve a relaxed yet alert state by focusing on a pleasant idea or thought or by chanting a phrase or special sound silently or aloud. The ultimate goal of meditation is to separate oneself mentally from the outside world by suspending the usual stream of consciousness. Some practitioners recommend two 15–20-minute sessions a day (Mayo Clinic, 2007).

Clinical trials have studied meditation as a way of reducing stress on both the mind and the body. Research shows that meditation can help reduce anxiety, stress, blood pressure, chronic pain, insomnia, and mood disturbance (Smith, Richardson, Hoffman, & Pilkington, 2005). A number of different types of meditation exist. Although step-by-step guides are available, most people benefit from an initial session with a therapist who is trained in teaching meditation skills (Mayo Clinic, 2007).

## Music Therapy

Music therapy is the supervised and therapeutic use of music to promote positive clinical outcomes (Bulfone, Quattrin, Zanotti, Regattin, & Brusaferro, 2009). Music therapy can be both active and passive. Active music therapy is based on improvisation between the therapist and the patient, and it requires the patient's actual participation in creating sound, lyrics, or other music. In passive music therapy, patients, individually or in a group, listen to music recorded or played with musical instruments by a therapist. During receptive music therapy, patients choose their favorite music to enhance therapeutic effectiveness. For each person, music is a unique experience, and preference is influenced by sex, age, culture, present mood, and attitude. It is vital for the therapist to enable the patient to find music that is acceptable and pleasant. Music with 60–80 beats per minute is typically restful, whereas faster beats can stimulate and give energy to depressive and melancholic people.

Music therapists design music sessions for individuals and groups based on their needs and tastes. Some aspects of music therapy include making music, listening to music, writing songs, and talking about lyrics. It also may involve imagery and learning through music. Music therapy can be done in different places, such as hospitals, cancer centers, hospices, at home, or anywhere people can benefit from its calming or stimulating effects. The patient does not need to have any musical ability to benefit from music therapy.

Music therapy may be used to encourage emotional expression, promote social interactions, and relieve symptoms (Clark et al., 2006). It can help to reduce pain and stress, relieve chemotherapy-induced nausea and vomiting, and provide an overall sense of well-being. Music therapy can lower heart rate, blood pressure, and breathing rate. Music therapy can improve comfort, relaxation, and pain control (Pelletier, 2004) and sometimes is used for distraction.

Music therapy that is provided by a professionally trained therapist can be therapeutic and is considered safe when used with standard treatment. Musical intervention by untrained people can be ineffective or even cause increased stress and discomfort (Bulfone et al., 2009). More information about professional licensed musical therapists is available through the American Music Therapy Association at www.musictherapy.org.

### Spirituality

Spirituality generally is described as an awareness of something greater than the individual self. It often is expressed through religion and/or prayer, although many other paths of spiritual pursuit and expression exist. Studies have found that spirituality and religion are very important to the QOL for some people with cancer and has been shown to improve QOL in people with cancer (Mayo Clinic, 2007). The psychological benefits of praying may include reduction of stress and anxiety, promotion of a more positive outlook, and strengthening of the will to live (Tinley, 2010).

Spirituality has many forms and can be practiced in many ways. Prayer, for example, may be silent or spoken out loud and can be done alone in any setting or in groups. Spirituality also can be practiced without a formal religion. Meditation, 12-step work (as practiced in Alcoholics Anonymous and similar groups), and seeking meaning in life all involve spirituality (Smith, 2005). Many medical institutions and practitioners include spirituality and prayer as important components of healing. In addition, hospitals have chapels and contracts with ministers, rabbis, clerics, and voluntary organizations to serve their patients' spiritual needs.

### Support Groups

Support groups present information, provide comfort, teach coping skills, help reduce anxiety, and provide a place for people to share common concerns and emotional support. For many patients, they can improve QOL (Goodwin, 2005). Many different kinds of support groups are available and vary in their structure and activities (Mayo Clinic, 2007). A self-help support group is fully organized and managed by its members, usually volunteers. It typically is facilitated by members who are affected by the same type of cancer. Professionally operated support groups are facilitated by professionals, such as nurses, social workers, psychologists, or members of the clergy, who do not share the problem of the members. The facilitator controls discussions and provides other managerial services. Professionally operated groups often are found in institutional settings, such as hospitals or outpatient clinics.

Some support groups are time-limited, while others are ongoing. Some groups are made up of people with the same type of cancer, while others include people who are having the same kind of treatment. Support groups are available for patients, family members, and other caregivers of people with cancer. The format of different groups varies from lectures and discussions to exploration and expression of feelings. Topics discussed by support groups are those of concern to the members and those the group leader thinks are important. Benefits include that most support groups involve little or no cost to the participants.

Support groups can enhance the QOL for people with cancer by providing information and support to overcome the feelings of aloneness and helplessness that sometimes result from a diagnosis of cancer. Some people with cancer are better able to deal with their disease when supported by others in similar situations (Penson, Talsania, Chabner, & Lynch, 2004).

Support groups vary in quality and focus. People with cancer may find the support group they have joined does not discuss topics of interest to them. Some people may find a support group upsetting because it stirs up too many uncomfortable feelings or because the leader is not skilled enough to provide direction to manage negative feelings. Information that is shared in some groups may not always be reliable (Zabalegui, Sanchez, Sanchez, & Juando, 2005). Internet support groups should be used with caution. This method cannot always ensure privacy or confidentiality, and the people involved may have no special training or qualifications, especially if found in unmonitored chat rooms.

### Tai Chi

Tai Chi is an ancient Chinese martial art. It is a mind-body, self-healing system that uses movement, meditation, and breathing to improve health and well-being. Tai Chi is useful as a form of exercise that may improve posture, balance, muscle mass and tone, flexibility, stamina, and strength in older adults. Tai Chi also is recognized as a method to reduce stress and can provide the same cardiovascular benefits as moderate exercise, such as lowered heart rate and blood pressure (Li et al., 2004; Mustian, Katula, & Zhao, 2006).

The slow, graceful movements of Tai Chi, accompanied by rhythmic breathing, relax the body as well as the mind. Each form contains 20–100 moves and can require up to 20 minutes to complete the movements, which are practiced in pairs of opposites. While doing these exercises, the person is urged to pay close attention to her breathing, which is centered in the diaphragm. Tai Chi emphasizes technique rather than strength or power, although the slow, precise movements require good muscle control.

Tai Chi has been associated with a sense of improved well-being and increased motivation to continue exercising. Many like Tai Chi because it is self-paced and noncompetitive and does not require large amounts of space, special equipment, or clothing (Mayo Clinic, 2007). Tai Chi is considered to be a relatively safe, moderate physical activity. It is important for patients to be aware of their physical limitations and to speak with their doctors before starting any type of therapy or exercise that involves the movement of joints and muscles.

### Yoga

Yoga is a form of nonaerobic exercise that involves a program of precise posture, breathing exercises, and meditation. It is a way of life that combines ethical standards, dietary guidelines, physical movements, and meditation to create a union of the mind, body, and spirit.

A typical yoga session can last between 20 minutes and 1 hour. A yoga session starts with the person sitting in an upright position and performing gentle movements, all of which are done very slowly while taking slow, deep breaths from the abdomen. Yoga requires several sessions a week for a person to become proficient. Yoga can be practiced in group classes or at home without a teacher. Many books and DVDs on yoga are available, and it often is offered through groups such as the Cancer Support Community (www.cancersupportcommunity.org).

Yoga can be used to control physical functions such as blood pressure, heart rate, breathing, metabolism, body temperature, brain waves, and skin resistance (Cohen, Warneke, Fouladi, Rodriguez, & Chaoul-Reich, 2004). This can result in improved physical fitness, lower levels of stress, and increased feelings of relaxation and well-being. Some yoga postures are hard to achieve, and injury can result from overstretching joints and ligaments. Patients should be instructed to check with their healthcare provider before initiating a program of yoga.

### Patient Education Regarding Complementary and Alternative Medicines

With CAM availability and use increasing, patients should receive help and support as they evaluate whether a particular CAM therapy is appropriate. Patient advocacy in the form of helping to evaluate the safety and effectiveness of CAMs is an important nursing responsibility. Assessment of medical and lifestyle history should include direct questioning about CAM use. If a patient uses CAM, it should be explored in more de-

tail to determine if it is safe for that individual. Researching the CAM therapy on the NCCAM Web site is an effective approach. Patients should be informed that CAM can be a useful adjunct to therapy, but only after discussing the safety in each individual situation. Many patients consider using dietary supplements such as vitamins, herbs, or any product made from plants as part of their cancer treatment. Currently, few governmental standards are in place to control the production and ensure the safety, effectiveness, and quality of dietary supplements. Patients must understand that dietary supplements, like medications, have potential risks and side effects. They usually can be used safely within certain dosage guidelines (Smith, 2005). But, unlike drugs, dietary supplements are primarily "self-prescribed," with little or no input from an informed healthcare provider. Often, reliable information about the safe use and potential risks of dietary supplements is lacking. The NCCAM Web site can be one reliable source of information. Healthcare providers should regularly assess if patients are using supplements and assist them in evaluating the safety of such supplements.

Patients also should receive guidance on selecting an appropriate CAM therapy and practitioner. Choosing a CAM provider should be done with the same care as choosing any other member of the healthcare team. Patients seeking a CAM practitioner should speak with their healthcare provider or someone knowledgeable about CAM regarding the therapy under consideration. The provider may be able to make a recommendation for the type of CAM practitioner the patient is seeking.

Before engaging CAM practitioners, the patient should ask basic questions about their credentials and practice. Where did they receive their training? What licenses or certifications do they have? How much will the treatment cost? CAM can be expensive. Patients should check with their insurer to see if the cost of therapy will be covered. Patients should contact CAM professional organizations to get names of practitioners who are certified, which indicates they have proper training in their field.

After selecting a practitioner, the patient should make a list of questions to ask at the first visit. Ideally, the patient should bring a friend or family member who can help ask questions and note answers. On the first visit, the patient should be prepared to answer questions about her health history, including injuries, surgeries, and major illnesses, as well as prescription medicines, vitamins, and other supplements. The patient should assess the first visit and decide whether the practitioner is a good fit. Things to consider include level of comfort, willingness to answer questions, and reasonableness of the treatment plan.

## Supportive Measures for Specific Problems

### Alopecia and Skin Changes

Alopecia is a side effect that can cause great distress during treatment for breast cancer. Cyclophosphamide and anthracyclines are commonly administered chemotherapeutic agents in breast cancers, and both are associated with a significant risk for alopecia. Thus, many women being treated with chemotherapy are likely to experience alopecia one or more times during the course of their care.

As part of the patient education about receiving chemotherapy, patients should be informed that hair loss is likely to occur. It is very important to be clear that this includes all hair, not just scalp hair (Nail & Lee-Lin, 2010). Patients also need to be prepared that this is not only a body image change but a functional change. Bald heads tend to get cold, and a runny nose may drip more suddenly; these issues can be managed by wearing a cap to prevent scalp heat loss and by carrying tissues. Patients can prevent scalp problems by protecting the bald scalp from sunburn when out in ultraviolet light and washing with a mild baby shampoo.

Although some women embrace hair loss as a symbol of their fight against the disease, others may feel self-conscious. Alopecia can be a traumatic event, and preparing patients for this occurrence may help with the adjustment. Some patients want to keep their own hair for as long as possible, preferring that it falls out gradually. Other patients adjust better by cutting their hair short prior to the time they will begin to lose it. Both of these choices can help patients to gain a little control over what feels like—and basically is—an uncontrollable event.

Many options exist for hair covering, including wigs, scarves, and hats. Patients may find it hard to see themselves without hair, and some women will wear a head covering even while alone. Patients should be supported in whatever choice they make.

Many resources are available to help women with adjusting to the hair loss of cancer therapy, as well as some of the other physical changes they may experience. "Look Good . . . Feel Better®" is a free program sponsored by the Cosmetic, Toiletry, and Fragrance Association Foundation in partnership with ACS and the National Cosmetology Association. The program's Web site (http://lookgoodfeelbetter.org) has helpful tips for hair and makeup and a program finder for classes where women can learn hair and makeup techniques while undergoing cancer treatment. The information is available in both English and Spanish, and specific information is available for teens.

Although the hair almost always grows back, it can be of a different color and texture. Sometimes it is also thinner. Women may be glad to have hair, but these differences can be distressing. Women need to be prepared for these changes.

Loss of pubic hair can be very distressing (Katz, 2007). Although it is seldom discussed, many women are very upset by this change in their physical appearance, and it ultimately has a negative effect on sexuality.

In addition to hair loss, some patients may experience skin changes from treatment. Radiation therapy can cause redness and irritation of the skin. Redness may occur early in treatment, whereas dry or moist desquamation occurs nearer to the end of the scheduled treatment; both may continue following treatment. Another possible side effect of radiation therapy is hyperpigmentation, and the darker pigmentation may remain following treatment. Radiated skin is more sensitive to exposure to ultraviolet light, and skin protection must continue indefinitely. Hyperpigmentation also may occur following administration of some chemotherapeutic agents. Skin color should be expected to slowly return to normal following chemotherapy.

## Weight Changes

For most people, food is a source of joy and comfort. However, for patients experiencing nausea, vomiting, and diarrhea, food can become a source of frustration. The question "What did you eat today?" can be a problem for the patient, the family, and the healthcare team. The weight loss that occurs is a visual reminder of the stress of eating and the resulting changes in body image, which can contribute to feelings of anxiety and depression. Nutritional supplements are available to improve calorie and protein intake for patients who are having difficulty with eating. The supplements come in many different forms, including powders, liquids, and semisolids. A nutrition consultation may be helpful for women experiencing weight loss and difficulty with eating.

Weight gain also can occur as a result of treatment for breast cancer and can have an impact on body image. Medications such as steroids used as part of a chemotherapy regimen can cause increased hunger and weight gain. Substantial evidence exists that weight gain often occurs in women after a breast cancer diagnosis. This increase in weight is most common among premenopausal women at diagnosis and those who receive chemotherapy as part of their treatment (Caan et al., 2008). The average weight gains have been reported to range from 3.9 to 9.7 pounds, with one-third of patients gaining more than 11 pounds (Caan et al., 2008). At a time when the patient may already have difficulty with body image because of the diagnosis of cancer, weight gain adds more stress and prevents some women from agreeing to therapy. Weight gain is associated with a negative impact on sexual function (Katz, 2007).

## Sexuality

Although altered sexuality is a psychosocial issue that should be addressed by oncology nurses, many times nurses are uncomfortable with or fail to address these issues (Katz, 2007). Nurses need to practice and take conscious steps to include sexuality as an important component of comprehensive cancer care. Some nurses may benefit from additional continuing education on the topic (Katz, 2007).

Women may feel uncomfortable initiating a discussion about sexuality at the time of diagnosis, a time when they feel the focus should be on the disease and treatment of the disease. In addition, discussing sexuality is frequently considered taboo. Following surgery for breast cancer, women may feel they do not want their partners to touch them in the same ways as prior to surgery, either because of emotional concerns of touching the surgical area or because of altered sensations in the breast from the treatment. Women should be encouraged to communicate their needs and feelings to their partners to lessen the physical and emotional discomfort for both of them. Two excellent resources include the ACS publication *Sexuality for the Woman With Cancer* (also available in Spanish) and *Woman Cancer Sex* (Katz, 2009).

In order to provide effective care, oncology nurses need to include sexual functioning as part of the nursing assessment. It is best carried out in a private environment. Nurses need to normalize the discussion and approach the topic directly. One way to begin is to state something such as, "I always ask patients if they have any questions or concerns regarding sexuality" (Katz, 2007). A model for assessment of sexual functioning is helpful for providing comprehensive care. A commonly used model is the PLISSIT. The first level involves *permission*; level two stands for *limited information*; level three refers to *specific suggestions*; and the fourth level refers to *intensive the*rapy (see Figure 10-8).

Potential changes in sexuality must be addressed for women with breast cancer. Concerns about sexuality begin at the time of diagnosis. Many women connect sexuality with their breasts, and the removal of the breast or any part of a breast may affect their sexual identity. Breast surgery can have significant emotional consequences for both women and their partners (Katz, 2007). Women who experience lymphedema may experience limited mobility, which also affects sexuality. Breast surgery forever alters the breast and breast sensation; even women who undergo reconstruction note that the breast is not the same. Women may benefit from seeing pictures of a reconstructed breast or a chest wall following mastectomy prior to surgery. This helps provide some anticipatory guidance and preparation. Some women also benefit from seeing prosthesis options before surgery. These interventions can help prevent later disappointment and adjustment problems (Katz, 2009).

Women may have trouble looking at the scar following breast surgery. Many women also do not know how to show the breast to their partner. Often, both the woman and the partner imagine the scar to be worse than it actually is; some need encouragement to look at the altered breast (Katz, 2009).

Currently, most women without a diagnosis of breast cancer can expect to live at least one-third of their life in the postmenopausal state. For women treated aggressively for breast cancer, its duration can be significantly longer. Hot flashes may be more troublesome to younger women diagnosed with breast cancer (Schultz, Klein, Beck, Stava, & Sellin, 2005). An estimated 53%–89% of premenopausal women experience ovarian failure and premature menopause after receiving multiagent chemotherapy (Rogers & Kristjanson, 2002). The older the woman, the higher the risk. When menopause occurs quickly, the symptoms may be more profound, including in-

---

### Figure 10-8. The PLISSIT Model

P—Permission giving
- The practitioner creates a climate of comfort and gives permission to clients to discuss sexual concerns, often introducing the topic of sexuality, thereby validating sexuality as a legitimate health issue and concern.
- "Women with breast cancer often experience sexual difficulties, such as a loss of desire or problems with enjoyment. Have you been affected by these types of problems?"

LI—Limited Information
- The practitioner addresses specific sexual concerns and attempts to correct myths and misinformation.
- "Once the sutures have been removed from the lumpectomy site, it is fine to gradually resume sexual relations. It is often helpful to tell your partner how you are feeling."

SS—Specific Suggestions
- After identification and clarification of the issues and how they have evolved over time, the nurse can offer the patient very specific directions on how to address the problem. The caregiver is responsible for providing the patient with honest, informative, and accurate answers to questions.
- A woman is experiencing vaginal dryness due to a premature menopause. The nurse suggests increased foreplay, the regular use of vaginal moisturizers, and lubricants.

IT—Intensive Therapy
- Referral to a therapist or specialist who provides specialized treatment in cases that are complicated by the coexistence of other complex life issues, including psychiatric diagnoses such as depression, anxiety disorders, obsessive-compulsive disorder, personality disorders, or substance abuse, or by interpersonal or intrapersonal conflict.
- After trying vaginal moisturizers, a woman with premature menopause still is having painful intercourse. The nurse refers her to a gynecologist for further evaluation and management.

*Note.* Based on information from Annon, 1976; Katz, 2007; Wilmoth, 2009.

---

creased and more severe mood swings, increased hot flashes, and vaginal dryness. The impact of these changes should not be underestimated and may have a negative effect on sexual functioning (Katz, 2007).

*Dyspareunia* refers to pain experienced during vaginal entry or intercourse. This symptom results from vaginal thinning that occurs following decreased estrogen levels (Nishimoto & Mark, 2010). In patients with breast cancer, it can be exacerbated by early menopause, chemotherapy, aromatase inhibitors, and hormonal manipulation.

The first step in the management of dyspareunia is patient education. Patients should be informed not only that this often happens but also that interventions are available to decrease the pain (Nishimoto & Mark, 2010). Patients should be instructed that they need to have honest communication with their partner, and they also need to have open communication with the healthcare provider so that the best management strategies can be implemented.

Vaginal dryness is an often-overlooked concern. The use of hormone replacement therapy is controversial. Alternate therapies that should be suggested include the use of vaginal lubricants such as K-Y® Jelly (McNeil-PPC, Inc.) or vaginal moisturizers such as Replens® (Lil' Drug Store Products) (Katz, 2009).

Many women also experience changes in libido. During treatment, as many as 64% of women report significant changes in libido (Katz, 2007). This can be a very distressing symptom that patients are reluctant to discuss. Risks for decreased libido include recent surgery, chemotherapy, fatigue, anxiety, depression, and nausea and vomiting. When one partner experiences decreased libido, it typically affects the relationship and ultimately both partners. Encouraging couples to communicate about their interests and needs is important because prolonged silence leads to more misunderstandings (Katz, 2009). Small steps, such as kissing and caressing, can lead to increased sexual desire later. It also is important to remind patients that good communication is critical. When something is pleasurable, this needs to be communicated; when something is uncomfortable, that also needs to be communicated (Katz, 2009).

## Fertility

Although breast cancer most often is diagnosed in mid to later life, it also can occur in younger women. Some of the options offered to treat the cancer may affect patients' fertility. Despite research efforts, few options are available to help these women with issues of infertility (Schover, 2008). Prior to a diagnosis of cancer, a woman who is at high risk for developing cancer of the breast or ovary may be offered genetic testing to assess her risk of developing cancer. At the time of the disclosure of her genetic results, she should be counseled regarding the options available to her, including earlier childbearing, egg harvesting, and storing fertilized embryos. Removal of the entire ovary for freezing is also a technique with a promising future for preserving fertility (Nishimoto & Mark, 2010). After the patient completes treatment, the embryos can be implanted into the woman, who may be able to carry a pregnancy to term. The type of tumor may affect patients' options for pregnancy, so complete knowledge of the tumor and the treatment that will be offered must be available prior to this discussion with patients. Estrogen and progesterone receptors may prevent women from carrying a pregnancy to term. Surrogacy and adoption are options that patients and their partners may need to consider if pregnancy is not possible.

The psychological consequences of infertility can be devastating to patients and may result in increased anxiety and depression. Younger women with breast cancer must cope not only with cancer at a young age but also with infertility, most likely caused by treatment for the breast cancer. Fertile Hope (www.fertilehope.org) is an organization designed to help patients with cancer to deal with fertility issues. It offers resources about options that are available prior to diagnosis, during treatment, and following treatment.

## Body Image

After surgery and treatment for breast cancer, women may perceive their body as disfigured and feel that they have lost part of their feminine identity (Vos, Garssen, Visser, Duivenvoorden, & de Haes, 2004). Vos et al. (2004) reported that five years after treatment, 25%–75% of the women still had disturbances with their body image. This is probably related not only to the surgery and other treatments but also to individual coping styles and patients' perceived level of support.

The adverse effects of breast cancer treatment vary based on treatment type. Mastectomy (with or without reconstruction) and lumpectomy have been associated with altered body image. Women who undergo mastectomy also may experience anxiety, depression, a decrease in sexual interest, or a decrease in perceived sexual attractiveness. Although breast reconstruction may alleviate some concerns related to disfigurement, reconstruction is associated with a loss of breast sensation (Herbenick et al., 2008). Women who undergo radiation therapy may feel bothered by radiation tattoos, changes in breast sensation, fatigue, or arm mobility. Tamoxifen therapy has been associated with pain, burning, or discomfort with intercourse, as well as vaginal tightness. All of these treatments can have a negative impact on body image (Herbenick et al., 2008).

Women need to be counseled about choices in breast restoration. This can include breast prosthetics (full or partial) or reconstructive surgery (see Chapters 5 and 6). This is important psychologically and physically. Psychologically, it helps women to feel better about themselves. Physically, weight replacement of the breast is important to prevent long-term shoulder and posture problems. Women should be encouraged to learn about all their options before making a choice. They should be reminded that one choice is not necessarily better than another. Women need to choose what is most comfortable for them and compatible with their lifestyle.

## Pharmacologic Management

The exact prevalence of depression, anxiety, and other mental health problems in women with breast cancer is not fully understood. It may be as high as twice the incidence seen in the general population (Burgess et al., 2005). Suggested risk factors include younger age at diagnosis, previous problems with depression, and lack of adequate psychosocial support. Pharmacologic management may be used to alleviate some of the psychosocial effects of cancer and its treatment.

### Anxiety

Anxiety is a common reaction to the diagnosis and treatment of cancer. An estimated 20%–47% of patients with cancer experience significant distress or anxiety (Sheldon, 2010). Anxiety can result in feelings of distress, tension, and apprehension.

For some patients, pharmacologic intervention is indicated, but it should be combined with psychosocial interventions. A variety of agents can be used, including anxiolytics, azapirones, antihistamines, antidepressants, and atypical neuroleptics (see Table 10-2).

## Depression

Up to 46% of patients with breast cancer experience depression (Sharp, 2010). It is a psychosocial concern that should not be ignored. In addition to other psychosocial interventions, some patients will benefit from antidepressant therapy. Antidepressants may help patients who feel extreme sadness, hopelessness, or a lack of interest in activities. Medications also may be used to help patients sleep, relax, and begin to cope with the diagnosis. As with any medication, the

potential side effects and interactions with current medications and medical treatments should be discussed. Common side effects of antidepressants or antianxiety medications include nausea, weight gain, sexual side effects, fatigue or insomnia, dry mouth, blurred vision, constipation, dizziness, mental slowing, and restlessness. The nurse should routinely evaluate the patient's response to these medications. See Table 10-3 for examples of commonly used antidepressants.

## Family and Social Issues

A diagnosis of breast cancer affects not only the woman but also her partner, children, and friends. Nurses provide care to the woman and to her social support system.

### Table 10-2. Medications for the Treatment of Anxiety

| Medication | Dosage | Route | Side Effects | Contraindications |
|---|---|---|---|---|
| **Benzodiazepines** | | | | |
| Lorazepam (Ativan®, Biovail Pharmaceuticals Inc.; Baxter Healthcare Corp.) | 0.5–2 mg every 8–12 hours | PO/IV | Central nervous system (CNS) depression, sedation, dizziness, weakness, transient memory impairment, disorientation, sleep disturbances, agitation, and abuse potential | Contraindicated in patients with acute narrow-angle glaucoma. Use with caution with opioids and other CNS depressants, including alcohol. |
| Diazepam (Valium®, Roche Laboratories Inc.) | 2–10 mg 2–4 times daily Increase gradually. | PO/IV | CNS depression, impaired coordination, fatigue, changes in libido and/or appetite | Contraindicated in patients with acute narrow-angle glaucoma. Use with caution with substance or alcohol abuse and depression. |
| Alprazolam (Xanax®, Pfizer Inc.) | Start at 0.25–0.5 mg TID. May increase every 4 days to 4 mg/day in divided doses | PO | CNS depression, fatigue, impaired coordination and memory, changes in libido and/or appetite | Contraindicated in patients with open-angle glaucoma. Use with caution in patients with suicidal ideation. Avoid abrupt cessation. |
| Clonazepam (Klonopin®, Roche Laboratories Inc.) | 0.5–1.5 mg/day | PO | Nausea, drowsiness, impaired cognition, irritability, impaired coordination and balance | Contraindicated in older adults, those at risk for falls, and patients with schizophrenia. Not recommended for those younger than 18 years. |
| **Azapirones** | | | | |
| Buspirone (BuSpar®, Bristol-Myers Squibb Co.) | 7.5 mg BID initially, then may increase by 5 mg/day every 2–3 days up to 60 mg/day | PO | Dizziness, nausea, headache, nervousness, dream disturbances, insomnia | Use caution with other CNS drugs and in patients with renal and hepatic failure. Do not use with concomitant monoamine oxidase inhibitors (MAOIs). Should not be taken with grapefruit juice. |
| **Antihistamines** | | | | |
| Hydroxyzine (Vistaril®, Pfizer Inc.) | 25–50 mg every 4–6 hours | PO/IV | Drowsiness, dry mouth, tremor, convulsions | Use with caution in older adults. |

*(Continued on next page)*

### Table 10-2. Medications for the Treatment of Anxiety *(Continued)*

| Medication | Dosage | Route | Side Effects | Contraindications |
|---|---|---|---|---|
| **Antidepressants** | | | | |
| Paroxetine (Paxil®, Glaxo-SmithKline) | Start at 20 mg/day and increase by 20 mg at one-week intervals up to 60 mg/day. | PO | Asthenia, sweating, decreased appetite, dizziness, somnolence | Contraindicated in patients with seizure disorder, cardiovascular disease, and narrow-angle glaucoma. |
| Sertraline (Zoloft®, Pfizer Inc.) | Start at 25–50 mg/day and increase at one-week intervals. | PO | Gastrointestinal (GI) upset, insomnia, sexual dysfunction | Contraindicated in patients with cardiovascular disease. Monitor for mania/hypomania and hyperglycemia. Use with caution in patients with seizure disorders. |
| Escitalopram (Lexapro®, Forest Laboratories, Inc.) | 10 mg/day May increase to 20 mg/day | PO | Nausea, insomnia, sexual dysfunction, fatigue | Do not use with concomitant MAOIs. Patients should avoid alcohol consumption. |
| Venlafaxine (Effexor®, Wyeth Pharmaceuticals) | 75 mg/day May start at 37.5 mg/day for 4–7 days | PO | GI upset, dizziness, somnolence, insomnia, headache, sexual dysfunction | Use with caution in patients with high blood pressure, heart disease, hypercholesterolemia, and seizure disorders. |
| Mirtazapine (Remeron®, Organon USA) | 15 mg/day May increase every 7 days up to 45 mg/day | PO | Visual hallucinations, increased appetite, nightmares, drowsiness, headache | Do not use with concomitant MAOIs. Patients should avoid alcohol consumption. Use with caution with benzodiazepines. |
| **Atypical Neuroleptics** | | | | |
| Olanzapine (Zyprexa®, Eli Lilly and Co.) | 5–10 mg/day | PO/IM | Tardive dyskinesia, dizziness, sedation, insomnia, orthostatic hypotension, weight gain | Avoid use in older adults with dementia. Not for IV use. |
| Risperidone (Risperdal®, Ortho-McNeil Pharmaceutical) | 1–3 mg/day Start at 0.5 mg/day in older adults. | PO | Extrapyramidal symptoms, dizziness, somnolence, nausea | Use with caution in older adults. Drug causes increased risk of cerebrovascular accident and death. Contraindicated in patients with hyperglycemia. |
| **Other** | | | | |
| Propofol (Diprivan®, Abraxis BioScience, Inc.) | Titrated IV dosage for sedation and anesthesia | IV | Airway obstruction, apnea, hypoventilation | Sedative hypnotic for anesthesia |

*Note.* Based on information from Swanson et al., 2008.

From "Anxiety and People With Cancer," by L.K. Sheldon in C.G. Brown (Ed.), *A Guide to Oncology Symptom Management* (pp. 58–59), 2010, Pittsburgh, PA: Oncology Nursing Society. Copyright 2010 by the Oncology Nursing Society. Reprinted with permission.

## Table 10-3. Antidepressant Medications

| Medication | Comments/Positive Effects | Common Side Effects/Concerns |
|---|---|---|
| **Selective Serotonin Reuptake Inhibitors (SSRIs)** | | |
| Fluoxetine (Prozac®, Eli Lilly & Co.) | Activating, good for patients with lack of energy, long half-life, good for forgetful or poorly compliant patients | Very long half-life, potent inhibitor of CYP2D6 iso-enzymes, not good for patients on multiple medications or medications that are anticipated to require frequent titration, sexual side effects |
| Sertraline (Zoloft®, Pfizer Inc.) | Low drug-drug interaction, good for patients with psychomotor retardation | Increased alertness, insomnia, weak inhibitor of CYP2D6 isoenzymes, diarrhea, sexual side effects |
| Paroxetine (Paxil®, GlaxoSmithKline) | Good for patients with comorbid anxiety disorder | Nausea, anticholinergic effects, dizziness, headache, may occasionally increase anxiety, increased half-life in older adults, weight gain, potent inhibitor of CYP2D6 isoenzymes, sexual side effects |
| Citalopram (Celexa®, Forest Laboratories, Inc.) | Low drug-drug interaction potential, few gastrointestinal (GI) side effects; good for older adults, those with agitated depression, and those with GI sensitivity | Hypersomnia, sexual side effects Use with caution in patients with renal impairment. |
| Escitalopram (Lexapro®, Forest Laboratories, Inc.) | Low drug-drug interaction potential, few GI side effects, good for older adults and those with agitated depression | Hypersomnia, sexual side effects Use with caution in patients with renal impairment. |
| **Serotonin-Norepinephrine Reuptake Inhibitors (SNRIs)** | | |
| Venlafaxine (Effexor®, Wyeth Pharmaceuticals) | Good for comorbid depression and pain | Hypertension at higher doses, constipation, vivid dreams, significant withdrawal syndrome requires slow taper, nausea and vomiting, headache, sexual side effects |
| Duloxetine (Cymbalta®, Eli Lilly & Co.) | Good for comorbid depression and pain | Nausea, constipation, major CYP1A2 and CYP2D6 inhibitor, sexual side effects Use with extreme caution in patients with heavy alcohol use or chronic liver disease. |
| Desvenlafaxine (Pristiq™, Wyeth Pharmaceuticals) | Does not interfere with most medications (except ketoconazole, desipramine, monoamine oxidase inhibitors, and midazolam), so is good for patients with polypharmacy | May worsen hypertension Increased risk of bleeding May activate mania |
| **Tricyclic Antidepressants** | | |
| Amitriptyline (tertiary amines) (Elavil®, AstraZeneca Pharmaceuticals) | Good for patients with peripheral neuropathy and insomnia | Sedating, dry mouth, constipation, dizziness, weight gain |
| Imipramine (tertiary amine) (Tofranil®, Tyco Healthcare) | Good for patients with chronic pain and comorbid depression Long-term use may be associated with an increased risk of breast cancer in women. | Hypotension, QT prolongation, drowsiness, dry mouth, dizziness, low blood pressure, thrombocytopenia, leukopenia, nausea, vomiting, weakness, blurred vision, constipation, urinary retention, may increase suicidality Adjust dose for older adults and patients with hepatic impairment and glaucoma. |
| Desipramine (secondary amine) (Norpramin®, Sanofi-Aventis) | Long-term use may be associated with an increased risk of breast cancer in women. | Dry mouth, drowsiness, urinary retention, constipation, dizziness |

*(Continued on next page)*

## Table 10-3. Antidepressant Medications *(Continued)*

| Medication | Comments/Positive Effects | Common Side Effects/Concerns |
|---|---|---|
| Nortriptyline (secondary amine) (Pamelor®, Tyco Healthcare) | – | Orthostatic hypotension, urinary retention, constipation, dry mouth, drowsiness |
| Protriptyline (secondary amine) (Vivactil®, Barr Laboratories, Inc.) | Used also for panic disorder | Long-term use may be associated with an increased risk of breast cancer in women. Dry mouth, drowsiness, urinary retention, constipation, dizziness |
| Doxepin (dibenzoxazepine derivative) (Sinequan®, Pfizer Inc.) | Good for anxious, depressed patients | Long-term used may be associated with an increased risk of breast cancer in women. Dry mouth, drowsiness, urinary retention, constipation, dizziness |
| **Other Antidepressants** | | |
| Mirtazapine (serotonin and alpha-2 receptor blocker) (Remeron®, Organon USA) | Good for patients with anorexia, insomnia, nausea, low drug-drug interaction | Weight gain, very sedating Reduce dose by 50% for hepatic impairment and 25% for renal impairment. |
| Bupropion (norepinephrine/dopamine reuptake inhibitor) (Wellbutrin®, GlaxoSmithKline) | Good for apathetic, low-energy depression, no sexual side effects, may be used in combination with SSRIs and SNRIs | May increase heart rate and lower seizure threshold Do not use if patient has history of seizure, substance abuse, bulimia, anorexia, or electrolyte disturbance. |
| Trazodone (triazolopyridine) (Desyrel®, Bristol-Myers Squibb Co.) | Good for insomnia | Used as adjunct for sleep but rarely used for depression because dose needed to treat causes oversedation |
| Nefazodone (serotonin-2 antagonist/reuptake inhibitor, triazolopyridine) (Brand name, Serzone, discontinued in the United States; only available as a generic.) | Good for anxious patients with insomnia | Fatigue, dizziness, sedation, weight gain, interactions with many common medications Black box warning: may cause hepatic damage/failure. Contraindicated with most statins, sildenafil (Viagra®, Pfizer Inc.), and pimozide; increases digoxin level; inhibits CYP3A3/4 |
| **Monoamine Oxidase Inhibitors** | | |
| Phenelzine (Nardil®, Pfizer Inc.) | Also used for bulimia | Avoid aged cheese, wine, and pickled meats, which can interact and cause severe hypertension. |
| Tranylcypromine (Parnate®, GlaxoSmithKline) | Same | Same as above |
| Isocarboxazid (Marplan®, Validus Pharmaceuticals, Inc.) | Same | Same as above |

*Note.* Based on information from Agency for Healthcare Research and Quality, 2007; American Psychiatric Association, 2000; *Epocrates Online*, 2008; Gutman & Nemeroff, 2002; Hentz, 2005; Khouzam, 2007; Newport, 2005; Oncology Nursing Society, 2007; Oquendo & Liebowitz, 2006; Schwenk et al., 2005; Sharpe et al., 2002; Valdivia & Rossy, 2004.

From "Depression," by K. Sharp in C.G. Brown (Ed.), *A Guide to Oncology Symptom Management* (pp. 161–163), 2010, Pittsburgh, PA: Oncology Nursing Society. Copyright 2010 by the Oncology Nursing Society. Reprinted with permission.

## Communication With Children

Helping children to understand what is happening to their family can help them to adapt throughout the process of breast cancer treatment and survivorship. Young children may believe a parent's illness is a result of their behavior and that they are being punished. Children also may have questions about how people get cancer and how it is spread, or they may be curious about why their mom is losing her hair. It is important to create an environment where children are able to ask questions and receive age-appropriate answers. Women with breast cancer who are in need of further support in talking to their children should be encouraged to seek help from a trained professional. Support groups exist that target the psychological needs of young children, teenagers, and partners. Family roles can shift rapidly during cancer treatment, and children may need to take on caregiver roles. Each patient will require different types of family support, and encouraging open communication allows for decision making regarding how that support can be given.

Younger women with breast cancer who are caring for children may be particularly stressed with the diagnosis. This stress may have negative effects on parenting (Sigal, Perry, Robbins, Gagné, & Nassif, 2003). Important mediators of this stress include the severity of the illness, the mother's adjustment to the illness, the stability of family relationships, and the children's coping style. A child may perceive a depressed mood in the mother as emotional inaccessibility. Constraints from the illness and treatment also may make the mother physically inaccessible for periods of time. Furthermore, the stressors of the illness may narrow the parent's attention, ability, and threshold to parent and address behavioral issues in the child. This reduction in parental attention may negatively manifest itself in the child as disruptive behavior, or the child may become saddened because of the losses in the relationship with the mother. During periods of recurrence and advanced or terminal disease, mothers may believe that caring for their children is more important than disciplining them (Kennedy, McIntyre, Worth, & Hogg, 2008).

Families with child-rearing concerns or children with concerns often benefit from services that are tailored to these needs. Mutual disclosure of fears, anxieties, and hopes among mothers, significant others, and children appears to have benefits for both patients and their families (Sigal et al., 2003).

Teenage children can have particular challenges and difficulty with accepting and adjusting to the diagnosis of breast cancer in their mother. Verbalizing their feelings and concerns with their parents and significant others, and perhaps another trusted adult, may be very helpful.

Children and teenagers should be encouraged to go to school, complete homework, and continue to participate in extracurricular activities and sports. Parents may need to rely on the assistance of others from time to time to enable children to continue participating in these activities. If a woman is unable to attend an activity with a child, she should make every effort to find out about it when the child comes home. Often, an event can be videotaped, and the parent can share in the activity with the child at a later point. Helpful interventions include preparing the children for what is going to happen in the immediate future and what the more distant future holds. For some, relationships are strengthened by the challenges imposed by breast cancer and its treatment. Open communication with children and honest answers to emotionally laden questions, including questions about death, in age-appropriate terms are important. Parents may need coaching and assistance with these issues. Open communication helps parents to understand children's worries and thoughts and can lead to increased understanding. Support should provide concrete strategies that are child appropriate and child oriented. Figure 10-9 provides specific suggestions for talking with children about cancer.

---

#### Figure 10-9. Tips for Parents on Talking With Children About Cancer

- Always be honest with children. If they ask a difficult question, think about it and then reply honestly but in as nonthreatening a way as possible.
- Assure children that they will be cared for no matter what happens during or as a result of treatment.
- Remind them that cancer is not universally fatal, and try to give them concrete examples of people they know and can relate to who are long-term survivors of the disease with good prognostic factors.
- Assure children of all ages that nothing they said, did, or thought could have led to the development of the cancer.
- Assure children that it is quite normal to be angry, scared, or sad when someone they love is diagnosed with cancer.
- Assure them that even though the appearance of their mother may change during treatment, they cannot "catch" the cancer.
- Recognize that it is sometimes helpful for children to participate in a support group with other children so that they realize they are not the only family experiencing a diagnosis of breast cancer.
- Help them to understand how and to what extent they should disclose information about what is happening in their family to others.
- Inform them that others may be reluctant to talk with them or, conversely, may seem like they are being overly kind and generous. Tell them this is a normal reaction because other people might not be sure of what to do or they may be really sad about the diagnosis as well.
- Be honest that home routines will probably be disrupted and that they may need to assume some extra responsibilities for a period of time and possibly permanently.
- Remind children that even if parents cannot attend a sports event or other activity, it does not mean they are not interested. Remind them that it usually saddens parents as well when they have to miss those types of events. Try to send someone else.
- Remind children that they are still expected to keep up with schoolwork and participate in extracurricular activities as before. The diagnosis is not an excuse to avoid studying.

## Family Relationships

Family members also have psychological needs. The diagnosis of a life-threatening illness for a family member creates fear of losing the loved one and concern about the suffering that might occur. Family members' psychological distress can be as severe as that of the patient. A meta-analysis of studies of psychological distress in both patients and their informal caregivers (predominantly spouses or partners) found that the psychological distress of patients and their informal caregivers generally was parallel over time, although when the patient received treatment, caregivers experienced more distress than the patient (Institute of Medicine, 2008).

Relationships are tested and challenged throughout the cancer diagnosis, treatment, and survival. The diagnosis may exacerbate problems in relationships already fraught with conflict. Even caring, committed relationships will be stressed by the diagnosis. Emotional distance may surface because of the inability to discuss feelings about grief, loss and potential loss, significant changes in body images or a sense of loss of femininity, and partners who want to protect the woman from other distressing situations or information. Women without a partner, close friends, or family may have significant distress because of a lack of support.

## Supporting Families During the Genetic Testing Process

In addition to coping with the diagnosis of breast cancer, many women must address a hereditary predisposition for developing cancer that puts their daughters and sisters at significantly increased risk for developing cancer. Genetic testing for breast cancer is becoming increasingly more available.

Families with a hereditary predisposition for developing breast or ovarian cancer should be referred to an expert in cancer genetics counseling and education. Many psychosocial ramifications are associated with testing and must be explored prior to ordering a test. Additional psychosocial needs often surface during and after the testing process. These women require services from a healthcare provider who takes and considers a detailed past medical and psychological history. Furthermore, these families need support about the meaning of the results, the possibility of inconclusive or uninformative results, and how to share the results of genetic testing.

For those who test positive, an underlying fear often exists of when and where the cancer will develop. Decisions about prophylactic surgery are complex and very personal, especially in areas related to body image and premature menopause. Also, those who test positive may have feelings of guilt that other relatives may have inherited the susceptibility gene. Those who test negative for a known mutation may experience "survivor's guilt" in that they did not inherit the predisposition.

## Financial, Employment, and Legal Concerns

All women, regardless of their socioeconomic situation, may eventually have financial, employment, and legal issues that are related to the diagnosis of breast cancer. Helping to address these issues often improves the QOL for these women. The costs associated with breast cancer treatment can be staggering. In addition to the healthcare costs for surgery, chemotherapy, and radiotherapy, treatment also carries many hidden costs. These include co-payments for appointments, transportation and parking costs for treatment, time away from work for the patient and perhaps a significant other, increased childcare costs, and other unreimbursed charges. Unemployment or time away from work can result in an inability to meet regular living expenses. These costs can easily and quickly deplete savings. In many cases, agencies and social service resources are available to assist families with these needs. However, patients often are unaware of these resources. Ongoing assessment in this area is essential, along with prompt referral when problems become evident.

The financial ramifications of a diagnosis of cancer cannot be overstated. In 2006, nearly one in five (12.3 million) people with chronic conditions lived in families that had problems paying medical bills; 63% of these individuals also reported problems in paying for rent, mortgage, transportation, and food as a result of medical debt (Institute of Medicine, 2008). The 2006 National Survey of U.S. Households Affected by Cancer found that 25% families in which a member of the household had cancer in the past five years said the experience led the patient to use all or most of his or her savings; 13% had to borrow money from relatives to pay bills, and 10% were unable to pay for basic necessities such as food, heat, and housing (USA Today/Kaiser Family Foundation/Harvard School of Public Health, 2006).

This financial stress is compounded when a patient suffers a job loss, is not working during periods of treatment, or lacks health insurance. An estimated 46 million Americans were without health insurance in 2008 (ACS, 2010). Family members (predominantly) and friends of individuals with cancer often provide substantial amounts of emotional and logistical support and hands-on personal and nursing care to their loved ones. The estimated value of their unreimbursed care and support exceeds $1 billion annually (Institute of Medicine, 2008). Furthermore, when their loved ones experience acute or long-term inability to care for themselves or to carry out their roles in the family, family members often step in to take up these roles. Taking on these responsibilities requires considerable adaptation (and readaptation as the course of the disease changes) on the part of family members. These experiences can add to the stress resulting from concern about the ill family member. Indeed, this stress, especially in caregivers who are compromised by morbidity accompanying their own aging, can be so substantial that caregivers are afflicted more by depression, other adverse health effects, and death than are patients themselves (Coughlin, 2008).

Lack of transportation is also a major stressor to some patients and can be a barrier to receiving adequate care. The inability to get to medical appointments, the pharmacy, the grocery store, health education classes, and other out-of-home resources can hinder health care, illness management, and health promotion.

Some women face multiple issues in the workplace during and after treatment, whereas others do not. Some women benefit from coaching and anticipatory preparation of what to expect when returning to work. Coworkers may not know how to approach a person who is newly diagnosed or returning to work after an absence. Sometimes employers may be unsure of how much a patient can or cannot do. They may not be aware of lingering fatigue, even after treatment is completed. Women with breast cancer need to anticipate what problems might occur and be prepared to address these issues. Women with breast cancer should be advised that it is illegal for employers to discriminate or treat them differently because of a cancer diagnosis. Some patients may need counseling about FMLA, which allows them to take unpaid leave to deal with medical problems.

In addition, women with breast cancer may need information about advance directives, wills and trusts, living wills, and durable power of attorney. Wills and trusts help to ensure that assets will be distributed to patients' heirs and others as desired. A living will helps people to know what type of medical care patients desire if they become unable to make that decision or to communicate their wishes. A durable power of attorney for health care is the person appointed to make health and medical decisions for patients if they are unable to do so. The person who is appointed power of attorney makes financial decisions for another individual when he or she is unable to make them.

## Conclusion

A diagnosis of breast cancer brings many psychosocial consequences. The diagnosis comes as a shock to most women and creates feelings of anxiety and depression. The treatments for breast cancer can be difficult, resulting in side effects and problems with adjustment. Hope is important but may change throughout the cancer experience. Healthcare professionals need to continually help patients and families to identify hope in different situations. For newly diagnosed patients, this might mean hope that the therapy will be effective. For survivors, it might mean hope for a new normalcy in their lives. For people in the terminal phases, it might mean hope for achieving good symptom management, finishing projects, or experiencing closure with loved ones. Although a diagnosis of breast cancer changes the life of anyone it touches, psychosocial support can enhance QOL for patients and their families throughout the journey.

A number of strategies exist that nurses can use to promote adjustment to the diagnosis of breast cancer and decrease dis-

tress throughout the cancer trajectory. The positive impact of these strategies on QOL should not be underestimated. Patients need enough information to make good decisions. This means information that is culturally sensitive and at an appropriate level to be understood. Once a decision is made, healthcare providers need to support patients and families in the decision regardless of whether they personally agree with it.

QOL is improved when problems are assessed and confronted directly. Nurses need to assess for symptoms that can be managed, such as pain, psychosocial distress, and fatigue. Nurses must try to explain to patients why the symptom is occurring, whether it is a common one, and what concrete steps are going to be taken to decrease the negative effects of the symptom. When symptoms are decreased, QOL usually improves.

NCCN (2010) noted that prompt and early intervention has many benefits in preventing and minimizing psychosocial distress. Ultimately, early intervention results in improved QOL. Communication with family members, significant others, and healthcare providers is significantly improved when distress is minimized. Finally, patients who have less distress are more likely to complete a full course of therapy on time.

## References

Agency for Healthcare Research and Quality. (2007, September 26). Comparative effectiveness of second-generation antidepressants in the pharmacologic treatment of adult depression: AHRQ executive summary. Retrieved from http://www.medscape.com/viewprogram/7793

American Cancer Society. (2010). *Cancer facts and figures 2010.* Atlanta, GA: Author.

American Psychiatric Association. (2000). *Diagnostic and statistical manual of mental disorders* (4th ed., text revision). Washington, DC: Author.

Annon, J.S. (1976). The PLISSIT model: A proposed conceptual scheme for the behavioral treatment of sexual problems. *Journal of Sex Education and Therapy, 2*(2), 1–15.

Arena, P.L., Carver, C.S., Antoni, M.H., Weiss, S., Ironson, G., & Durán, R.E. (2006). Psychosocial responses to treatment for breast cancer among lesbian and heterosexual women. *Women and Health, 44,* 81–102.

Astin, J.A., Shapiro, S.L., Eisenberg, D.M., & Forys, K.L. (2003). Mind-body medicine: State of the science, implications for practice. *Journal of the American Board of Family Practice, 16,* 131–147.

Aukst-Margetić, B., Jakovljević, M., Margetić, B., Bisćan, M., & Samija, M. (2005). Religiosity, depression and pain in patients with breast cancer. *General Hospital Psychiatry, 27,* 250–255. doi:10.1016/j.genhosppsych.2005.04.004

Azzone, V., Frank, R.G., Pakes, J.R., Earle, C.C., & Hassett, M.J. (2009). Behavioral health services for women who have breast cancer. *Journal of Clinical Oncology, 27,* 706–712. doi:10.1200/JCO.2008.16.3006

Baile, W.F., Buckman, R., Lenzi, R., Glober, G., Beale, E.A., & Kudelka, A.P. (2000). SPIKES—A six-step protocol for delivering bad news: Application to the patient with cancer. *Oncologist, 5,* 302–311.

Balmer, C. (2005). The information requirements of people with cancer: Where to go after the "patient information leaflet"? *Cancer Nursing, 28,* 36–44.

Bower, J.E. (2005). Fatigue in cancer patients and survivors: Mechanisms and treatment. *Primary Psychiatry, 12*(5), 53–57.

Brandenburg, D.L., Matthews, A.K., Johnson, T.P., & Hughes, T.L. (2007). Breast cancer risk and screening: A comparison of lesbian and heterosexual women. *Women and Health, 45,* 109–130. doi:10.1300/J013v45n04_06

Brown, J.P., & Tracy, J.K. (2008). Lesbians and cancer: An overlooked health disparity. *Cancer Causes and Control, 19,* 1009–1020. doi:10.1007/s10552-008-9176-z

Bulfone, T., Quattrin, R., Zanotti, R., Regattin, L., & Brusaferro, S. (2009). Effectiveness of music therapy for anxiety reduction in women with breast cancer in chemotherapy treatment. *Holistic Nursing Practice, 23,* 238–242. doi:10.1097/HNP.0b013e3181aeceee

Burgess, C., Cornelius, V., Love, S., Graham, J., Richards, M., & Ramirez, A. (2005). Depression and anxiety in women with early breast cancer: Five year observational cohort study. *BMJ, 330,* 702. doi:10.1136/bmj.38343.670868.D3

Caan, B.J., Kwan, M.L., Hartzell, G., Castillo, A., Slattery, M.L., Sternfeld, B., & Weltzien, E. (2008). Pre-diagnosis body mass index, post-diagnosis weight change, and prognosis among women with early stage breast cancer. *Cancer Causes and Control, 19,* 1319–1328. doi:10.1007/s10552-008-9203-0

Campenni, C.E., Crawley, E.J., & Meier, M.E. (2004). Role of suggestion in odor-induced mood change. *Psychological Reports, 94,* 1127–1136. doi:10.2466/pr0.94.3c.1127-1136

Chappy, S.L. (2004). Women's experience with breast biopsy. *AORN Journal, 80,* 885–901.

Chong, O.T. (2006). An integrative approach to addressing clinical issues in complementary and alternative medicine in an outpatient oncology center. *Clinical Journal of Oncology Nursing, 10,* 83–88. doi:10.1188/06.CJON.83-88

Clark, M., Isaacks-Downton, G., Wells, N., Redlin-Frazier, S., Eck, C., Hepworth, J.T., & Chakravarthy, B. (2006). Use of preferred music to reduce emotional distress and symptom activity during radiation therapy. *Journal of Music Therapy, 43,* 247–265.

Cohen, L., Warneke, C., Fouladi, R.T., Rodriguez, M.A., & Chaoul-Reich, A. (2004). Psychological adjustment and sleep quality in a randomized trial of the effects of a Tibetan yoga intervention in patients with lymphoma. *Cancer, 100,* 2253–2260. doi:10.1002/cncr.20236

Coughlin, S.S. (2008). Surviving cancer or other serious illness: A review of individual and community resources. *CA: A Cancer Journal for Clinicians, 58,* 60–64. doi:10.3322/CA.2007.0001

Deng, G., & Cassileth, B.R. (2005). Integrative oncology: Complementary therapies for pain, anxiety, and mood disturbance. *CA: A Cancer Journal for Clinicians, 55,* 109–116. doi:10.3322/canjclin.55.2.109

Donovan, T., & Flynn, M. (2007). What makes a man a man? The lived experience of male breast cancer. *Cancer Nursing, 30,* 464–470. doi:10.1097/01.NCC.0000300173.18584.37

*Epocrates Online.* (2008). Retrieved from http://www.epocrates.com

Ernst, G., Strzyz, H., & Hagmeister, H. (2003). Incidence of adverse effects during acupuncture therapy—A multicentre survey. *Complementary Therapies in Medicine, 11,* 93–97. doi:10.1016/S0965-2299(03)00004-9

Evens, K., & Eschiti, V.S. (2009). Cognitive effects of cancer treatment: "Chemo brain" explained. *Clinical Journal of Oncology Nursing, 13,* 1092–1095. doi:10.1188/09.CJON.661-666

Ezzo, J., Richardson, M.A., Vickers, A., Allen, C., Dibble, S., Issell, B.F., … Zhang, G. (2006). Acupuncture-point stimulation for chemotherapy-induced nausea or vomiting. *Cochrane Database of Systematic Reviews* 2006, Issue 2. Art. No.: CD002285. doi:10.1002/14651858.CD002285.pub2

Finlay, E., & Casarett, D. (2009). Making difficult discussions easier: Using prognosis to facilitate transitions to hospice. *CA: A Cancer Journal for Clinicians, 59,* 250–263. doi:10.3322/caac.20022

Ganz, P.A. (2008). Psychological and social aspects of breast cancer. *Oncology, 22,* 642–646, 650. Retrieved from http://www.cancernetwork.com/display/article/10165/1160706

Garofalo, J.P., Choppala, S., Hamann, H.S., & Gjerde, J. (2009). Uncertainty during the transition from cancer patient to survivor. *Cancer Nursing, 32*(4), E8–E14. doi:10.1097/NCC.0b013e31819f1aab

Goodwin, P.J. (2005). Support groups in advanced breast cancer. *Cancer, 104,* 2596–2601. doi:10.1002/cncr.21245

Gorman, L.M. (2006). The psychosocial impact of cancer on the individual, family, and society. In R.M. Carroll-Johnson, L.M. Gorman, & N.J. Bush (Eds.), *Psychosocial nursing care along the cancer continuum* (2nd ed., pp. 3–23). Pittsburgh, PA: Oncology Nursing Society.

Gutman, D., & Nemeroff, C.B. (2002). The neurobiology of depression: Unmet needs. Retrieved from http://www.medscape.com/viewprogram/2123

Hegel, M.T., Collins, E.D., Kearing, S., Gillock, K.L., Moore, C.P., & Ahles, T.A. (2008). Sensitivity and specificity of the Distress Thermometer for depression in newly diagnosed breast cancer patients. *Psycho-Oncology, 17,* 556–560. doi:10.1002/pon.1289

Hentz, P.B. (2005, June). Effective management strategies for depression. *Clinical Advisor Supplement,* pp. 15–20.

Herbenick, D., Reece, M., Hollub, A., Satinsky, S., & Dodge, B. (2008). Young female breast cancer survivors: Their sexual function and interest in sexual enhancement products and services. *Cancer Nursing, 31,* 417–425. doi:10.1097/01.NCC.0000339252.91194.6c

Hill, K.K., & Hacker, E.D. (2010). Helping patients with cancer prepare for hospice. *Clinical Journal of Oncology Nursing, 14,* 180–188. doi:10.1188/10.CJON.180-188

Hughes, M. (2009). Communication issues for oncology nurses at difficult times. In C.C. Burke (Ed.), *Psychosocial dimensions of oncology nursing care* (2nd ed., pp. 29–57). Pittsburgh, PA: Oncology Nursing Society.

Institute of Medicine. (2004). *Meeting psychosocial needs of women with breast cancer.* Washington, DC: National Academies Press.

Institute of Medicine. (2008). *Cancer care for the whole patient: Meeting psychosocial health needs.* Washington, DC: National Academies Press.

Jacobsen, J., & Jackson, V.A. (2009). A communication approach for oncologists: Understanding patient coping and communicating about bad news, palliative care, and hospice. *Journal of the National Comprehensive Cancer Network, 7,* 475–480.

Jacobsen, P.B., & Jim, H.S. (2008). Psychosocial interventions for anxiety and depression in adult cancer patients: Achievements and challenges. *CA: A Cancer Journal for Clinicians, 58,* 214–230. doi:10.3322/CA.2008.0003

Karten, C. (2007). Easy to write? Creating easy-to-read patient education materials. *Clinical Journal of Oncology Nursing, 11,* 506–510. doi:10.1188/07.CJON.506-510

Katz, A. (2007). *Breaking the silence on cancer and sexuality: A handbook for healthcare providers.* Pittsburgh, PA: Oncology Nursing Society.

Katz, A. (2009). *Woman cancer sex.* Pittsburgh, PA: Hygeia Media.

Kendall, A.R., Mahue-Giangreco, M., Carpenter, C.L., Ganz, P.A., & Bernstein, L. (2005). Influence of exercise activity on quality of life in long-term breast cancer survivors. *Quality of Life Research, 14,* 361–371. doi:10.1007/s11136-004-1468-5

Kennedy, C., McIntyre, R., Worth, A., & Hogg, R. (2008). Supporting children and families facing the death of a parent: Part 2. *International Journal of Palliative Nursing, 14,* 230–237.

Kerr, J., Engel, J., Schlesinger-Raab, A., Sauer, H., & Hölzel, D. (2003). Communication, quality of life and age: Results of a 5-year prospective study in breast cancer patients. *Annals of Oncology, 14,* 421–427. doi:10.1093/annonc/mdg098

Khouzam, H.R. (2007). Depression: Guidelines for effective primary care, part 2, treatment. *Consultant, 47,* 841–847.

Lally, R.M. (2009). In the moment: Women speak about surgical treatment decision making days after a breast cancer diagnosis [Online exclusive]. *Oncology Nursing Forum, 36,* E257–E265. doi:10.1188/09.ONF.E257-E265

Lee, C.O. (2003). Clinical aromatherapy. Part II: Safe guidelines for integration into clinical practice. *Clinical Journal of Oncology Nursing, 7,* 597–598. doi:10.1188/03.CJON.597-598

Li, F., Fisher, K.J., Harmer, P., Irbe, D., Tearse, R.G., & Weimer, C. (2004). Tai chi and self-rated quality of sleep and daytime sleepiness in older adults: A randomized controlled trial. *Journal of the American Geriatrics Society, 52,* 892–900. doi:10.1111/j.1532-5415.2004.52255.x

Loerzel, V.W., McNees, P., Powel, L.L., Su, X., & Meneses, K. (2008). Quality of life in older women with early-stage breast cancer in the first year of survivorship. *Oncology Nursing Forum, 35,* 924–932. doi:10.1188/08.ONF.924-932

Mayo Clinic. (2007). *Mayo Clinic book of alternative medicine: The new approach to using the best of natural therapies and conventional medicine.* New York, NY: Time.

Molckovsky, A., & Madarnas, Y. (2008). Breast cancer in pregnancy: A literature review. *Breast Cancer Research and Treatment, 108,* 333–338. doi:10.1007/s10549-007-9616-6

Mustian, K.M., Katula, J.A., & Zhao, H. (2006). A pilot study to assess the influence of tai chi chuan on functional capacity among breast cancer survivors. *Journal of Supportive Oncology, 4,* 139–145.

Nail, L.M., & Lee-Lin, F. (2010). Alopecia. In C.G. Brown (Ed.), *A guide to oncology symptom management* (pp. 17–27). Pittsburgh, PA: Oncology Nursing Society.

National Center for Complementary and Alternative Medicine. (2008). *The use of complementary and alternative medicine in the United States.* Bethesda, MD: Author.

National Comprehensive Cancer Network. (2010). *NCCN Clinical Practice Guidelines in Oncology™: Distress management* [v.1.2011]. Retrieved from http://www.nccn.org/professionals/physician_gls/pdf/distress.pdf

Newport, D.J. (2005). Family medicine and primary care: Working toward the 3 "Rs" for managing depression. Retrieved from http://www.medscape.com/viewprogram/3795

Nishimoto, P.W., & Mark, D.D. (2010). Altered sexuality patterns. In C.G. Brown (Ed.), *A guide to oncology symptom management* (pp. 423–455). Pittsburgh, PA: Oncology Nursing Society.

Oncology Nursing Society. (2007). Depression. Retrieved from http://www.ons.org/outcomes/measures/summaries.shtml#dep

Oquendo, M., & Liebowitz, M. (2006). The diagnosis and treatment of depression in primary care: An evidence-based approach. Retrieved from http://www.medscape.com/viewprogram/4571

Pant, K., & Dutta, U. (2008). Understanding and management of male breast cancer: A critical review. *Medical Oncology, 25,* 294–298. doi:10.1007/s12032-007-9034-y

Pelletier, C.L. (2004). The effect of music on decreasing arousal due to stress: A meta-analysis. *Journal of Music Therapy, 41,* 192–214.

Penson, R.T., Talsania, S.H.G., Chabner, B.A., & Lynch, T.J., Jr. (2004). Help me help you: Support groups in cancer therapy. *Oncologist, 9,* 217–225.

Robinson, J.D., Metoyer, K.P., Jr., & Bhayani, N. (2008). Breast cancer in men: A need for psychological intervention. *Journal of Clinical Psychology in Medical Settings, 15,* 134–139. doi:10.1007/s10880-008-9106-y

Rogers, M., & Kristjanson, L.J. (2002). The impact of sexual functioning of chemotherapy-induced menopause in women with breast cancer. *Cancer Nursing, 25,* 57–65.

Schnur, J.B., Montgomery, G.H., Hallquist, M.N., Goldfarb, A.B., Silverstein, J.H., Weltz, C.R., ... Bovbjerg, D.H. (2008). Anticipatory psychological distress in women scheduled for diagnostic and curative breast cancer surgery. *International Journal of Behavioral Medicine, 15,* 21–28. doi:10.1080/10705500701783843

Schou, I., Ekeberg, Ø., Sandvik, L., Hjermstad, M.J., & Ruland, C.M. (2005). Multiple predictors of health-related quality of life in early stage breast cancer. Data from a year follow-up study compared with the general population. *Quality of Life Research, 14,* 1813–1823. doi:10.1007/s11136-005-4344-z

Schover, L.R. (2008). Premature ovarian failure and its consequences: Vasomotor symptoms, sexuality, and fertility. *Journal of Clinical Oncology, 26,* 753–758. doi:10.1200/JCO.2007.14.1655

Schultz, P.N., Klein, M.J., Beck, M.L., Stava, C., & Sellin, R.V. (2005). Breast cancer: Relationship between menopausal symptoms, physiologic health effects of cancer treatment and physical constraints on quality of life in long-term survivors. *Journal of Clinical Nursing, 14,* 204–211. doi:10.1111/j.1365-2702.2004.01030.x

Schwenk, T.L., Terrell, L.B., Harrison, R.V., Shadigan, E.M., & Valenstein, M.A. (2005). Guidelines for clinical care: Depression. Retrieved from http://www.cme.med.umich.edu/pdf/guideline/depression04.pdf

Shaha, M., & Bauer-Wu, S. (2009). Early adulthood uprooted transitoriness in young women with breast cancer. *Cancer Nursing, 32,* 246–255. doi:10.1097/NCC.0b013e31819b5b2e

Sharp, K. (2010). Depression. In C.G. Brown (Ed.), *A guide to oncology symptom management* (pp. 153–171). Pittsburgh, PA: Oncology Nursing Society.

Sharpe, C.R., Collet, J.P., Belzile, E., Hanley, J.A., & Boivin, J.F. (2002). The effects of tricyclic antidepressants on breast cancer risk. *British Journal of Cancer, 86,* 92–97.

Sheldon, L.K. (2010). Anxiety and people with cancer. In C.G. Brown (Ed.), *A guide to oncology symptom management* (pp. 49–63). Pittsburgh, PA: Oncology Nursing Society.

Sherman, K.J., Cherkin, D.C., Eisenberg, D.M., Erro, J., Hrbek, A., & Deyo, R.A (2005). The practice of acupuncture: Who are the providers and what do they do? *Annals of Family Medicine, 3,* 151–158. doi:10.1370/afm.248

Sigal, J.J., Perry, J.C., Robbins, J.M., Gagné, M.A., & Nassif, E. (2003). Maternal preoccupation and parenting as predictors of emotional and behavioral problems in children of women with breast cancer. *Journal of Clinical Oncology, 21,* 1155–1160. doi:10.1200/JCO.2003.03.031

Sivesind, D.M., & Pairé, S. (2009). Coping with cancer: Patient and family issues. In C.C. Burke (Ed.), *Psychosocial dimensions of oncology nursing care* (2nd ed., pp. 1–28). Pittsburgh, PA: Oncology Nursing Society.

Smith, A. (2005). *American Cancer Society's complementary and alternative cancer methods handbook* (2nd ed.). Atlanta, GA: Author.

Smith, J.E., Richardson, J., Hoffman, C., & Pilkington, K. (2005). Mindfulness-based stress reduction as supportive therapy in cancer care: Systematic review. *Journal of Advanced Nursing, 52,* 315–327. doi:10.1111/j.1365-2648.2005.03592.x

Soden, K., Vincent, K., Craske, S., Lucas, C., & Ashley, S. (2004). A randomized controlled trial of aromatherapy massage in a hospice setting. *Palliative Medicine, 18,* 87–92. doi:10.1191/0269216304pm874oa

Stacey, D., Samant, R., & Bennett, C. (2008). Decision making in oncology: A review of patient decision aids to support patient participation. *CA: A Cancer Journal for Clinicians, 58,* 293–304. doi:10.3322/CA.2008.0006

Swanson, S., Dolce, A., Marsh, K., Summers, J., & Sheldon, L.K. (2008). *Putting evidence into practice: Anxiety.* Pittsburgh, PA: Oncology Nursing Society.

Theriault, R., & Hahn, K. (2007). Management of breast cancer in pregnancy. *Current Oncology Reports, 9,* 17–21. doi:10.1007/BF02951421

Thewes, B., Butow, P., Girgis, A., & Pendlebury, S. (2004). The psychosocial needs of breast cancer survivors: A qualitative study of the shared and unique needs of younger versus older survivors. *Psycho-Oncology, 13,* 177–189. doi:10.1002/pon.710

Tinley, S. (2010). Spiritual care from the oncology nurse. In C.G. Brown (Ed.), *A guide to oncology symptom management* (pp. 497–508). Pittsburgh, PA: Oncology Nursing Society.

USA Today/Kaiser Family Foundation/Harvard School of Public Health. (2006, November). National survey of households affected by cancer [Summary and chart pack]. Retrieved from http://www.kff.org/kaiserpolls/upload/7591.pdf

Valdivia, I., & Rossy, N. (2004, February 2). Brief treatment strategies for major depressive disorder: Advice for the primary care clinician. Retrieved from http://www.medscape.com/viewarticle/467185

Vallance, J.K., Courneya, K.S., Jones, L.W., & Reiman, T. (2005). Differences in quality of life between non-Hodgkin's lymphoma survivors meeting and not meeting public health exercise guidelines. *Psycho-Oncology, 14,* 979–991. doi:10.1002/pon.910

van Weert, E., Hoekstra-Weebers, J., Grol, B., Otter, R., Arendzen, H.J., Postema, K., … van der Schans, C. (2005). A multidimensional cancer rehabilitation program for cancer survivors: Effectiveness on health-related quality of life. *Journal of Psychosomatic Research, 58,* 485–496. doi:10.1016/j.jpsychores.2005.02.008

Vos, P.J., Garssen, B., Visser, A.P., Duivenvoorden, H.J., & de Haes, H.C. (2004). Early stage breast cancer: Explaining level of psychosocial adjustment using structural equation modeling. *Journal of Behavioral Medicine, 27,* 557–580. doi:10.1007/s10865-004-0003-z

Walsh, S.M., Martin, S.C., & Schmidt, L.A. (2004). Testing the efficacy of a creative-arts intervention with family caregivers of patients with cancer. *Journal of Nursing Scholarship, 36,* 214–219. doi:10.1111/j.1547-5069.2004.04040.x

Wasserman, L.S. (2008). Respectful death: A model for end-of-life care. *Clinical Journal of Oncology Nursing, 12,* 621–626. doi:10.1188/08.CJON.621-626

Williams, S.A., & Schreier, A.M. (2005). The role of education in managing fatigue, anxiety, and sleep disorders in women undergoing chemotherapy for breast cancer. *Applied Nursing Research, 18,* 138–147. doi:10.1016/j.apnr.2004.08.005

Wilmoth, M.C. (2009). Sexuality. In C.C. Burke (Ed.), *Psychosocial dimensions of oncology nursing care* (2nd ed., 101–124). Pittsburgh, PA: Oncology Nursing Society.

Wyatt, G., Beckrow, K.C., Gardiner, J., & Pathak, D. (2008). Predictors of postsurgical subacute emotional and physical well-being among women with breast cancer. *Cancer Nursing, 31*(2), E28–E39. doi:10.1097/01.NCC.0000305705.91787.55

Yeom, H.E., & Heidrich, S.M. (2009). Effect of perceived barriers to symptom management on quality of life in older breast cancer survivors. *Cancer Nursing, 32,* 309–316. doi:10.1097/NCC.0b013e31819e239e

Yoo, G.J., Aviv, C., Levine, E.G., Ewing, C., & Au, A. (2010). Emotion work: Disclosing cancer. *Supportive Care in Cancer, 18,* 205–215. doi:10.1007/s00520-009-0646-y

Zabalegui, A., Sanchez, S., Sanchez, P.D., & Juando, C. (2005). Nursing and cancer support groups. *Journal of Advanced Nursing, 51,* 369–381. doi:10.1111/j.1365-2648.2005.03508.x

# Building Breast Centers of Excellence Through Patient Navigation and Care Coordination

Elaine Sein, RN, BSN, OCN®, CBCN®

## Introduction

Patient navigation and care coordination have been showcased in health care for several years as a result of the fragmentation that commonly occurs among access, diagnosis, and treatment. It is essential that patients receive support and guidance to navigate the healthcare system and achieve the best possible outcome in care.

This chapter will provide background information and guidance for those who want to plan, initiate, and succeed in developing a breast center of excellence program using care coordination through patient navigation. Models of navigation and the importance of the multidisciplinary team in caring for patients with cancer, resources and tools for program development, and the delineation of the navigator's role will be reviewed.

## Definition and Rationale for Patient Navigation and Care Coordination

### History

Patient navigation in cancer care refers to the assistance offered to healthcare consumers to help them to access and then chart a course through the healthcare system while overcoming barriers to quality care (National Cancer Institute [NCI], 2005). Patient navigation and care coordination has its origination and early history in breast cancer management.

Harold Freeman, MD, considered the founder of the patient navigation concept, described navigation as a process to eliminate barriers to care, streamline care, ensure timely diagnosis and treatment, and provide resource support (Freeman, 2004). Freeman piloted the first patient navigation program in Harlem, New York, in the 1990s to assist underserved women to gain access to care and to navigate the healthcare system for the screening and diagnosis of breast cancer (Freeman, 2004). His goal was to pair "disadvantaged

patients who have had little experience with the healthcare system with a person who helps them navigate the often circuitous healthcare system" (Hede, 2006, p. 157). Evidence shows that in addition to unequal access to health care, racial and ethnic minorities and underserved populations do not always receive timely, appropriate advice and care when faced with a cancer diagnosis (Freeman, 2006). The navigation movement has slowly been gaining nationwide support since Freeman's program was first developed. The success of the Harlem Patient Navigation program sparked the development of similar programs across the United States and provided the impetus for federal support for patient navigation research looking at interventions to eliminate cancer disparities, particularly in minority and underserved populations (Freeman, 2006).

Care coordination takes patient navigation to a higher level, one that ensures not only guidance for access, screening, diagnosis, and treatment but also psychosocial care. The Institute of Medicine's (IOM's) report *Cancer Care for the Whole Patient* stressed the need that all cancer care should ensure the provision of appropriate psychosocial health services, facilitate effective communication, identify each patient's psychosocial needs, design and implement a plan that links the patient with needed psychosocial care, coordinate biomedical and psychosocial care, engage and support patients in managing illness, and systematically follow up on evaluating and adjusting the plan (IOM, 2008). The report brought cancer care coordination into the national spotlight and was a call to healthcare professionals to address patient needs throughout the continuum of care.

Care coordination is now a national initiative. In 2008, the National Quality Forum, through the National Priorities Partnership, developed a portfolio for care coordination that looked at preferred practices and performance measures, including structure, process, and outcome measures. According to its Web site,

> The Partners envision a healthcare system that
> guides patients and families through their health-

care experience, while respecting patient choice, offering physical and psychological supports, and encouraging strong relationships between patients and the healthcare professionals accountable for their care. (National Quality Forum National Priorities Partnership, n.d., "Vision" section)

Recently the Oncology Nursing Society (ONS), along with the Association of Oncology Social Workers and the National Association of Social Workers, published a joint position statement on patient navigation. This statement emphasizes the importance of collaborative multidisciplinary care (see Figure 11-1).

---

**Figure 11-1. Oncology Nursing Society Joint Position Statement on Patient Navigation**

It is the position of the Oncology Nursing Society, the Association of Oncology Social Work, and the National Association of Social Workers that

- Patient navigation processes, whether provided on-site or in coordination with local agencies or facilities, are essential components of cancer care services.
- Patient outcomes are optimal when a social worker, nurse, and lay navigator (defined as a trained nonprofessional or volunteer) function as a multidisciplinary team.
- Patient navigation programs in cancer care must address underserved populations in the community.
- Patient navigation programs must lay the groundwork for their sustainability.
- Nurses and social workers in oncology who function in patient navigator roles do so based on the scope of practice for each discipline. Educational preparation and professional certification play roles in regulating the practice of both disciplines.
- Nationally recognized standards of practice specific to the discipline and specialty also define safe and effective practice.
- Nurses and social workers in oncology who perform navigator services should have education and knowledge in community assessment, cancer program assessment, resolution of system barriers, the cancer continuum, cancer health disparities, cultural competence, and the individualized provision of assistance to patients with cancer, their families, caregivers, and survivors at risk.
- Additional research to explore, confirm, and advance patient navigation processes, roles, and identification of appropriate evidence-based outcomes measures must be supported.
- Ongoing collaboration to identify and/or derive metrics that can be used to clarify the role, function, and desired outcomes of navigators must be supported and promoted.
- Navigation services can be delegated to trained nonprofessionals and/or volunteers and should be supervised by nurses or social workers.

*Note.* From *Oncology Nursing Society, the Association of Oncology Social Work, and the National Association of Social Workers Joint Position on the Role of Oncology Nursing and Oncology Social Work in Patient Navigation,* by the Oncology Nursing Society, Association of Oncology Social Work, and National Association of Social Workers, March 2010. Copyright 2010 by the Oncology Nursing Society. Retrieved from http://www.ons.org/Publications/Positions/Navigation. Adapted with permission.

---

## Definitions of Navigation

The term *patient navigator* has become a healthcare buzzword as institutions strive to reduce system burdens generated by program inefficiencies. Navigators are being used to streamline and optimize patient care and assist with removing gaps in the healthcare system (Pedersen & Hack, 2010). Pedersen and Hack (2010) described five critical attributes of a patient navigator. A patient navigator is "an individual who (1) facilitates access to care, (2) is a skilled communicator and listener, (3) is knowledgeable of the cancer system and resources in which they work, (4) acts as an empathetic patient advocate, and (5) provides information and education" (Pedersen & Hack, 2010, p. 57).

A "patient navigator" or "navigator" is someone who, through knowledge of the healthcare system, helps a patient access and receive care (Freeman, 2004; Pedersen & Hack, 2010). The navigator may or may not be an active member of the healthcare system and may be a clinician or a layperson. A nurse who is a patient navigator is referred to as a *nurse navigator*. A complete description of navigators is presented later in Models of Navigation in Multidiciplinary Care.

Although patient navigators are becoming increasingly more common, hospitals have yet to reach a consensus as to the actual roles and responsibilities for the position. Certain core components are standard across many programs, such as providing access to community resources and patient education. Other less common roles identified in the research done by the Advisory Board Company Oncology Roundtable include symptom management and accompanying patients to appointments. Ultimately, the scope of the service is dictated by the goals of the program and the individual navigator's qualifications (Advisory Board Company Oncology Roundtable, 2008).

## Benefits of Navigation

The literature validates positive outcomes related to patient satisfaction in having navigator support during the cancer care journey, especially at high stress points. These points include the interval between the diagnosis and the first visit to the surgeon, the preoperative period, a few days after the surgery, and then at the conclusion of treatment, when interactions with clinical staff become less frequent (Cancer Care Nova Scotia, 2004).

Wells et al. (2008) performed a qualitative analysis of the research conducted on patient navigation through a PubMed literature search of 45 articles in 2007, 16 of which spoke to the efficacy of the navigator role. Two areas evaluated showed the efficacy of using a navigator in care coordination: improvement in timeliness to screening (10.8% to 17.1%) and improvement in adherence to diagnostic follow-up care (21% to 29.2%) (Wells et al., 2008).

As more hospitals and breast centers add patient navigators to their staff, opportunity exists for research on various navigator roles in specific settings. This research should ultimately provide information regarding the validation and efficacy of these roles.

# Models of Navigation in Multidisciplinary Care

The field of patient navigation has evolved from lay/survivor models to full clinical navigation with nurses and social workers. This section will review various models of navigation and provide resources for nurse navigators to begin or enhance clinical navigation programs.

## Nonclinical Navigation

### Lay/Cancer Survivor

Peer counselors are individuals with a diagnosis of cancer who function as lay navigators (Giese-Davis et al., 2006). These navigators are trained to provide emotional support and links to resources, as well as share their stories of recovery. Pedersen and Hack (2010) noted a program developed by Battaglia, Roloff, Posner, and Freund (2007) where the goal was to improve follow-up to abnormal breast cancer screening in an urban population by utilizing patient navigators. Battaglia et al. (2007) required patient navigators to have "previous experience caring for a diverse population and knowledge of the local health system" (p. 57) but did not require any specific training as a patient navigator.

Lay individuals also have provided assistance with follow-up of suspicious mammograms and screening promotion (Psooy, Schreuer, Borgaonkar, & Caines, 2004). In some centers, they provide practical information, schedule appointments, and offer a variety of resources, such as support groups. The strengths of a lay navigation program include that the navigators are familiar with local community resources, can assist clinical navigators, and cost much less than clinical navigators. The limitations of lay navigator programs include that the navigator has a lack of professional clinical knowledge and a restricted ability to provide patients with clinical information.

### Volunteer Navigators

Volunteer navigators may work within a community outreach program to assist with getting patients screened for breast cancer and promoting access to the healthcare system. Their strengths are the same as those of lay/cancer survivor navigators. Significant limitations of this model include the high level of turnover in volunteers and the impact on continuity of scheduling.

### American Cancer Society Patient Navigator Program

The American Cancer Society (ACS) Patient Navigator Program assists patients, families, and caregivers during the cancer journey by providing assistance to navigate the health-care system. Trained patient navigators provide personalized guidance, information, day-to-day assistance (resource referral), and emotional support to those diagnosed with cancer and their loved ones. ACS remains a well-recognized provider of patient education materials and community-based programs, but also provides assistance by optimizing the use of hospital services and other community-based resources. The ACS Patient Navigator Program is located in 133 cancer treatment facilities across the country, and services are provided free of charge. Patient navigators provide services to those diagnosed with cancer. Although everyone can benefit from navigation, ACS focuses particularly on assisting those most at need—medically underserved and newly diagnosed patients with cancer. In 2010, ACS provided services to more than 80,000 patients, families, and caregivers through this program. In addition to in-person, hospital-based navigators, ACS offers assistance and support through its 24-hour call center and Web-based applications for locating resources (personal communication, A. Esparza, February 9, 2011).

## Clinical Navigation

### Social Workers

Darnell (2007) stated that social workers are well suited to assume the responsibilities of patient navigators. She emphasized that social workers assist individuals and communities in obtaining services and stated that "patient navigation borrows from and advances many of the core social work functions" (p. 82). Social workers identify and refer patients with mental health issues, focus on care gaps, and ensure access to care. Counseling is inherent in their role, and they have excellent connections with community resources. For some institutions, incorporating patient navigation into the existing role of the social worker is less costly than employing a nurse navigator; however, social workers have limited clinical knowledge and still need to rely on nursing for the clinical piece of care.

### Registered Nurses

Nurses have long played a role in helping patients navigate the complexities of the healthcare system. The nurse navigator program is a relatively new model of care in which nurses follow patients through the trajectory of their cancer care from the initial diagnosis through survivorship. Nurse navigators provide patients with support in decision making, education, and supportive services (Sein & Keeley, 2009).

Nurses are also well suited to function as patient navigators (Doll et al., 2003; Fillion et al., 2006; Melinyshyn & Wintonic, 2006; Seek & Hogle, 2007). Breast centers and hospitals that employ nurse navigators stress the importance of triaging physical and psychological care needs in an empathetic manner (Fillion et al., 2006; Melinyshyn & Wintonic, 2006). Oncology nurses are effective as nurse navigators because they have leadership skills, are knowledgeable in performing comprehensive assessments, and are frequently engaged in health promotion activities that are vital aspects to navigation. "Nurses are best suited for assuming the patient navigator role because they are more likely to be available throughout the disease trajectory to educate and answer questions concerning pathology reports, treatment decision making, surgical options, and chemotherapy side effects" (Pedersen & Hack, 2010, p. 59).

### Advanced Practice Nurses

The strengths of having an advanced practice nurse (APN) in the role of the navigator include that some physicians find the APN background and clinical skills more advanced than those of the RN navigator, and APNs can run survivorship clinics and bill for services (Advisory Board Company Oncology Roundtable, 2008). The downside of using an APN as a navigator is the increased salary costs, which may be difficult to justify or recover. Some models use the RN navigator for the diagnostic and treatment phase of disease and the APN for surveillance care and a survivorship program (Advisory Board Company Oncology Roundtable, 2008).

When evaluating various programmatic models, it is important to remember that there is no right or wrong way to introduce patient navigation into a program. The foundation of all patient navigation programs is the provision of multidisciplinary care in a patient-centered approach. Each community, physician practice, and institution needs to develop a program that fits the strategic plan and culture of the organization.

## Building Multidisciplinary Disease Management Teams

Multidisciplinary care is the strategy of delivering healthcare services using interdisciplinary clinical teams, continuous analysis of relevant data, and cost-effective technology to improve health outcomes. Multidisciplinary disease management teams create an environment for a center of excellence program that will foster quality patient care, research, and collaborative teamwork. The teams are philosophically aligned using clinical guidelines; they improve health outcomes and provide a valuable service to the patient and the institution (Congressional Budget Office, 2004). The teams also reduce psychological morbidity associated with fragmented episodic care, which sometimes spans weeks. Disease teams foster collaborative treatment planning and an individualized approach to care. The nurse navigator is the glue of this team. The Advisory Board Company Oncology Roundtable (2008) reviewed various models to operationalize this care coordination approach.

### Prospective Treatment Planning Conference

The prospective treatment planning conference or tumor board is the foundation of all multidisciplinary care manage-

ment. A breast cancer–specific conference is usually the first step in formalizing a breast program. This provides a forum for consensus planning among the multidisciplinary team. The nurse navigator's role is to inform referring physicians that their patient is being presented at the case conference and to record the recommendations and research opportunities reviewed. In many institutions, the navigator is responsible for preparing the information about the cases presented at the breast cancer conference and obtaining slides, films, medical records, and any other items required.

## Virtual Navigation (Without Walls)

Most hospital-based clinical navigation programs are virtual programs (without walls) because the physicians who participate are in private practice and are not hospital employees. The goal is to combine multidisciplinary care through a "virtual clinic" setting where navigators work to facilitate timely multidisciplinary evaluation through coordinated appointments. A variety of flow maps are available that describe these programs; an example can be found in Figure 11-2.

## Multidisciplinary Clinic

This model provides a one-stop shopping experience for the patient and family. The patient is seen by the entire team in one visit and usually leaves with a plan of care established. The patient navigator coordinates these appointments and meets with the patient during the breast evaluation clinic appointment to ensure that the patient understands the information and treatment options that were reviewed. The navigator also provides education and referrals to additional support services, such as social work or pastoral care. This model allows a comprehensive review of the patient's case at the point of diagnosis with clear window of opportunity for enrolling the patient into a clinical research trial. Figure 11-3 depicts navigation from initial screening through survivorship using navigation throughout the trajectory of care.

## Community-Based Programs

Community-based programs usually are located within community health centers or clinic settings, and most of these programs have been funded by grants. Community-based programs often target the uninsured or underinsured populations, as well as patients who are not comfortable with the healthcare system. In partnership with community-based programs, the patient navigator develops site-specific presentations focusing on cancer awareness, prevention, and screening.

## Physician Office Practice

The patient navigator provides services to patients being seen in the private practice setting in order to intervene when a

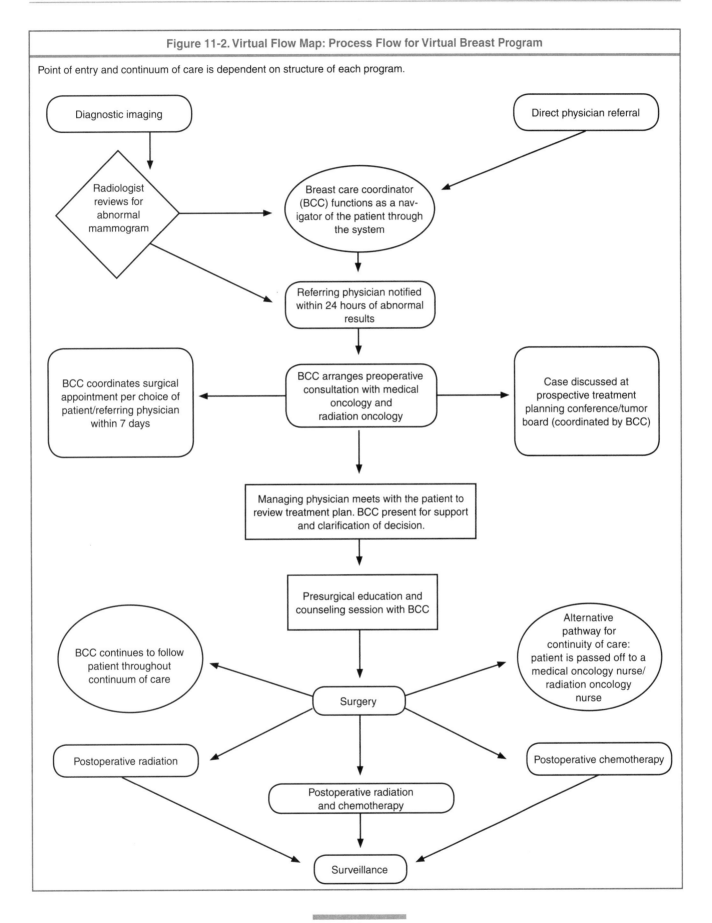

Figure 11-2. Virtual Flow Map: Process Flow for Virtual Breast Program

Point of entry and continuum of care is dependent on structure of each program.

## Figure 11-3. Multidisciplinary Clinic Model

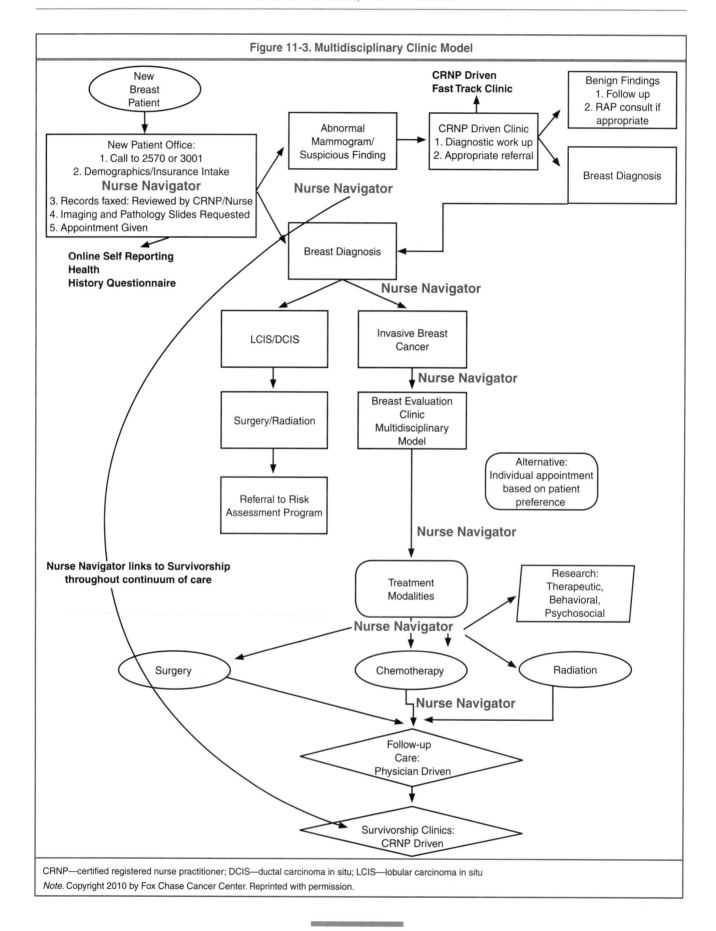

CRNP—certified registered nurse practitioner; DCIS—ductal carcinoma in situ; LCIS—lobular carcinoma in situ

*Note.* Copyright 2010 by Fox Chase Cancer Center. Reprinted with permission.

physician identifies a patient-specific need. An essential component to this model is to create a handoff/transfer of the patient care for the multiple treatment modalities and clinical expertise within the hospital setting while at the same time providing patients with the security of knowing that the navigator in their physician's office is there to provide overall coordination of care.

## Research and Funding of Navigation Programs

Several large funded studies evaluated the feasibility of the various models of navigation. The nonprofit organization C-Change (Collaborating to Conquer Cancer, www.c-changetogether .org) supports promoting and expanding the use of existing programs and new, well-planned, and evaluated national and community-based patient navigation programs using trained professional, nonprofessional, or volunteer navigators within the nation's oncology care network.

NCI addressed unequal patterns of access to standard care by creating the Patient Navigation Research Program. Its purpose was to "develop interventions to reduce the time of delivery of standard cancer services, cancer diagnosis, and treatment, after identifying an abnormal finding" from a cancer diagnostic procedure (NCI, 2005, "Key Points" section, para. 2). A survey conducted by NCI in 2003 found that 200 cancer programs nationwide had some sort of navigation program (Hede, 2006).

In 2005, NCI, with support from ACS, awarded $25 million in grants to nine pilot patient navigation programs through its Patient Navigation Research Program (PNRP). The goal of this funding was to assess the impact of patient navigators on the provision of timely, quality standard care, research collaborations and partnerships across the cancer care delivery systems, and organizations such as primary care facilities, community health centers, hospitals, and academic centers. This research project examined various disciplines carrying out patient navigation, including community health workers, medical assistants, telephone counselors, social workers, health educators, RNs, and APNs. The project is now in the evaluation phase of analysis and outcomes and, once published, will provide more evidence-based data on the efficacy of patient navigation programs (Freund et al., 2008). According to Dr. Steven Patierno, the principal investigator for the Washington, DC, PNPR site, which evaluated the efficacy of navigation services used to address breast cancer disparities, the NCI PNRP officially concluded its data collection on September 30, 2010. The intervention data for the nine PNRP projects will be made available sometime in 2011 (Broderick, 2010) and was not at the time of this writing.

In 2006, the Centers for Medicare and Medicaid Services (CMS) awarded four-year agreements to six demonstration sites to implement randomized trials to evaluate patient navigation programs designed to facilitate screening, diagnosis, and treatment for minority populations (CMS, 2008).

Most research to date has been involved in community-based programs that are looking at underserved populations. Dr. Freeman's research has proved that patient five-year survival rates went from 39% prior to the development of the navigator program to 70% (Healthcare Association of New York State, 2002). Additionally, Ell, Vourleskis, Lee, and Xie (2006) looked at a patient navigator program implemented with patients in a large, urban medical center. Patients with abnormal mammograms who worked with a navigator had a 90% adherence rate through diagnostic resolution, whereas the control group had a 66% adherence rate.

## Breast Centers of Excellence

The best way to manage patients with complex care is in a multidisciplinary team approach, which led to the concept and creation of multidisciplinary breast centers throughout the country since the 1970s. These outpatient centers treat benign breast disease as well as breast cancer. Evidence-based and consensus-developed standards have gained increasing acceptance and recognition.

Recently, the Joint Commission, NCI, the National Comprehensive Cancer Network, the American Society of Clinical Oncology, ACS, and ONS partnered in the National Accreditation Program for Breast Centers (NAPBC) and selected breast centers for the first subspecialty accreditation process through the American College of Surgeons. The NAPBC is a consortium of national professional organizations dedicated to improvement in the quality of care and monitoring outcomes for patients with diseases of the breast. NAPBC-accredited centers demonstrate the following services:

- A multidisciplinary, team approach to coordinate the best care and treatment options available
- Access to breast cancer-related information, education, and support
- Breast cancer data collection on quality indicators for all subspecialties involved in breast cancer diagnosis and treatment
- Ongoing monitoring and improvement of care
- Information about clinical trials and new treatment options. (American College of Surgeons, 2009, para. 2)

NAPBC Standard 2.2 requires that "a patient navigation process is in place to guide the patient with a breast abnormality through provided or referred services" (NAPBC, 2009, p. 27).

The Joint Commission offers disease-specific (including breast cancer) care certification. Since 2002, the Joint Commission has certified more than 1,400 clinical programs focused on a variety of disease states. Joint Commission certification requires a systematic approach to patient care, resulting in reduced variation and improved quality. All programs seeking certification must demonstrate compliance with consensus-based standards and national patient safety goals, implementation of evidence-based clinical practice guidelines, and collection and use of performance measure data. For additional information, e-mail the Joint Commission at DSCinfo @jointcommission.org or visit the Web site at www.joint commission.org.

## Breast Program Development

A breast program should be tied to the institution's overall mission, vision, and strategic goals. Figure 11-4 lists con-

---

**Figure 11-4. Considerations for a Breast Program Planning Task Force**

- Conduct an internal analysis to identify breast care service gaps and access to care; evaluate volumes in tumor registry, mammograms, breast imaging, and surgical procedures; identify clinical pathways, policies, and procedures currently in place; gain support from physicians and administration for investigation of the need for a breast program or actual breast center development; survey stakeholders (physicians, patients, and staff); and conduct focus groups to hear the voice of potential customers.
- Conduct a market share analysis of breast cases for the institution versus competing institutions. Part of this process is the identification of the needs of those who refer breast health services and those who provide breast health services. A market evaluation reviews the institution's primary service area, secondary service area, and out-migration data.
- Organize a breast program team by selecting a project facilitator; securing a physician champion; identifying key players; setting a framework, policies, and timeliness for program development; and establishing internal communication plan for policy and procedure development.
- Choose the model that fits the institution, and then define the responsibilities of all team members, as well as the nurse navigator.
- Educate all key stakeholders regarding the new process and their role in streamlining quality care for their patients.
- Implementation should occur in stages. Launch pilot program in stages by starting slowly and then adding services. It is important to correct any problems identified in the current process before moving forward.
- Market the breast program in stages. It is essential that all members of the program team are fully aware of their roles and responsibilities. It is helpful if the physician champion and the nurse navigator meet with key physician teams within the institution as a first step, followed by educating all members of the institution and then the referring physicians, with the rollout to the public occurring only after all key stakeholders understand and embrace the new process. This will set up the program for success.
- Define quality measures and benchmarks that will provide evaluation of the breast program, navigation services, and clinical quality. These quality measures provide the platform for carving out the details of the program and allow benchmarking against national standards and consensus on breast cancer care, and the processes to carry out that care.
- Evaluation should be built into the program plan so that the institution can monitor the success and roadblocks along the way and make necessary adjustments.

---

siderations for a task force during the planning process. Depending on the navigation model an institution implements, size and volumes may not allow for only one navigator to follow a patient through the entire journey.

Each institution needs to develop the nurse navigator's role to enhance clinical expertise, provide education, and foster program operations. Figure 11-5 provides a snapshot of the nurse navigator role in breast cancer management and can be used to develop a job description. It must be understood that each navigator position may encompass different responsibilities.

The Advisory Board Company Oncology Roundtable (2008) illustrates the various responsibilities a navigator may have in Figure 11-6, and they all revolve around patient-centered care.

## Nurse Navigator Role in Quality Improvement for the Breast Program

A successful breast program is crafted by choosing the right metrics that are institution-based and then building a breast center of excellence based on this platform for care. Comprehensive navigation programs have a clinical focus with ways to monitor and evaluate the successes and failures in the program. According to the American College of Surgeons Commission on Cancer (2009), "Quality or performance improvements are the actions taken, processes implemented, or services created to improve patient care" (p. 82).

The implementation of improvements demonstrates a program's continuous commitment to providing high-quality cancer care. The results of a study of quality provide a baseline to measure and improve patient care. Quality indicators encompass the continuum of care from screening and diagnosis to survivorship and patient satisfaction.

The nurse navigator's role is to assist the multidisciplinary team in choosing the outcome metrics to be monitored. These metrics can be patient focused, looking at the retention rate, the increase in patient volume, and patient satisfaction; physician focused, looking at the number of referrals to the program and physician satisfaction with the program; or focused on clinical quality, looking at the time to care, the number of patients participating in clinical trials, and care concordance with guidelines. Each institution needs to select the outcome indicators that are most important to the quality care in that particular institution, as well as the long-term sustainability of the multidisciplinary disease management program.

Various organizations are looking at quality measures for breast cancer programs. Their Web sites provide an overview of indicators that are currently tracked for breast cancer management (see Figure 11-7). An example of navigation-specific outcome measures from the Association of Communi-

---

**Figure 11-5. Nurse Navigator Responsibilities**

**Clinical Coordinator**
- Fosters a patient-centered care approach to disease-specific program development
- Plans, implements, coordinates, and evaluates the care of patients with cancer along with multidisciplinary team
- Follows patients and families through and across departmental lines as appropriate for the individual's care needs (e.g., inpatient, outpatient, cancer risk assessment, radiation therapy, home care, palliative care)
- Schedules interdisciplinary assessments, offers decision-making support, provides one-on-one counseling as needed
- Acts as a resource person for outside institutions and patients following discharge; helps patients connect with outside resources
- Provides the seamless coordination of care from diagnosis through treatment regardless of situation. The navigator is the glue of the disease management team.

**Educator**
- Conducts pre- and postoperative education
- Develops and maintains an oncology education resource center
- Facilitates breast cancer support group
- Seeks opportunities to participate in related community education activities
- Works both independently and with other healthcare disciplines/departments in developing, implementing, and evaluating breast oncology programs for patient, nursing, and community education

**Administrator**
- Participates in development of practice standards for the breast cancer program
- Participates in development and evaluation of program quality improvement metrics
- Acts as a change agent for the breast program through formulation of new standards and policies
- Collaborates with oncology program director to maintain navigation program operations within fiscal parameters
- Collaborates with marketing and public relations departments to develop and design materials for entire customer base, from physicians to consumers
- Evaluates potential funding opportunities to support the mission and goals of the breast program as it relates to breast disease

**Researcher**
- Promotes understanding of oncology clinical trials—clinical, behavioral, genetic, and prevention studies—to physicians and nursing staff as related to breast diseases
- Interprets, evaluates, and communicates pertinent research findings to nursing staff for integration into nursing care
- Participates in nursing evidence-based practice council
- Collaborates with both administration and nursing research in proposal development and data collection, analysis, and interpretation as needed as it relates to breast disease

**Consultant/Mentor**
- Partnerships and coalitions: Maintains strong community and professional linkages; builds relationships with all members of the medical team
- Acts as a resource person for staff to problem-solve potential complications that might arise in relation to specific therapies

**Professional Growth**
- Maintains and updates personal competency and continuing education (CE) through attendance at CE programs
- Participates in related professional and/or community organizations
- Strongly recommended certification as an oncology nurse
- Strives to contribute to nursing literature through submission of at least one article a year for publication

*Note.* From *Fox Chase Cancer Center/Fox Chase Cancer Center Partners Breast Care Coordinator/Navigator Orientation Manual* (pp. 13–14), by E. Sein and P. Keeley (Eds.), 2009, Philadelphia, PA: Fox Chase Cancer Center Partners. Copyright 2009 by Fox Chase Cancer Center Partners. Adapted with permission.

---

ty Cancer Centers (ACCC) *Patient Navigation: A Call to Action* resources is shown in Figure 11-8. The National Quality Forum has endorsed measures in Figure 11-9. These indicators are monitored in programs that are accredited through the American College of Surgeons Commission on Cancer. Figure 11-10 provides a list of various elements that can be obtained from patient satisfaction survey information.

The National Consortium of Breast Centers is currently engaged in a quality project for breast cancer management (the National Quality Measures for Breast Centers™). This is an interactive quality Internet model for breast centers to enter quality data points, filter for comparisons, and receive comparison reports on breast center quality measures established by the National Consortium of Breast Centers following quality measures suggested by the Advisory Board Oncology Roundtable. The immediate access to information allows participants to compare quality performance on select measures with other centers across the United States. International participation is now available. Additional information can be obtained at www.breastcare.org.

With funding from the National Philanthropic Trust Fund for Breast Cancer, the ONS Foundation has begun

## Figure 11-6. Nurse Navigator Roles

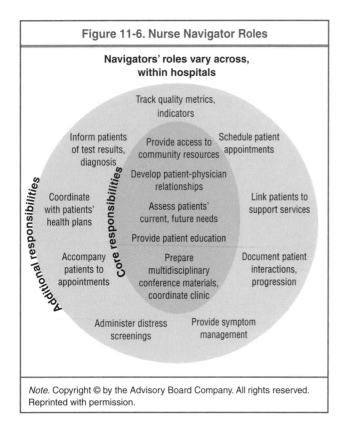

**Navigators' roles vary across, within hospitals**

Track quality metrics, indicators

Inform patients of test results, diagnosis

Provide access to community resources

Schedule patient appointments

Develop patient-physician relationships

Coordinate with patients' health plans

Assess patients' current, future needs

Link patients to support services

Provide patient education

Accompany patients to appointments

Prepare multidisciplinary conference materials, coordinate clinic

Document patient interactions, progression

Administer distress screenings

Provide symptom management

*Additional responsibilities*

*Core responsibilities*

## Figure 11-7. Quality Measure Resources

- Advisory Board Company Oncology Roundtable: www.advisoryboardcompany.com/content/clinical/oncology.asp
- American Cancer Society: www.acs.org
- American College of Surgeons: www.facs.org
- American Society of Clinical Oncology: www.asco.org
- Association of Community Cancer Centers: http://accc-cancer .org
- National Comprehensive Cancer Network: www.nccn.org
- National Consortium of Breast Centers: www.breastcare.org
- National Quality Forum: www.qualityforum.org
- Oncology Nursing Society: www.ons.org

work on developing patient-centered quality measures for breast cancer. Nursing-sensitive patient outcomes represent the impact of nursing interventions on areas such as patient symptom management, functional status, safety, quality of life, psychological distress, costs, and utilization of healthcare resources. ONS has contracted with the Joint Commission's Division of Quality Measurement and Research to complete the initial pilot testing of measures because of their broad experience in measurement development. These measures will look at symptom management for patients with breast cancer during the first year of treatment with chemotherapy. Pilot sites began testing measures in summer and fall of 2010 (ONS Quality Indicator Project Team for Breast Care, 2008). Figure 11-11 illustrates the first set of measures.

## Navigation Software

In addition to tracking the quality of care given to patients with a navigator, it is important to provide a mechanism that proves efficacy and sustainability of the navigator role. At the inception of most programs, navigators and administrators create spreadsheets to track patients with whom the navigator has interacted, as well as baseline timing metrics the program may be evaluating. This can be a very time-consuming aspect of the navigator role that takes time away from actual patient care. For this reason, many institutions have created their own homegrown navigation software with the assistance of their information technology department.

An example of a homegrown, Web-based, user-friendly database program that was designed to meet the needs of the institution is in use at Virtua Health in New Jersey. A database was created that captures the key touch points at which navigators typically intervene on their patients' behalf, such as after an initial chemotherapy treatment. This database captures key metrics that can be used both to monitor the success of the program and to document gained efficiencies to senior leadership. Queries can be run at any time so that quantitative improvement measures can be easily accessed and compared. It also allows for course corrections based on data trending. The system can send automated reminders/ticklers to the navigator indicating when it is time to carry out a task. Also incorporated into the database are automated patient itineraries and referring physician/primary care provider communication letters. The database eliminates some of the paperwork that can overwhelm navigators with a typical patient load of 150 clients, 60–90 of whom are in the active treatment phase. This internal database has also been made available to physicians, cancer registrars, cancer genetic counselors, and clinical oncology social workers within Virtua to enable them to track their patients through the cancer care continuum (personal communication, L. Shalkowski, Virtua Health, July 27, 2010).

However, this is not feasible for many institutions, and they need to find commercial navigation software programs. The few commercial programs developed organize the navigator's work flow and scheduling, including every point of contact the navigator has with the patient, education, and referrals. Some provide a secure message application so that the nurse and patient can e-mail each other. Administrators are able to run reports that speak to the number of patients the navigator is actively servicing, in follow-up, volumes, timing, and outmigration. These programs can be customized for each institution. Commercial navigation software programs can be costly; therefore, institutions need to investigate all possible resources to assist with creating an institution-specific tracking program that will fit their individual needs. Priority Consult and Nursenav are examples of commercial navigation software pro-

---

**Figure 11-8. Association of Community Cancer Centers'** *Patient Navigation: A Call to Action*

PATIENT NAVIGATION PROGRAM
SAMPLE OUTCOME MEASURES TOOL

This tool can help your organization identify outcome measures for your patient navigation program. Keep in mind, measures will be specific to individual programs.

**Patient Satisfaction**
1. Patient satisfaction score prior to implementation of navigation services (baseline score)
2. Patient satisfaction score 6–12 months after navigation program has unrolled. Continue to monitor scores on an ongoing basis.
3. Number of patients leaving the cancer center for treatment elsewhere prior to implementation of navigation services
4. Number of patients leaving the cancer center for treatment elsewhere 6–12 months after navigation program has unrolled
5. Number of patient referrals prior to implementation of navigation services
6. Number of patient referrals 6–12 months after navigation program has unrolled. Continue to monitor scores on an ongoing basis.
7. Patient satisfaction with navigation program. Continue to monitor scores on an ongoing basis.

**Patient Encounters**
1. Time to diagnostic mammogram BEFORE and AFTER implementation of navigation services
2. Time to needle biopsy BEFORE and AFTER implementation of navigation services
3. Time to diagnosis BEFORE and AFTER implementation of navigation services
4. BEFORE and AFTER implementation of navigation services, the time to initial treatment from (a) initial visit, (b) diagnostic mammogram, (c) diagnosis
5. BEFORE and AFTER implementation of navigation services, the time from diagnosis to consult with (a) breast surgeon, (b) plastic surgeon, (c) medical oncologist, (d) radiation oncologist, (e) genetic counselor
6. Time from OR to chemo/radiation BEFORE and AFTER implementation of navigation services
7. Number of referrals to (a) navigator, (b) genetic counseling, (c) nutrition, (d) social work
8. Number of underserved BEFORE and AFTER implementation of navigation services
9. Number of unavoidable admissions/ER visits BEFORE and AFTER implementation of navigation services
10. Length of hospital stay BEFORE and AFTER implementation of navigation services

**Programmatic Components and Performance Improvement**
1. Number of uninsured and underinsured patients navigated
2. Track tumor conference recommendations based on guidelines (e.g., National Comprehensive Cancer Network, American Society of Clinical Oncology).
3. Create standing order sets by disease site and measure use of tools.
4. Develop patient education programs and track outcomes of these programs.
5. Track percentage of patient provided with educational materials and information, BEFORE and AFTER patient navigation services.
6. Track percentage of patients given information on clinical trials and monitor percentage of patients put on clinical trials.
7. Create site-specific navigation programs.
8. Establish a Patient and Caregiver Advisory Committee.
9. Develop marketing materials and measure physician referrals BEFORE and AFTER implementation of navigation services.
10. Establish survivorship program, and measure patient satisfaction.
11. Develop end-of-treatment celebration, and measure satisfaction.
12. Create support groups and other educational programs, and evaluate.

ER—emergency room; OR—operating room

*Note.* Figure courtesy of the Association of Community Cancer Centers. All rights reserved. Reprinted with permission.

---

grams. For more information, go to www.priorityconsult.com and www.nursenav.com.

## Funding Navigator Positions

In most institutions, creating the funding to support the nurse navigator position is challenging. The average community hospital or breast center has to use institutional funds, as geographic areas limit grant funding from advocacy organizations for breast cancer. In some areas of the country, the local affiliate of Susan G. Komen for the Cure, the Avon Foundation, or the Lance Armstrong Foundation may provide some grant support. See Figure 11-12 for funding opportunities.

## Return on Investment and Sustainability of the Navigator Role

Research has shown that navigators have made a difference in helping patients to gain access to the healthcare system in a timelier manner for screening and diagnostic workups (Wells et al., 2008). This in turn captures the patient at diagnosis and usually leads to the patient staying within the health system for all aspects of cancer care. The trickle-down revenue for a patient with breast cancer spans from imaging, diagnostics, surgery, chemotherapy, and radiation, as well as additional services such as genetics and complementary medicine. The soft revenue is the patient's satisfaction with the care received, which in turn leads to a word-of-mouth testimonial regarding the care received by the navigator and the institution. Because administrators need to be able to prove the return on investment of the navigator role, a work team of finance and clinical team members should create a downflow revenue stream for patients with breast cancer before and after navigation was initiated. This assists in proving the value the navigator brings to the institution and also provides the leverage to hire another navigator, either in breast care or another cancer site.

---

### Figure 11-9. American College of Surgeons Breast Cancer Quality Metrics

- Breast-conserving therapy is followed by radiation to the breast in women younger than age 70.
- Combination chemotherapy is considered or administered within eight weeks of definitive surgery for women with hormone receptor–negative (estrogen receptor [ER] and progesterone receptor [PR]) breast cancer and greater than 1 cm in greatest diameter.
- Tamoxifen or third-generation aromatase inhibitor is considered for or administered to patients with hormone receptor–positive (ER+ or PR+) stage I (tumor size smaller than 1 cm and N0) and stage II/III (any tumor size and N+) disease.

*Note.* Based on information from the American College of Surgeons Commission on Cancer & National Quality Forum, 2007.

---

### Figure 11-10. Patient Satisfaction Survey Information

**Breast Care Services and Patient Satisfaction**

A key role in care coordination is the customer satisfaction you provide in navigating patients through the complex process of breast cancer diagnosis and treatment along the continuum of care.

The goal for any program is to provide the finest, most personal care possible. In order to improve the quality of services delivered, assessment of patient satisfaction is key.

The time invested in returning the survey will improve future experience with the institution, as well as improving the institution's performance.

**Elements to be Considered Across the Continuum of Care**

*Caveats*
- Friendly, courteous, helpfulness, responsive staff and physicians at every point of contact
- Accurate identification of patient
- Staff able to discuss procedures and treatments with patients and their support person in a manner they can understand
- Services are user-friendly
- Wait times are reasonable
  - Extended – acceptable – prompt
  - Kept informed of any delays
  - Environmental surroundings during wait time
- Cleanliness of facility, including bathrooms
- High-quality services provided
- Recommend to others
- Services meet or exceed expectations
- Designated breast care coordinator throughout continuum of care
- Explanation of role/expectations for each member of healthcare team

*Making Appointments*
- Call back within two or three hours if patient needs to leave message for appointment scheduling
- Date and time satisfactory
- Received information packet with directions to hospital and cancer center prior to appointment
- Information provided was helpful
- Web-based scheduling user-friendly

*Registration*
- Efficient
- Ease of navigating to appropriate departments, including use of elevators

*Mammography and Diagnostic Studies*
- Patient receives results of mammography and diagnostic studies within acceptable time frame
- Suspicious results reviewed with patient before leaving center
- Opportunity to receive satisfactory explanation of findings provided
- Optimal turnaround time to definitive diagnosis
- Received instructions for future mammograms
- Received education on breast self-examination (video, verbal, written)
- Received written information
- Opportunity to request additional educational resources offered
- Reason study was done at institution was identified: physician referral, recommendation of another, nearby location of facility, insurance capitation to facility

*Breast Care Coordinator/Navigator*
- Helpfulness of information provided before appointment
- Ability to address concerns
- Created atmosphere that encouraged questions
- Took concerns seriously
- Explanation of what to expect during visit
- Knowledge of facility and available resources
- Access to coordinator for support throughout continuum of care

*(Continued on next page)*

---

**Figure 11-10. Patient Satisfaction Survey Information** *(Continued)*

*Issues Important During Diagnostic Phase*

- Ability to have support person accompany patient to care conference
- Discussion of treatment options with physician
- Patient summary letter was helpful and understandable
- Access to a "buddy," professional counseling, and support groups for patient/significant other
- Receipt of information and education throughout process
- Role in decision making (active, collaboration, passive) and satisfaction with level of involvement
- Opportunity to discuss concerns and fears with physician

*Treatment Phase*

- Treatment received at same institution as diagnosis—if not, reason was given
- Education session/class offered to patient/significant other prior to each phase of treatment
  - High-risk assessment
  - Surgery
  - Radiation
  - Chemotherapy
  - Clinical trials
- Consideration/support provided regarding:
  - Right treatment decision by the patent
  - Use of medical jargon
  - Information overload
  - Financial issues discussed at intake
  - Self-care postoperatively—utilization of standardized postoperative instructions per physician is helpful
  - Unknowns in the surgical process
  - Side effects of anesthesia
  - Postoperative care in hospital
  - Comfort level with self-care at time of discharge
- Symptom/problem management related to treatment
  - Self-care for actual/potential problems
  - Pain
  - Distress
  - Communication
  - Coping with changes in body image
    * Available resources
  - Support group access for patient/significant others
  - Use of alternative/complementary therapies
    * Identification of currently used methods by patient
    * Discussion of risk/benefits
    * Recommendations for complementary therapies

*Recovery/Survivorship*

- Most stressful time identified:
  - Discovery of suspicious finding to diagnosis
  - Diagnosis to treatment
  - Treatment
  - Recovery
  - Recurrence
- Suggestions to improve services
- Any staff member who deserves special recognition and why
- Primary care physician kept informed during treatment
- Wish list (suggest potential improvements currently under consideration for the center such as a survivorship care plan where fear of recurrence is addressed)

*Demographics*

- Type of treatment/services received
- Age, age at diagnosis, race, zip code

*Note.* Based on information from Sein & Keeley, 2009. Copyright 2009 by Fox Chase Cancer Center. Used with permission.

## Navigator-Patient Ratio

Navigation programs vary across most institutions, physician offices, and community health centers. The nurse-patient ratio depends on the type of navigation program and where it is housed. A navigator who provides support with access to the institution and scheduling of appointments and referrals to other support services will be able to carry a larger active caseload than a nurse who will be providing ongoing education and decision-making support throughout the continuum of care. The Billings Clinic created an acuity scale to assist

with the nurse-patient ratio needed for nurse navigators to provide comprehensive care (see Table 11-1).

## Marketing the Nurse Navigator Position

The nurse navigator collaborates with the marketing department to market programs to physicians, patients, consumer, payers, coworkers, and community and outside agencies. By establishing these relationships, the navigator will provide a return on investment for the role. The nurse navigator is responsible for building physician relationships in the community, nurturing trust and a shared vision to improve patient care, and creating top-of-mind awareness to influence physician referrals. The nurse needs to meet with physicians to describe the navigator role and how developing standard operating procedures for patient referrals will create a seamless process for patient care. As the nurse navigator becomes established within the institution and the community, the physician practices should see an increase in patient volume.

It is important that the key stakeholders in the institution understand all the facts as well as the process for implementation of the nurse navigator position. Communication is the key to success. Phase one includes meeting with hospital subcommittees, which should touch on various disciplines throughout the institution. Phase two includes attending medical staff meetings for radiology, surgery, medical oncology, and radiation oncology. Phase three includes meeting with primary care physicians and obstetrics and gynecology physicians and any other referral base in order to clarify and promote the role and responsibilities of the nurse navigator. It is essential to prioritize short- and long-term goals and objectives and to evaluate response at specific junctures. The final phase is rolling out the nurse navigator program to the community.

Additionally, the nurse navigator can create awareness of the breast program and the navigator role by presenting at health fairs and women's church clubs, by lecturing on breast health and breast self-awareness (leave literature regarding quick access to appointments if needed), and by requesting that local businesses carry brochures regarding the program. Nurse navigators also can partner with physician offices,

---

### Figure 11-11. Oncology Nursing Society Nursing-Sensitive Quality Measures for Breast Cancer Care

- Assessment of distress, fatigue, and sleep-wake disturbances at least once between the time of breast cancer diagnosis and first intravenous chemotherapy treatment
- Continuing assessment of distress, fatigue, and sleep-wake disturbances at least once during each cycle of intravenous chemotherapy
- Intervention documented for moderate to severe distress or sleep-wake disturbances
- Exercise recommendation made prior to first intravenous chemotherapy infusion (intervention for fatigue)
- Assessment of chemotherapy-induced nausea and vomiting control at least once between the first and second intravenous chemotherapy infusions
- Education on neutropenia precautions, specifically on hand-washing and degree of fever that should initiate a call to the practice
- Colony-stimulating factors prescribed for chemotherapy regimens with a 20% or greater risk of febrile neutropenia

*Note.* Based on information from Oncology Nursing Society Foundation Quality Measures Project Team, n.d. For more information, visit www.ons.org/research/quality.

---

### Figure 11-12. Funding Opportunities: Grant Sponsors

- American Cancer Society: www.cancer.org
- Avon Foundation: www.avonfoundation.org
- Breast Cancer Alliance: www.breastcanceralliance.org
- Breast Cancer Research Foundation: www.bcrfcure.org
- Department of Defense Breast Cancer Research Program: http://cdmrp.army.mil/bcrp
- The Foundation Center: http://fdncenter.org
- GrantsNet, American Association for the Advancement of Science: www.grantsnet.org
- Howard Hughes Medical Institute: www.hhmi.org
- Lance Armstrong Foundation: www.livestrong.org
- National Breast Cancer Coalition:www.stopbreastcancer.org
- National Cancer Institute: www.cancer.gov
- Oncology Nursing Society: www.ons.org
- Oncology Nursing Society Foundation: www.onsfoundation.org
- Susan G. Komen for the Cure: www.komen.org

*Note.* Based on information from Sein & Keeley, 2009.

---

### Table 11-1. Billings Clinic Patient Navigation Acuity Scale

| Acuity Scale | Description |
|---|---|
| 0 | No navigation |
| 0.5 | Meet patient if referral received<br>Initial guidance/education/coordination as needed<br>Typically no follow-up required<br><br>Meet patient upon diagnosis<br>Initial guidance/education/coordination<br>Typically no follow-up required |
| 1.5 | Meet patient upon diagnosis<br>Coordination of multimodality treatment<br>Typically ongoing guidance/education for 3–4 months |
| 2 | Meet patient upon diagnosis<br>Coordination of multimodality treatment<br>Moderate intensity of needs<br>Typically ongoing guidance/education for 5–6 months or more |
| 2.5 | Meet patient upon diagnosis<br>Coordination of multimodality treatment<br>High intensity of needs, often inpatient hospitalizations associated with care<br>Typically ongoing guidance/education for 6–12 months or more |
| 4 | Meet patient upon diagnosis<br>Coordination of multi-modality treatment<br>High intensity of needs, often associated with care coordination outside of facility<br>Typically ongoing guidance/education for 6–12 months or more |

*Note.* Copyright © Billings Clinic. Used with permission.

especially surgical oncology and gynecologic oncology, for educational programs. Other options include chairing a hospital team for Relay for Life or Race for the Cure, calling local radio stations and volunteering for any breast cancer awareness month activities, and recruiting satisfied patients to be spokespeople for the program (Sein & Keeley, 2009).

## Training Programs and Resources for Navigation

The following training programs and resources are listed in alphabetical order. This is not a complete list of all known resources.

- The **Academy of Oncology Nurse Navigators** (www .aonnonline.org) is a national specialty organization dedicated to improving patient care and quality of life by defining, enhancing, and promoting the role of oncology nurse navigators for patients and their families, as well as cancer centers, hospitals, and community practices. This organization, which has more than 1,500 members, was founded in May 2009 to provide a network for oncology nurse navigators, patient navigators, oncology nurses, social workers, practice managers, patient care coordinators, and nursing administrators to better manage the complexities of the cancer care treatment continuum. Through the information provided by this academy, oncology nurse navigators have access to vast resources on patient care, continuing education, and dialogues with their peers.
- The **Association of Community Cancer Centers** (ACCC) Center for Provider Education provides ACCC members with Cancer Care Patient Navigation: A Call to Action, an online resource at http://accc-cancer.org/education/education-patientnavigation.asp. ACCC launched this project to identify barriers to access to care that patient navigation can address; increase successful implementation of patient navigation services; refine staffing models; establish effective metrics for measuring patient navigation services internally; and for benchmarking patient navigation services against other community cancer centers. ACCC offers many patient navigation resources and tools on its Web site, including standard operating procedures, intake forms, assessment forms, and surveys. See http://accc-cancer.org/education/education-patientnavigation.asp and use the links along the right of the page to view guidelines, tools, lectures, frequently asked questions, and other resources.
- *Becoming a Breast Cancer Nurse Navigator*, a book by Lillie D. Shockney, provides information on how to define the phases of diagnosis and treatment and manage patients through the course of their cancer care. It provides resources to nurses seeking administrative buy-in of a navigation program. Details may be found at www.jbpub .com.

- **C-Change** (http://c-changetogether.org) is an organization that comprises the key cancer leaders from government, business, and nonprofit sectors who publish resource information on patient navigation.
- The **University of Colorado Cancer Center** has partnered with Denver Health and the Colorado Community College System to train navigators through online and face-to-face education. For more information, visit http://patientnavigatortraining.org.
- **EduCare** (www.breasthealthcare.com) provides periodic training for nurse navigators. The site gives information on training sessions offered, including certification in breast health education and strategic planning of a breast health center.
- **Fox Chase Cancer Center/Fox Chase Cancer Center Partners Breast Care Coordinator/Navigators** with the support of the American Cancer Society's Making Strides Against Breast Cancer grant published an orientation manual for nurses who come from various practice backgrounds and are new to the role of nurse navigator in breast cancer care. The manual is not meant to be a textbook but rather a resource of the most current information regarding the role of the navigator. For more information, contact partners@fccc.edu.
- The **Harold P. Freeman Patient Navigation Institute** (www.hpfreemanpni.org), launched in 2007 with a $2.5 million grant from the Amgen Foundation, is the first certification and training program for patient navigators. Through a three-day training course, attendees are trained in patient navigation.
- The **National Consortium of Breast Centers** breast navigation certification program identifies navigation stages along the continuum of care for patients with breast cancer. The breast patient navigator's program content is based on each of these stages. The program includes national and regional lectures to prepare for the written examination. For more information, visit www.breastcare.org.
- The **National Coalition of Oncology Nurse Navigators** (NCONN) was conceived by five nurses who met while attending meetings of the Maryland/DC/Virginia Coalition of Breast Care Coordinators, a regional group of breast care nurse navigators who started to network and share information in 2003. This group believed it was important to share practice information by reaching other navigators; thus, NCONN was born. For more information, visit www.nconn.org.
- The **ONS Nurse Navigator Special Interest Group** was approved in 2010 and provides ongoing education and resources related to the nurse navigator role. For more information, visit http://navigator.vc.ons.org.
- The **NCI** *Patient Navigation Research Program Resource Manual* (http://ncipoetqa.cancer.gov/PatientNavigator/Index.cfm) was designed to provide a tool for patient navigators to use when sharing information with patients facing breast, cervical, prostate, and colorectal cancers. It pro-

vides a list of NCI documents, national organizations, and a place for navigators to insert a list of community resources available to their patients.

- **Pfizer** has an educational Web site (www.patientnavigation .com) specifically for patient navigation that provides free toolkits, updates, and educational resources.
- The **Smith Farm Center for Healing and the Arts** offers patient navigation services at six locations in the Washington, DC area. It offers five-day training to navigators as well. To learn more about the Smith Farm Center's program, visit www.smithfarm.com/patNav.html.
- Several **state navigation networks or programs** have been started; many have been offshoots of the state cancer control plan. This is one area where regional support for the navigator role may provide education and funding to support navigation projects. For more information, contact the state health department.
- Fox Chase Cancer Center, with funding from the Pennsylvania Department of Health, created *Your Resource Guide to Patient Navigation* for adopting or refining best practices in a patient navigation program. It can be accessed at www.fccc.edu/prevention/hchd/resources.

## Conclusion

This chapter provides a review of the basic elements of patient navigation, its historical context, literature to support the efficacy of the navigator's role in cancer care coordination, and the national healthcare position on the role of patient navigation in providing care to patients with cancer, especially the most vulnerable populations. Various disciplines provide patient navigation, and successful multidisciplinary breast program models for navigation exist. An important feature to this chapter is the toolbox of resources that can be used to develop a breast program of excellence through patient navigation and care coordination. This chapter has reviewed research related to the role that navigation plays in care coordination, efficiency, cost-effectiveness, and positive patient outcomes. As additional research is concluded, analyzed, and reported, patient navigation is expected to be embedded in comprehensive cancer care from screening through survivorship.

## References

Advisory Board Company Oncology Roundtable. (2008). Elevating the patient experience. Retrieved from http://www.advisory.com

American College of Surgeons. (2009, December 29). NAPBC accreditation application. Retrieved from http://accreditedbreastcenters .org/accreditation/application.html

American College of Surgeons Commission on Cancer. (2009). Cancer program standards 2009 revised edition. Retrieved from http://www.facs.org/cancer/coc/standards.html

American College of Surgeons Commission on Cancer & National Quality Forum. (2007). National Quality Forum endorsed Commission on Cancer measures for quality of cancer care for breast and colorectal cancers. Retrieved from http://www.facs.org/cancer/ qualitymeasures.html

Battaglia, T.A., Roloff, K., Posner, M.A., & Freund, K.M. (2007). Improving follow-up to abnormal breast cancer screening in an urban population: A patient navigation intervention. *Cancer, 109,* 359–367. doi:10.1002/cncr.22354

Broderick, J.M. (2010). Returning to the roots of patient navigation [Special NCONN section]. *OncNurse, 4*(6), 28–30.

Cancer Care Nova Scotia. (2004, March). Cancer patient navigation: Evaluation findings. Summary report. Retrieved from http://www .cancerpatientnavigation.ca/docs/Summary%20Evaluation%20report .pdf

Centers for Medicare and Medicaid Services. (2008, October 1). Cancer prevention and treatment demonstration for ethnic and racial minorities. Retrieved from http://www.cms.hhs.gov/ DemoProjectsEvalRpts/downloads/CPTD_FactSheet.pdf

Congressional Budget Office. (2004, October 13). *An analysis of the literature on disease management programs.* Washington, DC: Author.

Darnell, J.S. (2007). Patient navigation: A call to action. *Social Work, 52,* 81–84.

Doll, R., Stephen, J., Barroetavena, M.C., Linden, W., Poole, G., Ng, E., ... Habra, M. (2003). Patient navigation in cancer care: Program delivery and research in British Columbia. *Canadian Oncology Nursing Journal, 13,* 193.

Ell, K., Vourleskis, B., Lee, P.J., & Xie, B. (2006). Patient navigation and case management following an abnormal mammogram: A randomized clinical trial. *Preventive Medicine, 44,* 26–33. doi:10.1016/j.ypmed.2006.08.001

Fillion, L., de Serres, M., Lapointe-Goupil, R., Bairati, I., Gagnon, P., Deschamps, M., ... Demers, G. (2006). Implementing the role of the patient-navigator nurse at a university hospital centre. *Canadian Oncology Nursing Journal, 16,* 11–17.

Freeman, H.P. (2004, September/October). A model patient navigation program. *Oncology Issues, 19,* 44–46.

Freeman, H.P. (2006). Patient navigation: A community centered approach to reducing cancer mortality. *Journal of Cancer Education, 21*(Suppl. 1), S11–S14. doi:10.1207/s15430154jce2101s_4

Freund, K.M., Battaglia, T.A., Calhoun, E., Dudley, D.J., Fiscella, K., Paskett, E., ... Roetzheim, R.G. (2008). National Cancer Institute Patient Navigation Research Program: Methods, protocol, and measures. *Cancer, 113,* 3391–3399. doi:10.1002/cncr.23960

Giese-Davis, J., Bliss-Isberg, C., Carson, K., Star, P., Donaghy, J., Cordova, M.J., ... Spiegel, D. (2006). The effect of peer counseling on quality of life following diagnosis of breast cancer: An observational study. *Psycho-Oncology, 15,* 1014–1022. doi:10.1002/ pon.1037

Healthcare Association of New York State. (2002). HANYS Breast Cancer Demonstration Project™: Breast health patient navigator resource kit. Retrieved from http://www.hanys.org/bcdp/ resource_kits/upload/Complete-PNP-Kit-PDF.pdf

Hede, K. (2006). Agencies look to patient navigators to reduce cancer care disparities. *Journal of the National Cancer Institute, 98,* 157–159. doi:10.1093/jnci/djj059

Institute of Medicine. (2008). *Cancer care for the whole patient: Meeting psychosocial health needs.* Washington, DC: National Academies Press.

Melinyshyn, S., & Wintonic, A. (2006). The role of the nurse navigator in the Breast Assessment Program at Hotel Dieu Hospital. Retrieved from http://www.krcc.on.ca/pdf/The%20Role%20 of%20the%20Nurse%20Navigator%20in%20the%20Breast%20 Assessment%20Program.pdf

National Accreditation Program for Breast Centers. (2009). *Breast center standards manual.* Retrieved from http://accreditedbreastcenters .org/standards/2009standardsmanual.pdf

National Cancer Institute. (2005). NCI's Patient Navigator Research Program: Fact sheet. Retrieved from http://www.cancer.gov/cancertopics/factsheet/PatientNavigator

National Quality Forum National Priorities Partnership. (n.d.). Priorities. Retrieved from http://www.nationalprioritiespartnership.org/PriorityDetails.aspx?id=606

Oncology Nursing Society Quality Indicator Project Team for Breast Care. (2008). 2009–2011 Breast Cancer Quality Measures Project: Introduction and overview [Slide presentation]. Retrieved from http://www.ons.org/research/media/ons/docs/research/qualityinitiative.pdf

Pedersen, A., & Hack, T.F. (2010). Pilots of oncology health care: A concept analysis of the patient navigator role. *Oncology Nursing Forum, 37,* 55–60. doi:10.1188/10.ONF.55-60

Psooy, B.J., Schreuer, D., Borgaonkar, J., & Caines, J.S. (2004). Patient navigation: Improving timeliness in diagnosis of breast abnormalities. *Canadian Association of Radiologists Journal, 55,* 145–150.

Seek, A., & Hogle, W.P. (2007). Modeling a better way: Navigating the healthcare system for patients with lung cancer. *Clinical Journal of Oncology Nursing, 11,* 81–85. doi:10.1188/07.CJON.81-85

Sein, E., & Keeley, P. (Eds.). (with Miller, B., Masny, A., Vlahakis, P., Franke, M., & Brown, L.) (2009). *Fox Chase Cancer Center Partners breast care coordinators/navigators orientation manual.* Philadelphia, PA: Fox Chase Cancer Center Partners.

Wells, K.J., Battaglia, T.A., Dudley, D.J., Garcia, R., Greene, A., Calhoun, E., ... Raiche, P.C. (2008). Patient navigation: State of the art or is it science? *Cancer, 113,* 1999–2010. doi:10.1002/cncr.23815

# Index

*The letter* f *after a page number indicates that relevant content appears in a figure; the letter* t, *in a table.*

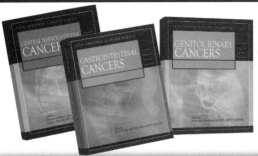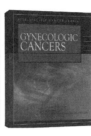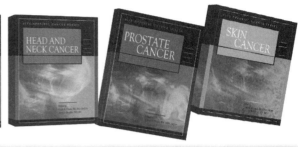